Preconceptional Health Care

PRECONCEPTIONAL HEALTH CARE

A PRACTICAL GUIDE

Second Edition

ROBERT C. CEFALO, MD, PhD

Professor
Department of Obstetrics and Gynecology
Division of Maternal and Fetal Medicine
University of North Carolina School of Medicine
Chapel Hill, North Carolina

MERRY-K. MOOS, BSN, FNP, MPH

Research Associate Professor
Department of Obstetrics and Gynecology
Division of Maternal and Fetal Medicine
University of North Carolina School of Medicine
Chapel Hill, North Carolina

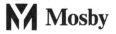 Mosby

St. Louis   Baltimore   Berlin   Boston   Carlsbad   Chicago   London   Madrid
Naples   New York   Philadelphia   Sydney   Tokyo   Toronto

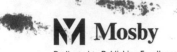
Mosby

Dedicated to Publishing Excellence

Editor: Susie Baxter
Developmental Editor: Ellen Baker Geisel
Project Manager: Mark Spann
Production Editor: Melissa Martin
Designer: David Zielinski
Manufacturing Supervisor: Kathy Grone

SECOND EDITION

Copyright © 1995 by Mosby–Year Book, Inc.

Previous edition copyrighted 1988

Printed in the United States of America
Composition by University Graphics
Printing/binding by Maple Vail

Mosby-Year Book, Inc.
11830 Westline Industrial Drive
St. Louis, Missouri 63146

Library of Congress Cataloging in Publication Data
                 Library of Congress Cataloging-in-Publication Data
Cefalo, Robert C.
   Preconceptional health care : a practical guide / Robert C. Cefalo, Merry-K. Moos.—
2nd ed.
      p.   cm.
   Rev. ed. of: Preconceptional health promotion. 1988.
   Includes bibliographical references and index.
   ISBN 0-8151-1638-1
   1. Prenatal care—Social aspects. 2. Health promotion. 3. Pregnancy—Complications—Prevention. I. Moos, Merry-K. II. Cefalo, Robert C. Preconceptional health promotion. III. Title.
   [DNLM: 1. Prenatal Care. 2. Pregnancy Complications—prevention & control. 3. Health Promotion. 4. Counseling. WQ 175 C389p 1994]
RG940.C44 1994
362.1′98—dc20
DNLM/DLC
for Library of Congress   94-10569
                                                CIP

94 95 96 97 98 / 9 8 7 6 5 4 3 2 1

Foreword

Throughout this century in most of the developed world there has been a decrease in perinatal mortality and an increase in life expectancy. In some segments of the U.S. population, however, the decline in the rates of premature births and perinatal mortality has slowed markedly, leaving our overall improvement well behind that of several other Western countries. Programs of prenatal and perinatal care, especially for the underprivileged, require further strengthening. Beyond this, there is a largely ignored field of prevention that is in need of adequate recognition—preconceptional counseling, the subject of this volume.

The potential for reducing the incidence of many handicapping conditions is expanding as epidemiologic and laboratory research provides new insights. Emphasis on programs for the prevention of disease and chronic disability is increasing steadily. For those involved in the promotion of optimal human development, each effort to prevent morbidity and mortality may be visualized as part of a continuum. Logic suggests that preconceptional counseling is an appropriate starting point, though it now reaches only a small portion of women in their childbearing years. It should become an essential component of health care services, addressing inadequate or inappropriate nutrition, smoking, alcohol intake, drug abuse, exposure to toxic substances in the workplace, maternal diabetes and other illnesses, and genetic conditions in either parent.

During pregnancy, adequate prenatal care must be available and utilized by all. Toxic environmental exposures must be avoided, and screening for such conditions as neural tube defects should be routine. Ultrasonography, amniocentesis, the developing technique of chorionic biopsy, and other means of prenatal diagnosis must be understood and employed when appropriate. As the time of delivery approaches, good perinatal care programs are needed; they should include intensive efforts to reduce the incidence of premature birth and to ensure the availability of delivery under optimal conditions. Newborn screening for metabolic disease, the availability of neonatal intensive care, and careful follow-up of high-risk infants are important.

The developing infant and child need adequate nutrition, protection from and prompt treatment of serious epidemic diseases, and protection from poisonous agents, serious trauma, and child abuse. Vigilance is needed in the implementation of immunization programs and mandatory motor vehicle restraint laws and protection from child abuse. Finally, health education in the public schools must address not only general health promotion but also the requirements for healthy pregnancies and the causes of infant mortality and morbidity. A better understanding of these issues can improve receptiveness to later preconceptional counseling. Thus the continuum of preventive approaches for mature adulthood comes full circle.

Giant strides have been made in some segments of this circle of prevention. Extensive immunization programs have eliminated smallpox and, in the developed nations, minimized the scourge of poliomyelitis and many other infectious diseases. In contrast, minimal attention has been paid to preconceptional counseling, even though adequate preconceptional health may be among the most important segments of the circle. Only in recent years have most health care providers, including obstetricians, realized that the initiation of care and guidance after conception may be too late for some patients.

The material covered by this book is thus of considerable importance. The authors not only present the broad scope of issues on which preconceptional counseling should focus but also incorporate comprehensive and specific directions for effective counseling. Carefully designed questions for the identification of potential or existing difficulties allow for both accurate data collection and extensive follow-up assessments of compliance rates and, hence, potential effectiveness.

In North Carolina and elsewhere, this approach has stimulated the interest of educational administrators at both state and local levels. Some health education curricula in the public schools have already been influenced by the program. This is a significant accomplishment, for it is in this segment of the circle of prevention that implementation is often most difficult.

The cost effectiveness of many programs to prevent handicapping conditions has been repeatedly demonstrated, and it can be convincingly predicted for many others. In a society that is facing difficult choices for the allocation of funds, even within the health care system fiscal reality demands a focus on prevention. For example, the expenses for the lifelong support of a single infant in whom phenylketonuria is not detected until severe retardation is inevitable can surpass the cost of running a state's newborn metabolic screening program for 1 year. The financial commitment required to achieve the survival of a tiny premature infant often exceeds $50,000 and may surpass $100,000 if the infant's course in the neonatal intensive care nursery is complicated. Among those infants with birthweights under 1,000 g who survive, approximately one-third are destined for permanent moderate or severe handicap. For many of these infants, thorough preconceptional counseling, as outlined in this volume and costing only a few dollars, would have led to improved care and to a normal full-term infant.

It is indeed encouraging that, throughout the United States, more and more new programs are being introduced in all areas of prevention. Curricula on health promotion and disease prevention are increasingly being established in medical schools, often in collaboration with schools of public health, dentistry, and nursing. Large-scale approaches to preventive health care require close collaboration not only among professionals in medical disciplines but also among experts in education, psychology, sociology, and other fields. This broad approach is frequently evident in the variety of professionals available to state committees or task forces on the prevention of handicapping conditions, usually associated with state councils on developmental disabilities. At the national level, the National Coalition on Prevention of Mental Retardation is becoming influential. The coalition includes the American Academy of Pediatrics, the American Association of University Affiliated Programs for Persons with Developmental Disabilities, the American Association on Mental Retardation, the National Association for Retarded Citizens, and the President's Committee on Mental Retardation.

Constant effort is needed in both the public and private sectors to promote preventive health care. Organized medicine at the national, state, and local levels should increase its involvement. State developmental disabilities councils that have stimulated and supported preventive activities must be certain that their limited resources are not entirely diverted to far more expensive programs for the amelioration of handicaps already present. Although treatment and management services are important for the many disabled in our society, increased emphasis on preventive measures is essential if we hope to reduce the prevalence of disease and handicap in future generations. Preconceptional counseling programs of the extent and quality described in this volume can contribute significantly to this emphasis.

One is reminded of the story of Marshal Lyautey, a famous French military leader, who, on finally retiring to his farm in Lorraine, approached his gardener about planting an orchard. "But," protested the gardener, "it will not bear fruit for 20 years."

"Then," replied the aging marshal, "we must plant it at once."

Harrie R. Chamberlin, M.D.
Professor Emeritus of Pediatrics
University of North Carolina at Chapel Hill

Preface

During the last decade, a quiet movement to expand the definition of prenatal care to encompass preconceptional counseling has gained momentum in this country. The United States Public Health Service, in its publication *Caring for the Future: The Content of Prenatal Care,*[1] endorsed preconceptional counseling as an integral component of care for all women contemplating pregnancy; the March of Dimes Birth Defects Foundation has recently recommended that annual preconceptional or interconceptional visits as well as a prepregnancy planning visit become standard components of care.[2] The Surgeon General, in the nation's health promotion and disease prevention initiatives, suggests that by the year 2000, 60% of primary care physicians should provide appropriate preconceptional care and counseling.[3] This level of interest indicates that preconceptional counseling has become an important focus for health promotion and disease prevention activity. However, this interest has preceded the establishment of a clear conceptual framework or standard philosophy for the provision of this service.

This book is offered to help health care providers who interact with women of reproductive age to understand the potential and limitations of preconceptional counseling and to develop a systematic and thorough approach to the service. The book is not intended to be the definitive word on preconceptional health care, because the field is evolving too quickly to achieve such an aim; instead, it is designed to be an initial and practical reference for the practitioner involved in women's health care.

Chapter 1 presents the rationale for including preconceptional health care in efforts to improve reproductive outcomes. The theoretical advantages and disadvantages of this approach to prevention and a framework for the organization of prepregnancy care are outlined. Subsequent chapters, such as Social History, Medical History, Family History, and Reproductive History, are organized around broad areas of interest in the patient's profile. The introduction to each chapter ends with appropriate screening questions to be asked of patients who desire counseling. To aid information gathering, Appendix A presents the screening questions in a cohesive format. Each chapter provides background information on proved and theoretical risks posed by specific diseases, patient behavior, or other patient characteristics targeted by the screening questions. Each chapter concludes with recommendations for patients who were identified through the screening process as having preconceptional risk factors, anxiety, or other concerns. Recommendations include patient education about risks and possible preventive steps that may be taken during the periconceptional period, appropriate consultations and referrals, and anticipatory guidance regarding problems that might arise during pregnancy.

One underlying philosophy is echoed throughout this book: All women deserve to have the information necessary to make informed decisions about their reproductive futures, because, as has been stated in a slightly different context, ''Ignorance renders the concepts of personal choice and responsibility meaningless.''[4]

References

1. Expert Panel on the Content of Prenatal Care: *Caring for the Future: The Content of Prenatal Care.* Washington, DC: US Public Health Service, 1989.
2. March of Dimes Birth Defects Foundation: *Toward Improving the Outcome of Pregnancy—The 90s and Beyond.* White Plains, NY: The March of Dimes Birth Defects Foundation, 1993.
3. US Public Health Service: *Healthy People 2000: National Health Promotion and Disease Prevention Objectives.* Washington, DC: US Dept. of Health and Human Services, 1991, DHHS publication No. (DHS)91-50212.P.
4. Enkin M, Chalmers I (eds): *Effectiveness and Satisfaction in Antenatal Care.* Philadelphia, JB Lippincott Co, 1987, p 285.

Writing is never an easy task, but the warm reception given the first edition of this book was both gratifying and stimulating. Positive feedback, constructive critique, and new developments in the area of preconceptional health care prompted our decision to update the original work. Many, many thanks to all who supported the current effort and most especially to Locke and Mary for their confidence that all things are possible.

MKM & RCC

Contents

1 Preconceptional Counseling for Informed Decision Making   1

2 Social History   11

3 Nutrition History   72

4 Medical History   98

5 Infectious Disease   165

6 Medication History   195

7 Reproductive History   205

8 Family History   224

9 Male Issues in Preconceptional Health   235

Appendix A   Preconceptional Health Assessment   243

Appendix B   Resources for Information on Reproductive Effects of Drugs and Chemicals   249

Appendix C   Estimates of Rates per Thousand of Chromosomal Abnormalities in Live Births by Single-Year Intervals   254

Appendix D   Nonmeat Protein Sources   257

Appendix E   Prenatal Nutrient Requirements   258

Appendix F   Food Sources of Iron   259

Appendix G   Iron Supplements   260

Appendix H   Food Sources of Calcium   261

Appendix I   Elemental Calcium Available in Some Over-the-Counter Supplements   262

Appendix J   Selected Drug, Vitamin, and Mineral Interactions   263

Appendix K   Caffeine Content per 5-oz Cup   265

Appendix L   Caffeine Content of Some Prescribed and
Over-the-Counter Medications   266

Appendix M   Standard Weight for Women and Deviations of
Weight for Height   267

Appendix N   Maternal Phenylketonuria (PKU) Collaborative
Study Contributing Centers   268

Preconceptional Health Care

Preconceptional Counseling for Informed Decision Making

. . . Ordered the maidens to exercise themselves,
with wrestling, running, throwing the quoit
and casting the dart,
to the end that the fruit they conceived might,
in strong and healthy bodies,
take firmer root and find better growth . . .

Plutarch[1]

Written more than 2,500 years ago, these words reflect the efforts of an ancient civilization to promote the health of its next generation. The Spartans' interest in improving the health of their nonpregnant women as a means of improving reproductive outcomes has received little attention in present-day societies. Medical research and a review of embryology indicate, however, that intervention during the preconceptional period may be a legitimate and overdue focus for modern obstetrics.

Although maternal and perinatal mortality rates have indeed declined significantly, spontaneous abortions, stillbirths, neonatal deaths, premature births, congenital defects, and maternal morbidity are costly reminders of lost or impaired human potential. Many of the successes achieved in reducing the infant mortality rate in the United States can be attributed not to the process of prenatal care, but rather to changes in socioeconomic conditions and to advances in neonatal technology. Remarkably little information is available about the extent to which routine antenatal care leads to the prevention or successful treatment of maternal or fetal disease.[2,3]

Two problems, low birthweight and congenital anomalies, have proved particularly resistant to current obstetric care. The incidence of low-birthweight babies in the United States has not changed significantly in more than 30 years, and the incidence of congenital malformation has not decreased appreciably since the beginning of the twentieth century. The absence of a national registry of birth defects coupled

1

with the availability of prenatal diagnosis and pregnancy termination make tracking the incidence of congenital anomalies nearly impossible. However, a study by the Centers for Disease Control (CDC) reports that the incidence of most of the 33 birth defects studied either increased or remained constant between 1970 and 1971 and between 1982 and 1983. The incidence of 11 of these defects (e.g., heart, urinary tract, and renal defects; congenital cataracts; congenital hip dislocation; and autosomal abnormalities) increased by 2% or more annually; the incidence of 17 birth defects was unchanged; and the incidence of 5 (anencephaly, spina bifida, exophthalmos, congenital rubella syndrome, and Rh hemolytic disease) decreased by a minimum of 2% annually.

Possible causes for the rising rates of congenital malformations include (1) the increasing numbers of women who are giving birth at the very beginning or very end of their reproductive years; (2) the current prevalence of alcohol abuse in women of childbearing age; (3) the increasing risk of chemical exposure; and (4) medical advances that allow women who had previously been unlikely to give birth because of chronic disease, such as phenylketonuria and diabetes mellitus, to carry a pregnancy to term. These theoretical explanations indicate a relationship between the eventual pregnancy outcome and the environment that maternal health and habits provide the conceptus. The significance of this link was first appreciated after the thalidomide tragedy of the 1960s and was then acted upon through the creation of the maternal-fetal subspecialty in obstetrics. A review of standard programs of obstetric care suggests, however, that awareness of the link has not changed basic principles of care.

The foundation of the maternal-fetal medicine subspecialty—prenatal care—is not as venerable as may be supposed. "Prevention in order to be truly preventive must be antenatal," wrote Ballantyne in 1902.[5] This treatise marked the beginning of a basic program of prenatal care that "has remained unchanged and largely unchallenged for well over half a century."[2(pxi)] By 1929, established minimal intervals for prenatal care included a first obstetric visit by 16 weeks, with subsequent visits at 24 weeks, every 2 weeks starting at 28 weeks, and weekly beginning at 36 weeks. At each visit, uterine size, fetal heart rate, and urine were assessed. Aside from efforts to move the initial visit to the first trimester, this formula for care is mirrored in today's obstetric practices. Therefore, in nearly 60 years, the basic approach to obstetric care has not changed. The persistent incidences of low birthweight and congenital malformation suggest that, despite Ballantyne's assertions, this approach is not preventive. The problem is that those who provide obstetric care are generally asked to enter the race to deliver a healthy baby only after the race has begun; all too often, they are placed in the uncomfortable position of practicing prenatal catchup rather than primary prevention.

The period of greatest environmental sensitivity for the developing fetus is between 17 and 56 days after fertilization. Cell organization, cell differentiation, and organogenesis take place during this period, and any insult, whether nutritional, drug-related, or viral, can jeopardize fetal development. In the first trimester, the fertilized ovum increases in mass by 2½ million times; during the second and third trimesters, the growth is only 230-fold.[6] By the end of the eighth week after conception and certainly by the end of the first trimester, any major structural anomalies in the fetus have already developed. Because many women do not have their pregnancies confirmed until this critical period of development is well under way or completed, the rapidly growing embryo is frequently subjected to potentially injurious stimuli during its most vulnerable developmental phase.

Women questioned about the impending birth of their child echo a common theme: "As long as it's healthy." This concern overshadows all other considerations, such as sex, familial characteristics, and labor anxieties. Most women are generally unaware of the critical significance of the weeks that precede the confirmation of a pregnancy, however. Unfortunately, the first time a woman traditionally receives information about the prevention of poor reproductive outcomes is the first prenatal visit. In many cases, this is too late. Data indicate that 25% of pregnant women in the United States in 1989 received either late care (defined as care initiated after the first trimester) or no prenatal care.[7] Although precise data are not available on the week of entry for those who received early care (defined as care initiated during the first trimester), it is the rare patient who has a first visit before organogenesis begins. Such a visit would require an appointment three days after the first missed menses. A modern obstetric challenge, therefore, is to educate women who are not yet pregnant about the potential influences of their lifestyle and health status on the earliest embryonic cells.

In its 1985 publication *Preventing Low Birthweight,* the Institute of Medicine addressed the logic of moving the traditional initiation of obstetric care to a period before pregnancy.[8] The report states:

> Much of the literature about preventing low birthweight focuses on the period of pregnancy—how to improve the content of prenatal care, how to motivate women to reduce risky habits while pregnant, and how to encourage women to seek out and remain in prenatal care. By contrast, little attention is given to opportunities for prevention before pregnancy. Only casual attention has been given to the proposition that one of the best protections available against low birthweight and other poor pregnancy outcomes is to have a woman actively plan for pregnancy, enter pregnancy in good health with as few risk factors as possible, and be fully informed about her reproductive and general health.

Thus the transcendent objective of obstetrics that every pregnancy be wanted and culminate in a healthy outcome for both mother and baby[9] suggests that obstetricians may find it necessary to redefine the time frame typically assigned to obstetrician-patient interactions. Leadership in efforts to prevent reproductive loss and perinatal death and morbidity is the responsibility of obstetricians, and increasing numbers of them are embracing the wisdom of preconceptional education and intervention as a means of achieving this goal.[10-13]

Preconceptional counseling serves a variety of purposes, but the overriding goal should be to provide each patient and, if desired, her partner with the information necessary to make informed decisions about future reproduction. An informed woman or couple can then decide to accept the increased risks that pregnancy may pose to the health of the woman or to the health of future children, to modify these risks, or to forgo childbearing. Geoffrey Chamberlain,[12] an early proponent of preconceptional counseling, noted that an important option for patients—avoiding pregnancy—has already been removed if care is not readily available until after conception.

Preconceptional counseling also allows patients to determine in advance whether recommendations that may be offered during pregnancy, such as changes in employment status, restrictions on maternal activity, or monitoring that extends beyond the perception of ''normal'' prenatal care, are acceptable to them. With counseling, prospective patients can confront the potentially difficult decisions they may face should pregnancy occur. Patients who have worked through before pregnancy the moral and ethical dilemmas associated with a diagnosis of fetal malformation and the alternative of abortion, for example, are more likely to be at ease with any decisions that they eventually make.

Another benefit of preconceptional counseling is the relief of anxiety about reproduction. Patients who have previously experienced poor outcomes are often left with guilt, fear, fantasies, and unresolved grief that affect their psychological motivations and readiness for a subsequent pregnancy. The counseling process allows concentrated time to be devoted to an exploration of the patient's and her partner's beliefs about previous losses and conflicts between their intellectual and emotional understanding. It is not unusual, for example, for a patient to report in detail the results of an autopsy yet to worry that a probably inconsequential action around the date of her delivery, such as rearranging her furniture, caused the loss. Explaining that the causes of most abnormalities are unknown and that the abnormalities were present early in the pregnancy and providing a genetic evaluation help such a patient to put aside her guilt and fear and to prepare for her next pregnancy with optimism. This role for preconceptional counseling is labor-intensive and involves none of the frequently comforting technologic props of modern obstetrics. The role is critical, however, because it acknowledges psychological readiness as an important precursor to a rewarding reproductive experience.

Although it may be tempting in the preconceptional counseling process to use a model that links a single pathologic event with a single antecedent, such a model not only implies clear preventive and remedial actions, but also may give the patient unrealistic expectations. In truth, most disease states, including most poor reproductive outcomes, result from a combination of several unfavorable events. For instance, not all women who abuse alcohol during pregnancy give birth to infants with fetal alcohol syndrome. The mother's physiologic response to alcohol, her nutritional status, the embryo's genetic susceptibility, and the timing of exposure probably all play a role in determining which infants will be born with irreversible retardation and which will be born without any discernible problems.

The multifactorial causation theory is well illustrated in the thalidomide tragedy. Some infants exposed in utero to as much as 100 mg daily of the teratogenic drug had no structural defects, while others exposed once to only 50 mg suffered lifelong consequences.[14] This model of causation suggests that some actions, such as following optimal nutritional guidelines and avoiding unnecessary exposures, can be taken to maximize the chances of an uncomplicated pregnancy and a healthy infant. On the other hand, prospective parents must understand that no pregnancy has a guaranteed perfect outcome. Miscarriage, congenital malformation, premature birth, behavioral disorders, cognitive defects, perinatal death, and maternal complications can occur even under optimal conditions.

It is important that patients prospectively understand the limitations of medical knowledge. It is equally important that they be aware of known risks and actions they can take to promote desired outcomes. Much of the energy behind preconceptional health promotion activities is based on theoretical advantages. This should be made clear to patients. However, proven or likely benefits of periconceptional activities should be explained. For example, discontinuation of category X drugs (e.g., gold, isotretinoin, and sodium warfarin [Coumadin]) before conception, avoidance of alcohol during organogenesis, and close control of maternal glucose levels in the periconceptional period have all been shown to benefit the developing embryo. Although the absolute advantages of other preconceptional and periconceptional interventions deserve study, it is unlikely that efforts to optimize the prospective mother's health and to provide her with the information she needs to make informed decisions about her future childbearing can have a negative impact on reproductive outcomes.

The provider of preconceptional care explains the knowns and unknowns to the patient and delineates actions that have the potential to benefit both maternal and fetal health, in the hope that a provider-patient partnership for health will evolve. Too often, patients externalize all responsibility. This perhaps understandable coping mechanism is well illustrated by the behavior of a woman who had been hospitalized for serial monitoring secondary to intrauterine growth retardation. During her hospitalization, she frequently railed against her employer, whom she held responsible for exposures of unknown significance. Despite repeated education on the documented hazards of maternal smoking to the fetus, the ash tray next to her bed was continually full. This patient had not incorporated the concept of shared responsibility into her approach to reproduction.

Although the advantages of preconceptional health promotion are numerous, careful thought must attend its adoption as a routine component of care. There are theoretical disadvantages. Such programs may heighten anxiety, suggest guarantees, reinforce guilt, and detract from, rather than enhance, personal decision making.

In general, women and couples should leave the counseling process hopeful about the likelihood of a successful pregnancy. Although the possible risks for maternal complications and perinatal death and morbidity must be determined individually, patients should recognize that a healthy baby is the rule rather than the exception. When specific risks are identified, care must be taken in discussing their potential significance in order to avoid creating unnecessary anxiety. This is particularly important for the patient who has already experienced a reproductive loss. Without sensitive phrasing of suggestions and, where appropriate, education about the multifactorial theory of causation, patients may assume that they could have prevented the previous outcome. Such an assumption serves no useful purpose.

If provided in an overzealous fashion, counseling may prompt conflicts in the provider-patient relationship. Too often, recommendations are phrased in a way that suggests guarantees. A statement such as "You'll have a nice healthy baby if you keep your blood sugar under control," offers an indefensible guarantee. A statement such as "If you continue to smoke, your baby will be too small to be healthy," sets the stage for a loss of credibility, because many babies of normal weight are born to smoking mothers.

Care must also be taken in preconceptional health promotion activities to ensure that values are not imposed on individual women. One geneticist states that

> it is now possible, with our present methods of prenatal diagnosis, to nearly eradicate neural tube defects, chromosomal disorders, hemoglobinopathies, inherited sex-linked recessive disorders, and many inborn errors of metabolism.[15]

Such statements, however well intentioned, require careful inspection and great caution. To place the emphasis on eradication of all disabilities, which may imply involuntary abortion or sterilization, rather than on responsible decision making is extremely dangerous. If the outcome of eradication is valued more than the process of informed decision making, society may come to embrace the belief that any means, including the loss of personal freedoms, justifies the end.

In a recent review of court cases involving maternal rights, Johnsen[16] notes that courts and legislatures are increasingly being called upon to restrict the autonomy of pregnant women by requiring them to behave in ways that others determine is best for their fetuses: "Though manifested thus far in a haphazard, even unthinking manner, the clear trend has been to expand 'fetal rights' at the expense of pregnant women." Johnsen adds that perhaps the most ominous aspect of the evolving legal recognition of the fetus is that it deprives women of their autonomy on the basis of their biologic success in achieving conception. Without careful attention, moving in the direction of preconceptional assessment and counseling could translate into a further encroachment on women's rights and a rebirth of the eugenics movement seen in the United States during the early decades of the twentieth century.[17]

The intent of preconceptional counseling programs should not be to make reproductive decisions for women; it should not be to encourage reproduction in one group and to discourage it in another. The intent of preconceptional counseling programs should be to provide enough information so that all women can make informed decisions about conception, lifestyle, and choices in medical care. Caregivers have a legal obligation to provide patients with accurate information on which to base decisions; they do not have the right to make those decisions for them.[18] Caregivers must respect the patient's decisions, whatever they may be.

From a clinical perspective, the process of preconceptional counseling has not failed if a woman makes an informed choice that potentially places her fetus at risk, such as choosing not to seek preconceptional control of her diabetes or choosing not to undergo testing for an autosomal recessive disorder. It has unquestionably failed, however, if a diabetic woman who delivers a malformed infant was unaware of the relatively poor reproductive outcomes associated with diabetes. It has failed if a child with a prenatally detectable autosomal recessive disorder is born to a patient who was unaware of the risk. These women did not have access to the information necessary to make active choices regarding the health of their future children.

Although opportunities for obtaining preconceptional information are not yet widely available, people who are considering pregnancy are eager for such information. The questions they pose in public forums on prepregnancy issues illustrate the range of their interests and concerns:

- Is there any adverse effect from the use of oil paints and turpentine during pregnancy?
- Could the use of hallucinogenic drugs by either prospective parent more than 10 years ago result in birth defects?
- What are the risks to a future child of parental exposure to video display terminals?
- Is paternal use of allopurinol harmful to the fetus?
- What effects do induced abortions have on future conception?
- Since my mother became diabetic at age 17, am I at increased risk of becoming diabetic during pregnancy or of passing the disease on to my child?
- What are the reproductive risks for a woman who has been exposed to diethylstilbestrol (DES), both for the woman and for her fetus?
- What are the consequences to the mother and fetus of large doses of aspirin for arthritis during various stages of pregnancy?
- What is the effect of alcohol on sperm?
- What precautions should a pet owner take?
- Can allergy shots affect pregnancy?
- Is it safe to drink alcohol during the first 14 days of the menstrual cycle?
- Is there any potential danger to the fetus if I continue to work with lead and stained glass in my hobby?

These thoughtful and sophisticated questions may suggest that only the well educated or affluent are concerned about the effect of their health status and lifestyle on a future pregnancy. A program of preconceptional health promotion in local health department family planning clinics in North Carolina indicates that such an assumption is erroneous. In these clinics, which predominantly serve persons of low socioeconomic status and limited formal education, the program was found to be of interest to 89% of the participants.

In a review of over 1,000 couples who sought preconceptional counseling at a tertiary facility in the United Kingdom, 91% were referred by obstetricians or other health care practitioners; only 9% were self-referred. Their concerns fell into three main categories: previous spontaneous abortion (44.5%); chronic maternal disease (22.3%); and previous fetal abnormality (19.6%). The remaining couples sought consultation related to complications during previous pregnancies, such as spontaneous preterm birth, unexplained intrauterine death, severe preeclampsia, and antepartum hemorrhage.[19]

A review of records in our preconceptional counseling clinic indicates that 50% of patients are self-referred and 50% are professionally referred. Two main questions prompt a woman's or couple's decision to seek preconceptional counseling: (1) What are the risks of pregnancy to my health? and (2) What are the risks to my (our) future child? Previous pregnancy losses and advanced maternal age are the leading concerns of women who initiate contact themselves, whereas medical conditions and previous pregnancy losses are the chief reasons for professional referral. Typical medical profiles of patients seen at our clinic include the following:

- hypertension, obesity, recent hepatitis (*Rx:* Maxzide)
- hypothyroidism, hypoparathyroidism, migraine (*Rx:* sodium levothyroxine [Synthroid], calcium, vitamin D, megavitamins)
- tuberous sclerosis, hyperprolactinemia (*Rx:* bromocriptine)
- diabetes, age 40, smoking (*Rx:* insulin)
- diabetes, hypertension, nephropathy, retinopathy (*Rx:* insulin, antihypertensives)
- lupus erythematosus, smoking (*Rx:* aspirin, hydroxychloroquine)
- leiomyomata uteri
- recurrent severe hyperemesis
- rheumatoid arthritis (*Rx:* gold injections)
- recurrent spontaneous abortion under 12 weeks

The range of these patients' medical conditions and the variety of drugs taken by them indicate that patients often have complex, multifaceted profiles that demand careful research and thoughtful response. As Chamberlain[20] noted in his experience with a London prepregnancy clinic, "Knowledge is not so important as the ability to know where to look for it." The information necessary to provide thoughtful responses is unlikely to be gathered and processed within the time and energy constraints imposed by a routine clinic schedule. Patients in our clinic are given an initial appointment for a one-hour visit. At this visit, they are frequently advised that specific recommendations cannot be made until the literature is reviewed and various experts in the field are consulted. Follow-up contact is arranged, which, depending on the specific issues under consideration, may include written communication, telephone conversation, or return visits.

Providers from several medical specialties may contribute to the care of many women who seek preconceptional counseling. For example, a nephrologist, endocrinologist, ophthalmologist, internist, and gynecologist may all be involved in the care of a single patient. If the gynecologist referred the patient for preconceptional counseling, the endocrinologist may be unaware of the action or of the patient's desire to become pregnant, although the endocrinologist remains involved in related aspects of the patient's care. To ensure that patients need not sort through competing recommendations from various medical specialists, the preconceptional counselor should communicate with other key providers, particularly if preconceptional recommendations require adjustment to an existing medical regimen.

Preconceptional counseling is properly directed by specialists in the field of obstetrics and gynecology, but it should be a multidisciplinary effort if its goals are to be fully achieved. Many obstetricians do not have the time or training, for example, to assess the adequacy of protein in a vegetarian's diet, to offer specific risk information on complex patterns of inheritance, or to provide the psychosocial services to help patients end addictions. When a circumstance occasionally arises in preconceptional counseling that requires expertise beyond the scope of traditional obstetric training, the counselor should feel comfortable seeking consultation or offering referral.

Experience in our preconceptional clinic underscores the value of a thorough and systematic assessment of risk. For example, questioning and examination of the patients who sought counseling at our clinic because of advanced maternal age revealed that 66% had additional risk factors, including birth defects in the husband's family, uterine leiomyomata, a positive reaction to a purified protein derivative (PPD) test for tuberculosis, Jewish ancestry with the associated risk of Tay-Sachs disease, the ingestion of vitamin supplements in megadoses, and elevated copper levels in the household drinking water. By focusing only on the immediate concern, these potentially significant problems could easily have been overlooked. To facilitate a comprehensive approach to the counseling process, Appendix A provides a tool for obtaining a full health history of the woman or couple beginning the preconceptional counseling process. Use of this tool will help in systematically identifying important features of the patient's profile and in maximizing the opportunity for timely education.

In summary, programs of preconceptional health promotion should include three components: (1) the systematic and comprehensive identification of individual risks; (2) the provision of personalized, nonjudgmental education; and (3) the ready access to complementary services, such as in-depth genetic and nutritional counseling and behavioral modification programs. Routinely providing these services to all women of reproductive age can make childbearing a more fully informed process and, in so doing, improve opportunities for successful reproduction in the United States.

References

1. Plutarch: *Lycurgus* 14 (trans. John Dryden), New York, Random House, 1932; 59-60.
2. Enkin M, Chalmers I (eds): *Effectiveness and Satisfaction in Antenatal Care.* Philadelphia, JB Lippincott Co, 1982.
3. MacLennan AH: Is traditional antenatal care worthwhile? *Healthright* 1986;5: 22-27.
4. Edmonds LD, James LM: Temporal trend in the incidence of malformation in the United States, selected years, 1970-71, 1982-83. *MMWR* 1985;34:1-3.
5. Ballantyne JW: *Manual of Antenatal Pathology and Hygiene* (vol. 1). Edinburgh, William Green and Sons, 1902.
6. Preconception clinics, editorial. *Br Med J* 1981;283:685.
7. National Center for Health Statistics. *Advance report of final natality statistics,* 1989. Monthly Vital Statistics Report. Vol. 40, No. 8 (supplement) Hyattsville, MD: NCHS, 1991.
8. Institute of Medicine: *Preventing Low Birthweight.* Washington, DC, National Academy Press, 1985, p 119.
9. Pritchard JA, MacDonald PC, Gant NF (eds): *Williams Obstetrics,* ed 17. Norwalk, Conn, Appleton-Century-Crofts, 1985, p 1.
10. Moos MK, Cefalo RC: Preconceptional health promotion: A focus for obstetric care. *Am J Perinatol* 1987;4:63-67.
11. Hollingworth DR, Jones OW, Resnik R: Expanded care in obstetrics for the 1980's: Preconception and early post-conception counseling. *Am J Obstet Gynecol* 1984;149:811-814.
12. Chamberlain G: The use of a prepregnancy clinic. *Matern Child Health,* August 1981, pp 314-316.
13. Queenan JT: Preparing for pregnancy, editorial. *Contemp Ob/Gyn,* June 1985, pp 11-12.
14. Robe LB: *Just So It's Healthy.* Minneapolis, CompCare Publications, 1982, pp 101-103.
15. Shaw MW: When does treatment constitute a harm? In McMillan RC, Engelhardt TH, Spicker SF (eds): *Euthanasia and the Newborn.* Boston, D. Reidel Publishing Co., 1987, pp 132-133.
16. Johnsen D: A new threat to pregnant women's autonomy. *Hastings Cent Rep,* August 1987, p 35.
17. Stevenson RE: Reproductive fitness. *Semin Perinatol* 1985;9:263-272.
18. Annas GJ: Righting the wrong of wrongful life. *Hastings Cent Rep,* February 1981, pp 8-11.
19. Cox M, Whittle MJ, Byrne A, et al: Prepregnancy Counselling: Experience from 1075 cases. *Br J Obstet Gynaecol* 1992; 99:873-876.
20. Chamberlain G: The prepregnancy clinic. *Br Med J* 1980;281:29-30.

2

Social History

The preconceptional social history helps the counselor to identify behaviors and exposures that may compromise reproductive outcome. The counselor should determine, at a minimum, whether the patient

- drinks beer, wine, or hard liquor
- smokes cigarettes or uses any other tobacco products
- uses marijuana, cocaine, or any similar drugs
- uses lead or chemicals at home or at work
- participates in an exercise program

A positive response to any of these questions necessitates a more detailed history. When potentially risky habits or exposures are identified, appropriate education should be provided and, if necessary and desired, behavioral changes facilitated.

Alcohol Use

R esults of the 1990 National Household Survey on Drug Abuse reveal that up to 73% of women between the ages of 12 and 34 expose their fetuses to alcohol at some time during pregnancy.[1] A study of 1,336 women randomly selected to represent a birth cohort from Maryland, the District of Columbia, and Northern Virginia found that 63% used alcohol at some time during pregnancy, with 29% quitting for at least some portion of the gestational period. Abstinence was associated with younger maternal age, black race, and moderate household income.[2] Another recent study indicates that the prevalence of alcohol consumption among pregnant women steadily declined from 32% in 1985 to 20% in 1988, with no decline observed among the less educated or those under the age of 25 years.[3] The varying numbers most likely reflect differing methodologies. The latter study, for instance, specifically targeted alcohol use during the preceding month and was, therefore, unable to determine what percentage of women had consumed alcohol at some point during their pregnancies.

In 1982, one third of the nation's alcoholics were women, compared with only 12.5% in 1950.[4] The reasons for this dramatic increase are complex, but the effect of this change in women's drinking behavior on reproductive outcomes is cause for concern.

Alcohol abuse during pregnancy is recognized as the third leading cause of mental retardation, following neural tube defects and Down syndrome.[5] Of these, only alcohol-related impairments are entirely preventable. Malformations, intrauterine death, prenatal and postnatal growth retardation, low birthweight, central nervous system abnormalities, and behavioral deficits have also been associated with maternal drinking,[6] as have spontaneous abortion[7,8] and abruptio placentae.[9] In addition, animal models indicate the possibility of chromosomal damage.[10]

BACKGROUND

Since ancient times, women have been warned about using alcohol during pregnancy. Whether these warnings have been the result of observed defects in children born to women who consumed alcohol during pregnancy or the result of a societal proscription against female drunkenness has been debated.[11] In the late nineteenth century, it was suggested that there was an empiric link between maternal drinking and infant outcomes after an observation that women alcoholics at the Liverpool jail had a fetal and infant death rate more than twice that of their relatives.[6] Lemoine and associates,[12] in a 1968 French journal, described a number of similarities among children born to alcoholic women, including growth deficiencies, psychomotor disturbances, and dysmorphic facial features. Five years later, these similarities were identified as the components of fetal alcohol syndrome (FAS),[13] and a rush of research activity commenced to determine the range of reproductive effects associated with maternal alcohol abuse. Current clinical, epidemiologic, and experimental evidence establishes a link between maternal alcohol ingestion and poor neonatal outcomes. Researchers have reached a consensus that maternal alcoholism places exposed offspring at risk for fetal alcohol syndrome and that the chronicity of maternal drinking is a major factor.

The Effects of Maternal Alcohol Abuse

Criteria for the diagnosis of fetal alcohol syndrome include
- prenatal or postnatal growth retardation (i.e., below 10th percentile in body weight, length, and head circumference)
- at least two of three characteristic facial anomalies
  - microcephaly
  - microphthalmia
  - underdeveloped philtrum, thin upper lip, and maxillary hypoplasia
- central nervous system dysfunctions, including neurologic abnormalities, mental deficiencies, or developmental delays[14]

The average reported intelligence quotient (IQ) of children with fetal alcohol syndrome is 68 (mildly retarded), but scores ranging from 16 to 106 have been recorded.[15] The overall incidence of fetal alcohol syndrome ranges from 0.4 to 3.1 per 1,000 live births, depending on the population studied and the methodologies employed.[16,17]

If some, but not all, of the diagnostic criteria for fetal alcohol syndrome are met, the appropriate diagnosis may be fetal alcohol effects (FAE). In such instances, maternal alcohol abuse during pregnancy must be established before the diagnosis is made because there are marked similarities among the signs of fetal alcohol effects, fetal hydantoin effects, and other conditions (e.g., Noonan and De Lange syndromes).[18] The incidence of partial expression of fetal alcohol syndrome ranges from 1.7 to 90.1 per 1,000 live births.[16]

Abel[11] placed the average minimal incidence of fetal alcohol syndrome at 1.1 cases per 1,000 live births and the average minimal incidence of fetal alcohol effects at 3.1 cases per 1,000 live births. Using a series of computations, Abel[11(p81)] estimated that between 1,800 and 4,400 infants are born annually in the United States with fetal alcohol syndrome, and between 6,550 and 11,000 are born with partial expression.

The Effect of Consumption Levels on the Fetus

A question of particular concern is whether alcohol in any amount has a detrimental effect on a fetus. Currently, there is no consensus. Data published in 1978 indicate that 19% of the children born to women who consumed more than 4 drinks per day had features consistent with fetal alcohol syndrome, as did 11% of those born to women who consumed 2 to 4 drinks daily.[19] In a British study published in 1982, researchers report that the incidence of fetal alcohol syndrome was 44% among offspring of "heavy drinkers"; 91% of the offspring were small for gestational age.[20] Researchers did not attempt to definitively quantify consumption levels. Another study indicates that a maternal alcohol intake of fewer than 14 drinks per week did not increase the risk of any adverse outcome, except the risk of placenta previa.[9] The latter risk was apparent with an intake of 2 or more drinks per day, with some increased risk at levels of 1 drink per day.

Research in human beings on the reproductive effects of maternal alcohol consumption presents numerous methodologic problems. It is difficult to quantify reliably the amount of alcohol consumed and to identify precisely the patterns of consumption, because both determinations depend on self-report. Self-declaration is likely to result in underreporting, however, and asking for averages is likely to obscure patterns of drinking. For example, a woman may accurately report an average of 1 drink daily to reflect 7 drinks on one occasion during that week. This reporting phenomenon is problematic for establishing accurate human dose-response curves, which are important because animal research indicates that the fetal effects of alcohol exposure depend on a combination of dose and timing.[21] Other research problems are raised by the fact that smoking, paternal alcoholism, other drug use, and parity may contribute to the ill effects of alcohol use on the fetus.[6]

In addition, researchers vary in their definitions. In three major studies, the term *heavy drinking* was variably defined as consuming at least 45 drinks per month with at least 5 drinks on one occasion[22]; an average of 1 or more ounces of absolute alcohol per day (equivalent to 2 or more drinks of beer, wine, or liquor)[23]; and more than 1.5 ounces of absolute alcohol daily (equivalent to 3 drinks).[16] In one review, it was found that "heavy" drinking in pregnancy had been reported at percentages varying from 0.1% to 9% of pregnant women.[11(p51)] In American studies, the median percentage of "heavy" drinking among pregnant women is reported as 2%.[11(p53)] This figure is considerably lower than the percentage reported for all women in the general population. Of these women, 9% drink 2 drinks per day and 60 or more drinks per month, and 3% drink 4 drinks per day and 120 or more per month.[24] The inconsistency in gravid and nongravid habits is explained by the finding that during pregnancy many women develop a distaste for alcohol that sharply decreases the quantity consumed.[8(p54)]

Studies tend to indicate that drinking early in pregnancy hampers fetal growth but not to the degree associated with drinking in later pregnancy. In a prospective study published in 1977, Little[23] found that an average ingestion of 1 ounce of absolute alcohol before pregnancy resulted in an average decrease in birthweight of 91 g; the same intake in late pregnancy was associated with a decrease of 160 g. These findings were independent of smoking, but maternal pregravid weight and subsequent weight gain were not assessed. In a more recent study, Little and associates[25] considered maternal weight in their analysis and concluded that an average consumption of approximately one drink daily in the week before conception was related to a 225-g decrease in infant birthweight. A difference of 710 g was found between infants born to women labeled "infrequent" drinkers (an average of one or two drinks per week) and infants born to "regular" drinkers (an average of 2½ drinks per day). No attempt was made in this study to control for drinking behaviors in later pregnancy. Similarly, investigators who collected data on the drinking behaviors of more than 31,000 pregnant women at their entrance into prenatal care concluded that, after an adjustment for other risks, alcohol exposure during early pregnancy was associated with a reduction in mean birthweight ranging from 14 g in those infants born to women who have less than one drink per day to 165 g in those infants born to women who have three to five drinks per day.[26] Although these studies appear to indicate that maternal drinking early in pregnancy may have a detrimental effect on birthweight, attempts to establish causality between early pregnancy alcohol intake and diminished fetal growth are hampered by the failure to control for maternal alcohol consumption throughout pregnancy.

In an attempt to assess the effects of changes in maternal drinking behavior during pregnancy, one group of investigators found that heavy alcohol use sustained throughout pregnancy was associated with an increased incidence of growth retardation in weight, length, and head circumference and with an increased incidence of malformation but that heavy drinkers who reduced their consumption before the third trimester had infants similar in size to the infants of the infrequent and moderate drinkers. Infants of the heavy drinkers who had reduced their consumption had an increased incidence of abnormalities.[22]

Mental retardation, hyperactivity, and developmental delays are associated with maternal alcohol abuse. The long-term consequences to the child of mild to moderate alcohol exposure during pregnancy have received little study, however. One of the few existing studies on this issue was an attempt to determine the long-term effect of alcohol exposure by correlating the behaviors of 4-year-old children with their mothers' prenatal drinking habits.[27] Researchers found that the offspring of moderate drinkers (equivalent to or slightly less than one drink daily during pregnancy) were more likely to display behavior associated with hyperactivity or attentional deficit syndrome than were the offspring of occasional drinkers or nondrinkers. Although the home environments of all the subjects in this study were comparable, the authors suggest that causality is extremely difficult to establish because of the possibility that postnatal rather than prenatal factors are partially responsible for variation in observed outcomes. This possibility is particularly troublesome in efforts to assess the developmental outcomes of children born to heavy drinkers. Known antecedents of mental retardation are derived, in part, from environmental factors, and children of alcoholics are likely to be at increased risk of exposure to suboptimal environments.[28]

A 10-year follow-up study of 60 children diagnosed with FAS in infancy or childhood found that persistent mental retardation is the major sequela of intrauterine alcohol exposure and that characteristic craniofacial malformations tend to diminish over time.[29] The study recorded catch-up growth in height and weight, but 65% of the children continued to be microcephalic at follow-up, compared with 88% at diagnosis. At the time of data collection, all but two of the children were receiving their care from persons other than the biologic mother. The authors note that improvements in domestic circumstances did not ameliorate the effects of FAS to the degree expected. A study by Streissguth and associates[30] compared longitudinal IQ scores of 40 patients diagnosed with FAS or FAE. Scores obtained at approximately age 8 were compared with scores from adolescence (mean age 16.6). No significant change in IQ was observed for patients with either FAS (mean IQ 66.7; s.d. 15.7) or FAE (mean IQ 82.3; s.d. 15.4).

Two reports link drinking during pregnancy to increased rates of spontaneous abortion. One retrospective study indicates that even moderate consumption of alcohol during pregnancy may contribute to the risk of spontaneous abortion.[4] This conclusion is based on the finding that 17% of the women studied who had a spontaneous abortion drank a mean of 1 ounce of absolute alcohol (equivalent to two drinks) at least twice a week, whereas only 8% of the women who delivered after 28 weeks of gestation reported an equivalent intake. Based on a computed odds ratio, the authors estimate an abortion rate of 29.3% for women who drink this amount at least twice a week and 13.6% for women who drink less frequently. The sample included only women of low socioeconomic status, and the investigators undertook an analysis of other factors (e.g., demographics; previous spontaneous abortions; and tobacco, marijuana, and caffeine use). The second frequently quoted study in which alcohol use is linked to spontaneous abortion is a large prospective study that included an analysis of demographics, smoking behavior, and previous abortions.[5] The authors of this study concluded that women who reported drinking at least one alcoholic drink a day were two to three times more likely than nondrinkers to have spontaneous abortions. The studies indicate a dose-response effect.

Alcohol passes freely across the placental membrane,[3] but the mechanism by which it causes the fetal alcohol syndrome and related effects remains unclear. One theory is that the syndrome results from deficiencies in zinc and magnesium in the mother or fetus. Both minerals are necessary for normal RNA and DNA synthesis, and deficiencies, particularly in zinc levels, have been shown to cause fetal malformations.[31] A 1985 Finnish study shows that women who drank during pregnancy had normal zinc concentrations throughout pregnancy, even those who subsequently gave birth to infants with the fetal alcohol syndrome, but that reduced zinc levels were present immediately after delivery in the infants of the women who reported prenatal alcohol use.[32] The authors postulate that alcohol or some alcohol-induced mechanism may decrease the placental transport of zinc and that the decrease may be a factor in fetal alcohol syndrome if it occurs at a crucial period of organogenesis.

It is unknown whether fetal alcohol effects are a direct result of alcohol or are related to alcohol metabolites. Some authorities think that acetaldehyde, an alcohol metabolite that is more toxic than alcohol itself,[8(p40)] is the teratogenic agent in fetal alcohol syndrome.[33] Majewski[33] speculates that progressive alcohol dependence results in progressively disturbed acetaldehyde metabolism, as chronic alcoholics have higher concentrations of the metabolite. This theory would explain why the later children of women who are chronic alcoholics are more likely to be affected and why women who consume equal amounts of alcohol do not experience equal reproductive effects. Other researchers disagree with this theory, suggesting that alcohol itself is the fetotoxic agent. Indeed, alcohol has been found to decrease embryonic growth in vitro where no acetaldehyde is produced.[8(p207)]

Just as it is not known whether the causative agent is a deficiency in some trace mineral, elevated acetaldehyde concentrations or alcohol levels, or some combination of these, the pathophysiology by which the fetus is affected is unclear. After reviewing various theories, Henderson and associates[31] concluded that the most established concept is that alcohol interferes with protein synthesis and that this could account, at least in part, for the growth retardation associated with fetal alcohol syndrome. Others have suggested that changes in blood flow associated with alcohol ingestion are responsible for growth retardation.[8(p210)] Alcohol consumption results in the release of catecholamines that cause vasoconstriction and thereby reduce blood flow. This effect could produce not only necrosis, which could lead to spontaneous abortion or congenital malformation, but also intrauterine growth retardation. Other biochemical theories have also been suggested, including alterations in cerebral neurotransmitter balance, deviations in fetal growth hormone, fetal acidosis, and changes in cellular membranes.[3,31]

Although the precise effects of maternal alcohol use during pregnancy have not been quantified nor the mode of action explained, there is enough evidence to conclude that maternal alcohol consumption has a variety of negative reproductive effects. The most agreed-upon conclusion is that women who drink during pregnancy at a level consistent with a clinical diagnosis of alcoholism are at significant risk of producing children with fetal alcohol syndrome. The *Journal of the American Medical Association* states:

> Certain differentials in alcohol-related deficits may well depend on the stage of fetal development, with the first trimester of pregnancy apparently critical for dysmorphology, the second for fetal loss, and the third for impaired intrauterine growth.[34(p2519)]

The influence of preconceptional counseling on the incidence of fetal alcohol syndrome and related effects has not been studied, but some studies indicate that preconceptional counseling could be beneficial. A study in Seattle showed that mothers of infants whose features suggested fetal alcohol syndrome had a higher average intake of absolute alcohol in the month before confirmation of pregnancy and in the first 5 months after confirmation than did a control population.[19] The authors conclude that ''the strongest relationship between maternal consumption and fetal outcome seems to exist for drinking behavior in the month preceding recognition of pregnancy."[19(p460)] Because the quantity and timing of alcohol ingestion during the earliest weeks of pregnancy have important implications for fetal growth and development, the investigators recommend advising women to reduce their alcohol intake before conception.

Although a decrease in alcohol consumption at any time during pregnancy may reduce fetal effects, particularly growth retardation, interventions aimed only at women already pregnant are unlikely to eliminate all the adverse reproductive outcomes associated with maternal alcohol ingestion. In July 1981, the Surgeon General's Advisory on Alcohol and Pregnancy advised "women who are pregnant or considering pregnancy not to drink alcoholic beverages and to be aware of the alcohol content of food and drugs."[35(p99)] Health professionals were "urged to inquire routinely about alcohol consumption by patients who are pregnant or considering pregnancy and to include this information in their medical records."[35(p10)] Efforts to prevent fetal alcohol syndrome should emphasize increased public awareness of the syndrome and the identification and interruption of maternal drinking before conception.

In a 1991 survey, primary care physicians were asked about counseling and referral behaviors for patients suspected or known to abuse alcohol. Of 113 obstetric/gynecologic practitioners, only 38.7% routinely counseled or referred at-risk patients. The study did not include information on what percentage of patients were actively evaluated for risk status.[36]

PRECONCEPTIONAL COUNSELING

Given the prevalence of alcohol use in the United States, an alcohol consumption history should be a routine component of health care. Because problem drinkers cannot be identified by appearance or by socioeconomic characteristics,[37] all women, regardless of the provider's index of suspicion, should be asked about their alcohol use. A preconceptional counseling session is an optimal time for the provider to explain the dangers of alcohol consumption in pregnancy. During such sessions, the preconceptional counselor should

- systematically assess the drinking behavior of the woman
- explain the effects of alcohol on pregnancy outcomes
- suggest that the woman limit her drinking
- avoid guilt-provoking criticisms or scare tactics
- follow up on progress
- refer the woman to a specialized treatment program if she is unable to limit her intake
- document diagnosis and referral
- identify and address associated risks for poor reproductive outcomes, such as marginal nutritional status, tobacco exposure, and the use of psychotropic drugs[38]

Such an approach helps the patient to develop trust in the provider as a nonthreatening and nonjudgmental source of information.

Tools for Identifying and Assessing Alcohol Use

Because no amount of alcohol intake has been proved safe during pregnancy, the preconceptional visit should involve systematic assessment for all women of both alcohol exposure and indicators of abuse.

To determine exposure, a matter-of-fact series of specific questions about her use of beer, wine, and hard liquor is necessary. The Ten-Question Drinking History (TQDH), designed for use in pregnancy, provides a framework for asking about the frequency and quantity of alcohol use (Figure 2-1). This tool was designed to aid in identifying problem drinking[37] but is a useful tool to determine exposure. If no use is uncovered and is consistent with the clinical impression, the woman should be advised that her decision to avoid alcohol is the safest choice as she prepares for pregnancy and that this decision should be maintained.

To identify women who may have difficulty moderating their alcohol use before and during pregnancy, it is useful to screen for indicators of alcohol abuse in all women who use alcohol. Several relatively quick screening tools have been developed, including the Michigan Alcoholism Screening Test[39] and the CAGE.*[40] Sokol,[41] who has conducted research on the clinical identification of obstetric/gynecologic alcohol use, believes a screening tool is enhanced by investigating a patient's tolerance to the inebriating effect of alcohol. According to Sokol,[41(p93)] ''Most women of reproductive age begin to feel high after two or three drinks.'' He suspects that this approach produces less defensiveness and is, therefore, more reliable in identifying women who have an alcohol problem or are at risk of developing one.

To this end, Sokol[42] modified the CAGE and named the new tool the T-ACE

---

*Desire to cut down; annoyed by criticism; guilt about inebriated actions; use of eye opener

Beer: How many times per week? _____
               How many cans each time? _____
               Ever drink more? _____

Wine: How many times per week? _____
               How many glasses each time? _____
               Ever drink more? _____

Liquor: How many times per week? _____
               How many drinks each time? _____
               Ever drink more? _____

Has your drinking changed during the last year?

Figure 2-1 Ten-question drinking history. (Adapted from The American College of Obstetricians and Gynecologists: *Obstet Gynecol* 1981;57:1–7.)

T   How many drinks does it take to make you feel high? (TOLERANCE)
A   Have people ANNOYED you by criticizing your drinking?
C   Have you ever felt you ought to CUT DOWN on your drinking?
E   Have you ever had a drink first thing in the morning to steady your nerves or get rid of a hangover? (EYE-OPENER)

Figure 2-2 The T-ACE questions. (From Sokol RJ, Martier SS, Ager JW: The T-ACE questions: Practical prenatal detection of risk drinking. *Am J Obstet Gynecol* 1989;160:863-870.)

(Figure 2-2). Like the CAGE, the T-ACE comprises only four questions. Unlike the CAGE, however, the T-ACE has a weighted scoring system. The tolerance question is considered to be positive if a woman indicates that she must have more than two drinks to feel high; a positive response receives two points. Each of the other questions is worth one point. A total score of two or greater is considered a positive test.

Because of the lack of biologic markers for use and abuse before the onset of advanced alcoholism, screening tests for alcohol abuse are difficult to validate. Sokol[42] attempted validation of the T-ACE, reporting a sensitivity of 69%, a specificity of 89%, and a positive predictive value of 23%. Confirmation of these findings through additional testing has not been reported. Because it is unlikely that women will exaggerate their alcohol intake, women who have a positive T-ACE should be considered at risk for alcohol-related adverse reproductive outcomes.

In asking about alcohol and other drug use, it is important for the health care provider to use tact and sound judgment in the interview and to integrate the queries as much as possible into the overall history. Any embarrassment or defensiveness on the part of the provider is clear to the patient and is likely to interfere with the development of trust and with the accuracy of reported consumption.[43] Indeed, some patients may become angry when their drinking histories are explored, and this anger should alert the counselor to potential abuse problems.

Types of Problem Drinking

According to Rosett and colleagues,[37] one reason that physicians often fail to inquire about alcohol use is their lack of knowledge about the appropriate treatment if a problem is encountered. They found a classification of problem drinking useful in designing treatment plans.[38] Classifying alcohol use according to motivating factors rather than quantity or duration of use, they note three types of problem drinking: (1) social problem drinking, (2) symptom problem drinking; and (3) alcohol dependence or alcoholism.

Women who drink primarily because of social pressures are likely to report that alcohol is an essential ingredient of their marriages, friendships, and social positions in the community. Rosett and his colleagues found that women in this group are likely to stop drinking for the duration of their pregnancies if they receive brief supportive and educational guidance, including an explanation that they may improve their chances of having a healthy child if they avoid alcohol. The attitudes of the partner or family members are important motivational factors. The latter observation supports the wisdom of including partners in preconceptional counseling sessions.

Women who are symptom problem drinkers are psychologically dependent on alcohol to alter their mood and to relieve such emotions as fear or depression. These women are likely to be sensitive to the attitudes that others have toward them and often misinterpret comments of the staff. Such women require extensive counseling and support.

Alcohol dependence implies a physiologic tolerance for alcohol. Frequently, alcohol-dependent women consume between 0.5 and 1 liter of alcohol each day and have medical complications secondary to alcohol abuse. These women require intensive support and treatment, sometimes through alcohol treatment centers, halfway houses, Alcoholics Anonymous, or drug therapy. The preconceptional counselor should offer drug therapy only after a careful assessment of a woman's contraceptive history and disclosure of potential risks to fetal development should pregnancy occur. Disulfiram (Antabuse), for instance, is a potential teratogen that has been associated with limb anomalies.[37] It should not be prescribed for pregnant women or for women likely to become pregnant while taking the drug.

The research of Rosett and colleagues is specific to pregnant women. They note that a motivator of these women is the health of their future infants; there is no reason to believe that the same motivator would not work with women who are planning a future pregnancy. Rosett and associates indicate that primary care providers who are interested, knowledgeable, and accepting have the skills needed to initiate supportive therapy for women in all three categories and that, for some patients, such management is preferred. They recommend, however, that women who fail to respond within 2 weeks of care be referred to specialized treatment centers.[38]

Therapy and Treatment Sources

To make the proper referral for treatment of alcohol abuse, the preconceptional counselor must be familiar with local resources. As Sokol and colleagues point out,[44] a physician would not tell a patient at risk for genetic disease simply to get in touch with someone at a genetics center. Similarly, it is inappropriate to suggest to the alcohol-abusing patient simply that she call Alcoholics Anonymous. Rather, the provider should refer the patient to a specific alcohol counselor or program or to specific Alcoholics Anonymous meetings, arrange contacts for the patient, and generally facilitate the treatment process.

Some patients may refuse treatment when initially offered. It is important, however, for the provider to maintain contact with these patients and to demonstrate a continuing interest in their drinking behavior. Sokol and associates[44(p16)] report, ''We found that patients with alcohol problems are often distressed if we do not ask how they are doing in controlling their alcohol intake.''

Patients are likely to inquire about safe levels of alcohol consumption in preconceptional counseling sessions. Although it is agreed that there is a dose response to alcohol consumption, no universal threshold has been unequivocally established. Patterns of consumption, timing of fetal exposures, genetic variations in response, and the presence of other risk factors (e.g., marginal nutrition or the use of tobacco) probably determine individual thresholds. Because thresholds for the various alcohol-related reproductive outcomes cannot be prospectively determined by individual patients, their safest choice is to avoid alcohol consumption whenever they suspect that they are pregnant. Patients should know that there is, to date, no measurable risk associated with an occasional drink during pregnancy; this reassurance prevents panic in patients who have had an occasional drink in the early stages of unsuspected pregnancies.

Tobacco Use

Maternal smoking has been identified as the most important single preventable determinant of low birthweight and perinatal mortality in the United States.[45] Associations have been found between smoking and (1) infertility; (2) menstrual disorders; (3) spontaneous abortions; (4) ectopic pregnancies; (5) low birthweight; (6) placental irregularities; (7) infant mortality; and (8) infant and childhood morbidity. Long-term effects on the physical, emotional, and intellectual development of children born to women who smoke during pregnancy have also been reported.

BACKGROUND

Physicians first suggested that there is an association between tobacco exposure and poor reproductive outcomes in the mid-nineteenth century, when they observed that women who were working in tobacco factories appeared to be more prone to spontaneous abortions than were nonexposed women.[46] Little additional attention was paid to the consequences of maternal smoking until Simpson, in her 1957 landmark study, linked cigarette use to premature delivery.[47] Simpson's work stimulated research on the effects of smoking on a spectrum of pregnancy outcomes. Cigarette smoking is currently recognized as a major reproductive risk; a 1980 publication, *The Health Consequences of Smoking for Women,* contains a list of more than 160 references that deal with the effects of smoking on pregnancy outcomes.[48(pp239-249)]

Prevalence of Smoking

The relationship between smoking and reproductive outcome becomes an even greater concern when smoking prevalence data are reviewed. Approximately 26% of women in the United States currently smoke.[49] The lowest prevalence is for Hispanic women (18.7%) followed by that for whites (25.7%) and blacks (27.8%). The rate of smoking varies not only with race but also with age, cultural background, and socioeconomic status. Women ages 25 to 44 are most likely to smoke (29.7%); nearly 30% of women without formal education beyond high school smoke, compared with 23.5% of those who attended some college and 14.6% of women who have a college degree. Data collected in conjunction with the National Health Interview Survey indicate that 32% of women smoked before pregnancy, with 21% quitting during their gestations.[50] A related study determined that one third of white women ages 20 to 44 smoked cigarettes before pregnancy and that the cessation rate during gestation was 40%; 70% to 80% of these women resumed smoking within a year of delivery.[51,77] It is generally estimated that 25% of women continue to smoke during pregnancy.[52]

Effects of Smoking on Pregnancy and Its Outcome

Estimates of the effect of smoking on pregnancy outcome vary. Lincoln[53] reports estimates that smoking results annually in 50,000 fetal deaths and 4,000 infant deaths; Feldman[54] states that approximately 14,000 infant deaths could be prevented annually if pregnant women did not smoke. Maternal smoking has been demonstrated to increase perinatal mortality by 20% in women who smoke less than one pack per day and by 35% in women who smoke more.[55] In a review of five studies, involving nearly 113,000 births in the United States, Wales, and Canada, it was found that 21% to 39% of the births of low-birthweight babies were attributable to maternal cigarette smoking[48(p191)]; 14% of preterm deliveries were related to maternal tobacco use.[54] Compared with the nonsmokers, a woman who smokes has, on the average, twice the risk of giving birth to an infant who weighs less than 2,500 g.[55,56] Smokers' babies are 150 to 250 g lighter than are nonsmokers' babies, or 8 to 9 g lighter for each cigarette smoked on a daily basis.[53] It is generally accepted that the relationship between maternal smoking and reduced birthweight is direct and causal and that there is a clear dose-response relationship between the number of cigarettes smoked and the birthweight deficit.[48(p193),53] One frequently quoted study indicates that maternal smoking of less than one pack per day increases the risk of having a low-birthweight baby by 53%; smoking one pack or more per day increases the risk by 130%.[55]

Studies have shown that women who smoke have an increased incidence of spontaneous abortion[48(p206)] and that the risk of abortion is dose-dependent.[48(p206),53,57] The spontaneously aborted conceptuses of women who smoke tend to be chromosomally normal.[57] This finding, together with the observation that abortions of women who smoke occur later in gestation than do those of nonsmokers, suggests that spontaneous abortions in women smokers are due to complications of pregnancy and to placental factors rather than to abnormalities of the embryo or fetus.

Reports of the incidence of congenital anomalies in the offspring of women who smoke are inconsistent. Some studies have shown no difference in the incidence of congenital anomalies in the children of smokers and those of nonsmokers.[48(p209)] A 1978 study, however, indicates that the risk of abnormalities for the children of smokers is 2.3 times that for the children of nonsmokers, depending on maternal age, pregnancy history, and other factors.[58] Increases have been reported in the incidence of cleft lip and palate,[59] as well as in the incidence of cardiovascular and urogenital anomalies.[58] Other studies have indicated that, although the spontaneously aborted conceptuses of women smokers are more frequently chromosomally normal, they are also more frequently congenitally malformed.[45,53] This observation has prompted the theory that women who smoke are more likely to have malformed fetuses but that their fetuses are more frequently aborted.

Placental complications, including placenta previa, abruptio placentae, and vaginal bleeding, occur more frequently in women who smoke. The risk of placenta previa increases 25% for light or moderate smokers (those who smoke less than one pack per day) and 92% for heavy smokers (those who smoke in excess of one pack per day); the incidence of abruptio placentae increases 24% and 68% for light and heavy smokers, respectively.[55] These findings can be linked to the high perinatal mortality statistics associated with pregnancy in women smokers, as 27% of pregnancies complicated by abruption and 11% of pregnancies complicated by placenta previa result in fetal or infant death, compared with 2% of pregnancies complicated by neither.[55]

Maternal smoking habits either do not affect placental weights or affect them less than they affect birthweights.[48] Because of dose-related reductions in birthweights, the ratio of placental weight to birthweight tends to be larger for smokers than for nonsmokers.[60] The placentas of women who smoke have numerous pathologic abnormalities. They are thinner, have a larger diameter, and manifest various abnormalities of the microcirculation.[61] The latter observation may prove significant in the increased occurrence of placental abruption in women who smoke. Moreover, the larger placental diameter may account for the increased incidence of placenta previa.[56] Another possible explanation for the occurrence of placenta previa in women who smoke is that the placenta may implant itself near the cervix because this area tends to be vascular despite the vasoconstrictive properties of tobacco smoke.[61]

Cigarette smoking may delay conception. In one study, the fertility of smokers was estimated to be 72% of the fertility of nonsmokers, and smokers were found to be 3.4 times more likely to take longer than 1 year to conceive.[62] Another study showed that the risk of tubal infertility among current smokers was 2.7 times that of nonsmokers; for heavy smokers, the risk was 4.2 times greater. Women who smoked and used an intrauterine device (IUD) experienced tubal infertility 6.7 times more often than did their nonsmoking counterparts.[53]

The long-term consequences of maternal smoking for children born to women who smoked during pregnancy are difficult to assess, because they are obscured by the effects of passive smoking during infancy and childhood. The British perinatal mortality study has provided longitudinal data on 17,000 children born in Great Britain in 1958.[60] A multifactorial analysis of these data showed that, at age 11, the children of smokers were an average of 1 cm shorter than those of nonsmokers and were behind an average of 3 to 5 months in reading, mathematics, and general abilities. The deficits that had been noted when these children were 7 years old had neither increased nor decreased during the intervening years. Children of women who smoke during and after pregnancy have more respiratory infections, more hospitalizations, and more visits to the physician.[45,53] Several studies have linked maternal smoking with sudden infant death syndrome (SIDS).[48(p225)] In one report, the relative risk of SIDS for the infants of smokers versus the infants of nonsmokers was shown to double from 2.3 per 1,000 to 4.6 per 1,000.[63] To date, the relative contribution of prenatal and postnatal exposures has not been determined.

Mechanisms of Action of Cigarette Smoke

The mechanisms by which cigarette smoke affects reproductive outcomes are not fully understood. Tobacco smoke contains between 2,000 and 4,000 chemicals, including nicotine, carbon monoxide, thiocyanide, plutonium, resins, tars, polycyclic aromatic hydrocarbons, cadmium, and vinyl chloride. While it would be simplistic and naive to ascribe all the reproductive consequences of smoking to a single factor,[45] the most significant exposures currently appear to be those to nicotine, to the polycyclic aromatic hydrocarbons, and to carbon monoxide.[48(pp229-235)] These substances are absorbed through the alveoli into the bloodstream. By means of simple diffusion, facilitated diffusion, and active transport, the chemicals cross the placental membrane.[54]

Nicotine is known to be a vasoconstrictor that affects the central nervous system, skeletal muscles, and sympathetic and parasympathetic ganglia much as acetylcholine does. The vasoconstrictive properties of nicotine have been associated with decreased uterine blood flow and diminished placental perfusion. Vasospasm of the umbilical and peripheral fetal vascular circulations may also occur, resulting in decreased oxygen exchange and tissue hypoxia.[45] Inhalation of nicotine is an unnecessary precursor to these physiologic effects. Blood levels of nicotine that follow the use of smokeless tobacco are similar to those that follow cigarette smoking,[64] and there is evidence to link the maternal use of smokeless tobacco to deficits in neonatal weight and length.[65]

The amount of tobacco smoked determines the concentrations of polycyclic aromatic hydrocarbons found in the placenta. These substances, which result from the incomplete combustion of organic material, have been implicated in the disruption of normal maternal-fetal transport systems.[48(p233)]

Approximately 4% of cigarette smoke is carbon monoxide.[66] After displacing the oxygen carried in hemoglobin, carbon monoxide joins with hemoglobin to form carboxyhemoglobin. The concentration of carboxyhemoglobin is approximately 1% in nonsmoking women and increases by 4% to 5% per pack smoked per day.[45] Elevated concentrations of carboxyhemoglobin have been associated with numerous physiologic alterations in adults, and fetal carboxyhemoglobin concentrations are generally 10% to 15% higher than maternal levels.[67] The effects on the fetus are not fully understood, but elevated fetal concentrations have been associated with decreased fetal blood oxygen tension and chronic hypoxia.[68]

Sources of Information on the Hazards of Smoking

Pregnant women have reported obtaining information about the hazards of smoking during pregnancy from the following sources: 84% from television, 52% from posters and leaflets, 37% from their husbands, 34% from books and magazines, 16% from their physicians, and 9% from nurses.[53] Physicians are important relayers of information, and many studies indicate that a physician's advice to stop smoking can influence a patient to do so. Minimal physician advice has been reported to cause 10% to 30% of pregnant women to stop smoking for 1 year.[69] In a recent study, however, only 44% of all smokers could recall that a physician had ever advised them to stop smoking.[70] Another recent survey reveals that only 48.6% of 113 obstetric/gynecologic physicians routinely counseled or referred the smokers in their practices.[71]

PRECONCEPTIONAL COUNSELING

The goal of preconceptional counseling regarding tobacco use is to educate the woman and her partner about the general health risks of tobacco use and the effect of smoking on reproductive outcomes. The counselor should make a firm statement about the wisdom of ceasing to use tobacco preconceptionally. Should the patient accept this recommendation, the counselor should explain the various techniques that have helped others to stop smoking. This action verifies the commitment of the provider and gives the patient specific tools with which to make the transition from smoker to ex-smoker. Although very little has been written about cessation strategies for smokeless tobacco, information drawn from available resources on cigarette smoking should be applicable to other tobacco habits.

Preparation for Smoking Cessation

Physicians generally report a lack of success in motivating patients to change their tobacco habits but have indicated that their success rates would improve with appropriate support, such as referral information, patient literature, risk factor questionnaires, and education in behavior modification.[72] In addition, physicians should remember a number of principles when counseling the cigarette smoker. For example, they should recognize smoking as a complex, addictive behavior influenced by physical, emotional, and social factors.[69] Not only are smokers psychologically dependent on the habit, but they also have a chemical dependency on nicotine that can create a sensation of pleasure, relaxation, and sedation while diminishing anxiety, regulating mood, and improving performance on certain types of tasks.[54]

The creation of guilt or anxiety is not an effective strategy to help patients stop smoking. This fact is of particular importance in counseling the woman who is contemplating a pregnancy following the poor outcome of an earlier pregnancy. The emphasis should be on the prevention of future problems rather than the causation of past outcomes.[73]

Current evidence indicates that those who stop smoking have typically been unsuccessful in earlier attempts to do so. With repeated attempts, however, 60% of self-quitters succeed.[69] Many smokers are unaware of this and interpret past failures as a sign of the futility of any future effort. Therefore, the counselor should emphasize the positive nature of past attempts while exploring the circumstances that surrounded relapses. When past obstacles to quitting are identified (e.g., lack of social support, poor timing, limited plans for dealing with stress), strategies for future attempts can be more thoughtfully designed.

Many smokers think that they will automatically gain weight if they give up their cigarette habit. This common fear should be explored, and patients should be reassured that nearly 70% of those who stop smoking do not gain weight.[74] For those who do gain weight, the average gain is 5 to 8 pounds. A preventive visit to a nutritionist may prove beneficial for those patients who plan to stop smoking.

The preconceptional counselor should acknowledge that withdrawal symptoms are real and unpleasant, although as many as 40% to 50% of ex-smokers in several surveys reported no withdrawal effects.[75] Patients should understand that their withdrawal symptoms are likely to be intense for only 1 to 2 weeks and that cigarette cravings last 3 to 5 minutes—whether or not a cigarette is smoked. The fact that the body rids itself of nicotine in 3 to 7 days may account for the reported severity of withdrawal symptoms in the first week. It is recommended that the counselor prepare all prospective quitters for the common withdrawal symptoms, such as craving, coughing, and light-headedness, and inform them that these symptoms indicate the body's ability to overcome the previous effects of smoking. Patients should be encouraged to plan ways to cope with withdrawal symptoms (e.g., exercising, chewing gum, or drinking water). To reduce the intensity of withdrawal symptoms, some practitioners advocate brand-switching to cigarettes that are progressively lower in nicotine over several weeks before quitting and then quitting abruptly rather than tapering.[69,74]

Successful Intervention

One authority reports that 90% of smokers in the United States want to quit.[69] The preconceptional counselor can make use of that motivation by helping the patient to learn and practice effective quitting skills and to mobilize her social support system. It is wise to include the patient's partner in the preconceptional visit. Questions regarding the hazards of secondary smoke, if the partner is a smoker, can also be addressed at this time.

Successful practitioner interventions for smoking behavior consist of four basic components: (1) documenting the patient's history; (2) setting a quit date (which should be determined by the patient and then noted in her record); (3) encouraging the involvement of friends and family; and (4) reinforcing the message while monitoring progress.[52,72] The latter can be achieved through telephone calls, letters, or clinic visits.

The patient should be given an opportunity to choose the technique that she will use to stop smoking. Among her options are quitting on her own; undergoing hypnosis; participating in an organized group method, such as those sponsored by the Seventh Day Adventists, the American Cancer Society, the American Lung Association, and others; or using nicotine replacement therapy. The latter approach has been demonstrated to increase the effectiveness of smoking cessation programs by approximately 50% when the patient is evaluated 6 months after the intervention.[76] Success with nicotine replacement therapy is markedly enhanced when combined with other supportive therapies, such as social support. Nicotine gum is contraindicated during pregnancy, and the manufacturers' inserts for transdermal patches advise that pregnant women not use them except under the guidance of their physician. These precautions are taken because nicotine is considered to be an important contributor to the adverse reproductive effects associated with smoking. Identifying women who smoke and facilitating cessation before conception, with or without nicotine replacement therapy, will result in a timely reduction of reproductive risk.

In no instance should the motivated patient leave her counseling session without a specific plan and written information to enable her to implement it. For example, the American Lung Association, the American Cancer Society, and the American Health Foundation publish self-help guides; such resources should be available for loan from the preconceptional counseling clinic. If the patient's plan involves an organized group, she should not leave the clinic until she has the name and telephone number of a person to contact.

Some patients may not wish to stop smoking, or they may be unable to stop. Explaining that the adverse effects of tobacco use on reproduction appear to be dose-related and that any decrease in exposure is beneficial, the practitioner should encourage these patients to taper their habit to the fewest cigarettes possible each day, with a goal of fewer than ten. However, patients should be reassured through attitude and action that the practitioner's regard for them will not be adversely affected by uneven progress or a lack of success. To imply otherwise is to invite a lack of candor in their reporting or a loss of contact with them regarding other important preconceptional issues.

Finally, considerable evidence shows that women who stop or decrease smoking during pregnancy resume their old habits postnatally. Approximately 50% of women who stop smoking during pregnancy resume the habit within 3 months of giving birth, and 70% to 80% do so by 12 months postpartum.[51,77] It seems appropriate, as a general health promotion effort, to flag the charts of women who have changed their habits before and during pregnancy and to provide them with structured support and education as they near their delivery date and later as they return for postpartum evaluations. Their past success will most likely prove a helpful motivator.

Illicit Drug Use

In taking routine histories, health care providers often do not include specific queries about the use of illicit drugs. Mounting evidence suggests that these substances have serious reproductive consequences. Recent reports document that 7.3% to 13.3% of pregnant women use cocaine, marijuana, or opiates. Women seeking prenatal care through private practices are likely to be underdiagnosed for illicit drug use. One study found no significant difference in the prevalence of illicit substance use between public and private patients.[79]

BACKGROUND

Statistics on the prevalence of illicit drug use are understandably scarce and of questionable reliability. Data from the 1990 National Household Survey on Drug Abuse identify marijuana as the most common illicit drug used in the United States; 20.7% of women ages 18 to 25 and 14.9% of women ages 26 to 35 reported having used the drug at least once during the previous year.[83] Estimates derived from the survey indicate that 17.4% of pregnant women between the ages of 12 and 34 used marijuana at some time during their pregnancies.[84(p21)]

The second most frequently used drug is cocaine. The prevalence of cocaine use appears to be declining, with 6.6 million persons reporting use in a 1990 survey, compared with 12 million in 1988.[85] The 1990 National Household Survey reports that 4.8% of women ages 18 to 25 and 4.5% of women ages 26 to 34 admitted to cocaine use in 1990.[83] Several institutional and geographic surveys estimate the use among pregnant women at widely varying levels, ranging from 0.3% to 36%.[84] The disparity most likely represents the diversity of populations studied and methodologies used. Estimates based on the 1990 Household Survey indicate that a realistic estimate for cocaine use during pregnancy is 4.5%.[84]

Effects of Marijuana Use

In 1982, researchers at Carleton University in Ottawa collected data on the marijuana use habits of 420 predominantly middle-class pregnant women.[86] They found that, in the 12 months preceding conception, 82% had not used marijuana; 13% had been irregular users, meaning that they had smoked one joint or fewer per week or had been exposed to the exhaled smoke of others; 2% had been moderate users, meaning that they had smoked two to five joints per week; and 3% had been heavy users, meaning that they had smoked more than five joints per week. Three of the 344 prepregnant nonusers reported irregular use during pregnancy. The percentage of women in each of the other prepregnancy categories decreased after conception, although nine women continued to be heavy users throughout gestation.

When the researchers at Carleton University compared the women classified as moderate to heavy users with nonusers, they observed no differences in the rates of miscarriage, complications at birth, length of labor, or medication requirements.[86] Regular use (i.e., moderate to heavy use), however, was associated with shorter gestations, decreased maternal weight gain, and a decreased likelihood that the offspring would respond to light stimuli. The offspring also exhibited heightened tremor and startle responses. One third of the regular users had infants with the high-pitched cry that has been observed in neonates undergoing narcotic withdrawal. By 1 year of age, the offspring of users and nonusers had similar motor, mental, and behavioral characteristics. The heavy and moderate users were more likely to smoke cigarettes and to drink alcohol than were the irregular users and nonusers, but the numbers in the study were too small to allow for an analysis of the relative contribution of each of these habits on the observed outcomes.

The findings of subsequent studies have been inconsistent. Three reports indicate a relationship between prenatal marijuana exposure and fetal anomalies,[87-89] but most human evidence indicates that prenatal use does not by itself cause abnormalities. It is possible, however, that marijuana has an additive effect on the teratogenic potential of other substances, such as alcohol.[88,90(p26-27)] Some researchers have voiced concern that the psychoactive ingredient in marijuana, tetrahydrocannabinol (THC), causes genetic damage; however, no evidence of chromosomal damage to cells incubated with THC has been found in either animal or human studies.[90(p25)]

Marijuana, like tobacco, reduces the amount of oxygen and increases carbon monoxide levels in maternal blood; both of these effects decrease the oxygen available to the fetus, which should, theoretically, have a negative effect on fetal growth. However, studies on humans have been unable to demonstrate consistently an association between marijuana use and birthweight. A study by Zuckerman and associates[91] indicates that misclassification of users may have resulted in negative findings. In their study of 1,266 women, 16% of the 331 women who used marijuana denied use during interviews but tested positive in urine assay. After controlling for potentially confounding variables, including pregravid weight, prenatal weight gain, alcohol, tobacco, and other drug exposures, infants of the women known to have used marijuana prenatally, by history, testing, or both, had a 79 g decrease in birthweight ($p = 0.04$) and a 0.5 cm decrement in length ($p = 0.02$), compared with a control group. Gestational length was unaffected. When outcomes for women identified as marijuana users only by self-report were examined, there was no birthweight association. The authors note that had they relied on self-report to ascertain marijuana use, as is typical of most studies, their findings would have been obscured.

Researchers have examined the behavioral consequences of prenatal marijuana exposure. Infants exposed in utero have been noted to have increased jitteriness during the neonatal period.[86,92] A longitudinal study is under way to compare children known to have been prenatally exposed to marijuana with children who have no history of exposure. Comparisons are made at yearly intervals; data for the first 4 years are currently available.[93,94] Testing during the first 3 years demonstrated no negative effect of marijuana exposure on mental or linguistic development. Testing at 4 years of age, however, revealed poorer performance in memory and verbal skills. The children will continue to be studied through age 6.

A small study conducted in California indicates that users of marijuana may have more problems during labor, such as meconium staining; precipitate, prolonged, or arrested labors; and manual removal of the placenta; but differences between users and nonusers generally were not statistically significant.[95]

As these studies show, it is difficult to ascribe outcome to particular behaviors. Maternal behaviors such as drinking, smoking, and using marijuana or other psychoactive drugs are difficult to quantify reliably because measurement requires self-reporting. Underreporting, which may be particularly problematic in assessing the use of illegal substances, is a serious concern because it obscures real effects.[96] Furthermore, maternal use of alcohol, tobacco, and recreational drugs is likely to be interrelated, necessitating multivariate analysis to assess the relative contribution of any given behavior to an outcome.

Although current data conflict, until marijuana is proven to have no negative consequences women should be counseled to avoid this unnecessary exposure.

Effects of Cocaine Use

In recent years, the relationship between cocaine use and pregnancy outcomes has been studied a great deal. In a landmark study conducted in 1985 at Northwestern University, Chasnoff and associates[97] compared and contrasted pregnancy outcomes for 12 women who conceived while using cocaine; 11 women who conceived while using both cocaine and heroin; 15 women who conceived while using heroin, but not cocaine; and 15 women who were not drug abusers. The groups were matched for maternal age; number of previous pregnancies; and cigarette, marijuana, and alcohol use. The heroin users were placed on methadone maintenance. Women in the first two groups (i.e., those who used cocaine) reported contractions and increased fetal movement within minutes of using cocaine. Four women in the two groups experienced the onset of labor and abruptio placentae immediately after a cocaine injection; the drug's association with hypertension and vasoconstriction may be responsible for the high incidence of abruption.

No statistically significant differences were found in birthweights, lengths, or head circumferences among the infants from the four groups.[97] However, infants exposed to cocaine in utero had a significant depression of interactive behavior and a poor organizational response to environmental stimuli. Only one infant in the entire sample had an anomaly. This child, who had prune-belly syndrome, was born to a woman who reported heavy use of cocaine at 5 weeks' gestation but no other use until the third trimester.

Subsequent studies have indicated stronger associations between in utero cocaine exposure and congenital anomalies. In one study, 50 infants born to women who used cocaine were compared with 30 infants born to polydrug, noncocaine-using women. The two groups of women were similar in age, gravidity, and race; all women were entered into the study during the first trimester of pregnancy. The infants were similar in mean birthweight. Seven of the cocaine-exposed infants were found to have genitourinary tract malformations, and two were diagnosed with biliary atresia, whereas no such defects were identified in the comparison group. The authors speculate that the vasoconstrictive effects of cocaine might explain the difference.[98] The study, however, lacks statistical power to establish clearly a relationship between cocaine use and anomolous development. A large case-control study compared 276 infants with congenital urinary tract anomalies, 4,315 infants with other birth defects, and 2,637 healthy infants. The neonates with urinary tract anomalies were significantly more likely to have been exposed to cocaine.

In addition to congenital anomalies, cocaine has been associated with many other maternal-fetal risks. A recent review article summarizes findings from the plethora of studies undertaken in the late 1980s.[99] Maternal risks include placental abruption, abnormal labor, spontaneous abortion, and premature rupture of the membranes. Fetal and infant effects include low birthweight, shortened gestation, poor fetal growth, behavioral abnormalities, congenital anomalies, sudden infant death syndrome, necrotizing enterocolitis, and cerebrovascular accidents. In addition, cocaine use provides risks to users irrespective of gravid status: myocardial and vascular toxicity, cerebrovascular accidents, subarachnoid hemorrhage, hypertension, seizures, hyperpyrexia, intestinal ischemia, pulmonary edema, and sudden death. Risks not included in this review but well recognized include malnutrition, sexually transmitted diseases, including hepatitis B and the human immunodeficiency viruses, and related addictions.[100]

The long-term effects of cocaine on the developing child have caused a great deal of concern and speculation. The popular press and many professional articles have promulgated the belief that the majority of infants exposed to cocaine in utero suffer neurodevelopmental effects that are incompatible with normal social functioning or educational achievement. These sentiments are not based on scientific study. As one commentary notes, ''Valid concern about the high rate of cocaine use among pregnant women has resulted in an apparent rush to judgment about the extent and permanency of specific effects of intrauterine cocaine exposure on newborns.''[101] To date, the scientific literature regarding cocaine exposure has been characterized by numerous methodologic problems, and no prospective, longitudinal study of the consequences of intrauterine cocaine exposure has been published in the peer-review literature.[101] Until conclusive data are available on the long-term effects of cocaine exposure, care must be taken not to represent these children as irretrievably damaged, because such attitudes could themselves prove equally damaging.

Effects of the Use of Other Illicit Drugs

Female heroin addicts often experience menstrual abnormalities and anovulatory cycles. They are relatively infertile, but they have high rates of sexual activity and do become pregnant.[102] Detoxification and methadone maintenance are the two safest options in the prenatal care of these women.[103] Abrupt abstinence during pregnancy has undesirable effects on the fetus, because the withdrawal may lead to hyperactivity, intrauterine convulsions, passage of meconium, or stillbirth.[104] Addicts who are on methadone maintenance programs are less likely to have complicated pregnancies, although this may result from more frequent contact with the health care system rather than from changes in drug exposure. Infants exposed in utero to methadone tend to have better intrauterine growth patterns, but the neonatal withdrawal syndrome is more severe and prolonged than that of heroin-exposed infants.[105]

Neither heroin nor methadone has been associated with physical abnormalities in prenatally exposed infants. After birth, however, children exposed to either drug typically suffer from the neonatal withdrawal syndrome characterized by a high-pitched cry, tremors, increased muscle tone, vomiting, loose stools, fever, tachypnea, nasal stuffiness, disturbed sleep, and a voracious appetite.[104,106] The infants require days to weeks of pharmacologic and physical support to overcome the effects of their withdrawal.

Both heroin and methadone are believed to be behavioral teratogens that lead to hyperactivity and short attention spans in children exposed to them prenatally.[107] Because children born to addicts are likely to have been exposed prenatally to many negative influences (e.g., alcohol, tobacco, numerous other abused drugs, and poor nutrition) and because they are frequently raised in suboptimal environments, it is difficult to prove cause-and-effect relationships between heroin or methadone and behavior. However, animal models support the hypothesis that these drugs adversely affect long-term behavior.

Phencyclidine (PCP or ''angel dust'') was a commonly used illicit substance during the 1970s, when it was involved in approximately 25% of psychedelic drug use.[108] Its relatively low cost makes it attractive to drug users, particularly to adolescents, but the current prevalence of its use is unknown. In utero PCP exposure results in detectable amounts of PCP in the neonate's urine and in characteristic newborn behaviors similar to those of the neonatal withdrawal syndrome.[108] Like adults intoxicated with the substance, exposed newborns may have sudden bursts of agitation and rapid changes in levels of consciousness.[109] Short-term follow-up of exposed children has indicated that the effects are self-limiting.[109] Occasional case reports have suggested that PCP may be a teratogen; however, most women exposed to PCP are polydrug users, and large, carefully designed studies that take into account all such exposures must be conducted before the teratogenicity of PCP can be confirmed. There is no evidence in mice that the drug is a teratogen at levels of ingestion nontoxic to the mother.[109]

Similarly, it is not yet possible to draw definitive conclusions about the teratogenicity of lysergic acid diethylamide (LSD). Although there have been case reports of limb and nervous system defects associated with LSD exposure, causation has not been established.[110] In at least one study of chromosomal breakage in association with LSD use, no increase in chromosomal damage was uncovered in 41 infants whose parents had used LSD.[111]

PRECONCEPTIONAL COUNSELING

The goals of preconceptional counseling in regard to illicit drug use are to identify women with a past or current history of use; to educate them and, when they wish, their partners about the personal and fetal risks of exposure; and to screen them for associated high-risk conditions.

Because of the apparent prevalence of drug use across the socioeconomic spectrum, routine and matter-of-fact inquiries about exposures should be made of all patients who seek preconceptional counseling. The line of questioning can be adapted from either of the tools used to investigate a patient's alcohol use (see Figures 2-1 and 2-2), or it can follow a tool specifically designed to explore drug use (Figure 2-3). Whichever approach is used, all patients should be asked questions relative to the most commonly used drugs, cocaine and marijuana; clinical judgment determines whether it is necessary to explore the use of other drugs.

The rationale for the questions should be explained to all women, whether their responses are positive or not. A statement such as "Cocaine and marijuana have become very common in our society, but we know that they can have harmful effects on pregnancy and on the newborn," may relax patients during this series of questions and provide health information to those unwilling to reveal their exposures.

The American Council for Drug Education suggests criteria for categorizing marijuana and cocaine use patterns (Table 2-1).[112] Women with low exposure may benefit from a single educational encounter on the reproductive effects of the drug

1. Have you ever tried _____ ?
2. How old were you when you first used _____ ?
3. When did you most recently use _____ ? (If you quit, why?)
4. How much do you usually use now?
5. Do you ever use more? How much?
6. Have you ever had problems associated with _____ ?
7. Do you plan to quit? How?
8. Do you ever take any other drugs, including alcohol, with _____ ?

Figure 2-3 Questions useful in exploring drug use. (Adapted from *Drugs and Pregnancy: It's Not Worth the Risk*. American Council for Drug Education, 1986.)

Table 2-1 Categorizing drug use patterns

DRUG	HIGH EXPOSURE	MODERATE EXPOSURE	LOW EXPOSURE
Marijuana	1 or more joints/ day or 2 or more joints/occasion	1-2 joints/week and no more than 1 joint/occasion	Occasional use and no more than ½-1 joint/ occasion
Cocaine	Use 3 times/week or more	Less than weekly use	Occasional use— monthly or less

Adapted from *Drugs and Pregnancy. It's Not Worth the Risk.* American Council for Drug Education, 1986.

that they use, coupled with reinforcement at subsequent visits. Women with moderate exposure may benefit from additional group education that is, ideally, available in the community; preconceptional counselors should investigate the availability of such services so that they can provide specific information, including hours, costs, telephone number, and name of a contact person, to women who wish to modify their drug exposures. The women with high exposure should also be offered these services but are likely to require individual counseling in a substance abuse treatment program. Again, the preconceptional counselor should be prepared to make an appropriate referral to a specific program. Several sessions may be necessary before the woman with high exposure is sufficiently motivated to seek referral. These sessions should include a review of the various actions that she has already taken for the health of her future child and an explanation of the additional benefits that she and her child would gain through abstinence from unnecessary drugs.

An important intervention to prevent the use of hazardous drugs during pregnancy and, presumably, before conception is a strong practitioner-patient alliance that is focused on the delivery of a healthy baby and based on a genuine mutual respect.[112] Recognizing the importance of this strategy in behavioral modification, the practitioner should be willing to commit the time necessary to develop rapport with the patient and to establish useful interventions. It is also helpful in counseling the drug-abusing woman to determine the reasons for her drug use (e.g., pressure from friends or partner, depression). Should the patient be able to provide such insights, the plans for intervention can be personalized to address the specific issues involved in her illicit drug use.

It is unlikely that a woman addicted to heroin will seek preconceptional counseling. If an addict does seek counseling, however, the goal should be to enroll the patient in a program of supervised withdrawal to be completed before conception. In this way, both the fetal and neonatal effects of heroin and methadone exposure can be avoided.

In women with a history of intravenous cocaine or heroin use, related high-risk factors (e.g., infection with the human immunodeficiency virus [HIV] and hepatitis B virus) should be evaluated. Women who have not used intravenous routes of drug administration but are admitted or suspected illicit drug users may also be at risk for infection with these viruses through their sexual activity. Current or former sexual partners of drug users are more likely than is the general population to have been involved in the drug culture and, thus, to have been infected through the intravenous route.

Women who have a history of illicit drug use are more likely to use alcohol, smoke cigarettes, and be at nutritional risk. All of these factors should be carefully assessed and appropriate interventions offered during the preconceptional counseling process.

Environmental Exposures
at Home and at Work

A t least one third of the babies born each year have a work history before their delivery. Chemical exposure is not, however, limited to those women who work outside the home; it can safely be said that every woman is exposed daily to many chemicals found in her environment. Nonchemical exposures at work and at home may also be of concern. The effect of various maternal environmental exposures on reproductive outcomes is generally unknown, although it has been stated that those birth defects related to environmental agents are potentially the most preventable.[113]

BACKGROUND

In a recent book devoted to chemically induced birth defects, Schardein[114(p565)] writes:

> As recently as 1980, an estimate by the United States Environmental Protection Agency indicated that there were 55,000 chemicals in use. Approximately 10% of this number are produced in quantities exceeding 1 million pounds per year. More than 35,000 pesticides are registered with the EPA, some 3,600 food additives are approved for use by the FDA and more than 1,500 chemicals are listed as common ingredients in cosmetics. Over 1,200 additional compounds are incorporated into countless household products.

Estimates of the incidence of congenital malformation secondary to environmental exposures vary. One report states that 3% of anomalies may be attributable to drugs or chemicals.[115] Another indicates that 5% to 10% of all birth defects can be ascribed to teratogens and that an additional 60% to 65% may result from multifactorial influences, including an interplay between environmental exposures and genetic features; of those birth defects caused by environmental agents, 4% to 6% are reportedly linked to chemical exposures.[113]

Congenital anomalies are not the only adverse reproductive outcomes associated with environmental exposures. For example, anesthetic gases have been implicated as a cause of infertility and spontaneous abortion, as well as malformation[116]; inorganic lead has been associated with sterility, spontaneous abortion, fetal and neonatal losses, low birthweight, and disorders of the central nervous system in the offspring.[117] Other outcomes that have been associated with maternal exposures to various chemicals include menstrual disorders, genetic alterations, and childhood developmental and behavioral problems.

Effects of Toxic Exposures

Toxic agents may act as mutagens, teratogens, or carcinogens. Mutagens disrupt the genetic material of living cells; they can affect both male and female germ cells and thus have a subsequent effect on reproduction. Teratogens affect embryonic development after maternal exposure. Teratogenic exposure may result in a lethal insult to the conceptus if it occurs between days 1 and 17 of embryogenesis, in structural anomalies if it occurs between days 17 and 56 of embryogenesis, or in no discernible effect at all. Should the pregnancy continue after a toxic exposure or should the exposure occur later in gestation, the result may be a functional rather than a structural impairment.

Substances that increase the incidence of cancer in the offspring of the exposed woman have been termed *transgenerational carcinogens.*[118] Interest in transgenerational carcinogens has focused on those with transplacental effects, the most widely known of which is diethylstilbestrol (DES). Adverse outcomes theoretically may result from either parent's exposure to transgenerational carcinogens if the increased susceptibility to cancer is secondary to chromosomal breakage, point mutation, or abnormalities in gametogenesis or fertilization. Transgenerational carcinogens are extremely difficult to identify because the latency period for tumor formation in affected offspring appears to be 5 to 18 years.[119]

The result of a potentially toxic exposure depends on a number of factors, including:

- the ability of the toxin or agent to alter normal processes
- the susceptibility of the target tissues as determined, in part, by the stage of development of the embryo or fetus
- the intensity of the exposure
- the host's resistance, which may relate to maternal or embryo/fetal genotype[115,120]

Because of these variations, only a fraction of the pregnancies exposed to embryotoxic or fetotoxic substances are adversely affected.

The effect that a potentially toxic substance will have on a conceptus cannot be extrapolated from experiences with adult populations. The embryo or fetus may be more susceptible to the toxic effects of environmental exposures than are adults because of its rapid cell division, a relative lack of metabolic detoxification and excretion mechanisms, and relatively poor immunosurveillance.[121] It is not uncommon, for instance, for fetal methylmercury poisoning to occur in the offspring of asymptomatic women.[117]

Identification of Toxic Exposures

Unfortunately, knowledge that makes it possible to associate specific chemicals with specific reproductive outcomes is severely limited. Because much of the available information is based on anecdotes and inference, its validity is subject to change.[122] In 1973, for example, a study that linked industrial exposure to adhesive sprays with increased chromosomal breaks and birth defects led to a ban on these sprays; nine women elected to terminate their pregnancies as a result of this action, only to see the ban lifted 6 months later because the association could not be confirmed by further experiments.[117] History is replete with cases of inappropriate anxiety created by the media as a result of suggestive findings; the media generally do not give equal attention to follow-up data that refute the original report.[123]

Prospective parents themselves may promote considerable anxiety. Rumors that the incidence of spontaneous abortion, for example, is unusually high when women or their partners are exposed to certain substances or situations sometimes run rampant in occupational settings. Because the public is generally uninformed that approximately 20% of all conceptions result in spontaneous abortion, emotionally fueled conclusions are drawn. Such rumors require epidemiologic investigation by impartial observers before they are presented or accepted as fact.

In 1981, researchers at Columbia University who undertook a comprehensive review of the literature found that, of the 10 occupational exposures that had been investigated for their effects in humans after maternal exposure, five (50%) were associated with poor reproductive outcomes.[124] Of 15 paternal exposures, seven (47%) were associated with poor reproductive outcomes. The paucity of data in human populations makes it necessary to rely on animal research in assigning risk. Over 800 chemicals have been demonstrated to be teratogenic in laboratory animals,[113] whereas only one nondrug substance, organic mercury, has been conclusively proved teratogenic in humans.[114(p619),125] (It is of note that the one chemical proved teratogenic in humans is not associated with exposure in the workplace but rather with contamination of the food chain.[114(p574)])

Care must be taken, however, before it is said that substances demonstrated to be teratogenic in animals are also teratogenic in humans. Karnofsky's law, accepted by most teratologists, is that any drug given in large enough doses at a sensitive time during pregnancy will affect embryonic or fetal development.[123] The law also applies to chemicals. Warnings of potential teratogenicity or other poor outcomes are, in some cases, based on the administration of substances to laboratory animals in amounts 1,000 times the therapeutic or normal dose.[123] On the other hand, all the known teratogens, with the exception of the coumarin anticoagulants, are also teratogenic in one or more laboratory species. Unfortunately, in almost every instance, the teratogenicity of drugs and environmental agents has been discovered in humans before it has been discovered in animals.[114(p27)]

To identify a new teratogenic agent in humans, it is necessary to observe:
- an abrupt increase in a particular defect or association of defects
- a coincidental increase in a known environmental factor
- a recognized exposure to the environmental factor early in pregnancy
- the absence of other factors common to all the pregnancies that resulted in infants with the characteristic defect[126]

Add to these criteria the variability in embryo and fetal response to exposure, the likelihood of multiple maternal exposures to chemicals at work and at home, and the number of women who behave in ways that have known adverse reproductive effects (e.g., use alcohol or tobacco), and it is easy to understand why it is difficult to reach definitive conclusions about the reproductive risks of individual agents.

Providers should routinely assess exposures so that they can give patients prudent education or advice. The education and recommendations should be based on up-to-date information such as is available through a number of resources (Appendix B). As a starting reference, general categories of environmental exposures, reported reproductive effects, and common modes of exposure are provided in Table 2-2. Of

Table 2-2 Selected effects reported for various environmental exposures

Hazard	Types	Associated Outcomes	Sources of Exposure
Metals	Lead	Abnormal sperm, menstrual disorders, spontaneous abortions, stillbirths, mental retardation	Solder, lead pipes, batteries, paints, ceramics, smelter emissions
	Mercury	Impaired fetal motor and mental development	Thermometers, mirror coating, dyes, inks, pesticides, dental fillings (for those who prepare the filling material)
Solvents	Trichloroethylene Chloroform Benzene Toluene	Birth defects	Dry cleaning fluids, degreasers, paint strippers, drug and electronics industries
	Carbon disulfide	Decreased fertility, increased spontaneous abortion rate	Textile industry
Vinyl monomers	Vinyl chloride	Decreased fertility, chromosomal aberrations, spontaneous abortions, stillbirths, birth defects	Plastic manufacturing

Continued

Table 2-2 Selected effects reported for various environmental exposures—cont'd

Hazard	Types	Associated Outcomes	Sources of Exposure
Pollutants	Polychlorinated biphenyl (PCB) Polybrominated biphenyl (PBB)	Low birth rate, stillbirths	Pesticides; carbonless copy paper; rubber, chemicals, and electronics industries; fire retardants; food chain
Pesticides	2,4,5-T 2,4-D organophosphates (e.g., malathion)	Birth defects, spontaneous abortions, low birthweight	Farm, home, and garden insect sprays; treated wood (for outdoor buildings)
Gases	Carbon monoxide	Low birthweight, stillbirths	Automobile exhausts, furnaces, kerosene heaters, cake ovens, cigarette smoke
	Anesthetic gases	Decreased fertility, spontaneous abortions, birth defects	Dental offices, operating rooms, chemicals industries
Radiation	X-rays	Sterility, birth defects	Medical and dental offices, electronics industries
Drugs	Antineoplastics (e.g., cyclophosphamide, doxorubicin, and vincristine)	Fetal loss	Pharmacies, medical offices, hosptials

particular note is the fact that, for many categories of chemicals, exposure may be through activities other than employment. For example, refurbishing an old house may expose a woman to excessive levels of lead; a woman heavily involved in gardening may come into close contact with pesticides; and persons who use kerosene heaters may be exposed to high levels of carbon monoxide.

Sources of Exposures

Frequently overlooked sources of potentially toxic substances are the materials used in hobbies. A 1975 poll indicated that approximately 56.7 million people in the United States engage in woodworking, weaving, pottery, ceramics, or other crafts and that approximately 21.8 million people engage in painting, drawing, or sculpture.[127] Although some of these people are professional artisans, the vast majority are hobbyists who may be at increased risk for adverse exposures because they lack knowledge about safety precautions. Potentially toxic art materials in common use include lacquer and paint thinners, paint and varnish removers, cleaning solvents, lead, plastics, and adhesives.[127] Even though causal relationships between each of these substances and poor reproductive outcomes have not been established, it seems prudent to advise women to minimize or modify their exposures to these substances whenever possible. If it is necessary to use these substances, women should take precautions, such as ensuring excellent ventilation and wearing gloves.

Ionizing Radiation

Investigation of environmental factors that may affect reproductive outcomes should not be limited to chemical compounds. For example, parental exposure to ionizing radiation has been associated with genetic damage, increased cancer risks, and malformations in their offspring. The broad definition of radiation, which is the movement of energy from one location to another, includes sound waves, heat waves, and electromagnetic waves (e.g., infrared, visible, and ultraviolet light waves; x-rays; and microwaves).[128] Ionizing radiation, which is radiant energy that can add or subtract electrons, comes from x-rays and radioactive materials. Microwaves and ultrasound waves are nonionizing.[129]

Understanding data relevant to the effects of ionizing radiation is complicated by the terminology involved. Exposure dose is expressed in roentgens (R), and absorbed radiation is measured in rads. *Rem* refers to roentgen equivalents in humans. For practical purposes, the roentgen, rad, and rem may be considered equivalent in quantifying human exposures.[130(p251)] To further confuse the issue, the terms *gray* (1 Gy equals 100 rad) and *sievert* (1 Sv equals 100 rem) have been introduced. Exposure to ionizing radiation is continuous, with the typical dosage from background or environmental radiation in the United States estimated at 0.08 rads in the eastern and western states and 0.15 rads in the mountain states.[129] Sources of background radiation are cosmic, terrestrial, and internal radioactivity. In addition to these ubiquitous sources of ionizing radiation, people may be exposed through occupational and radiodiagnostic contact. An individual's average total exposure to ionizing radiation in the United States from background, occupational, and medical sources is 0.2 rads (200 mrads) per year.[129] The significance of this degree of exposure can be drawn from reported threshold effects: skin erythema (300 to 1,000 rads), cataract formation (250 rads), fertility reduction (100 rads), and depression in the concentration of white blood cells (25 rads). The amount of exposure necessary to reach these levels is placed in context by considering that victims of the bombings in Hiroshima and Nagasaki averaged an exposure of 14 rads.[131] During its development, the human fetus receives 60 mrads from background sources.[130(p251)]

Definitive thresholds for genetic effects, fetal malformation, and cancer induction will most likely never be determined. A probable threshold for fetal malformation has been suggested as 10 rads with exposure during the period of organogenesis.[129] Mossman and Hill[132(p240)] report that a dose of 10 rads or less to the embryo "probably results in little, if any, increase in the incidence of congenital malformation, growth retardation, or fetal death, but significant teratogenic or mutagenic effects are possible." Yamazaki and Shull[133] recently reevaluated evidence of fetal effects associated with the atomic bomb attack on Hiroshima. At that time, fetuses were exposed to at least 10 to 19 rads. The researchers found the most sensitive fetal period to be 8 to 15 weeks' gestation, when exposure was associated with microcephaly and mental retardation. After 15 weeks, milder effects were evident. Interestingly, exposures in the 10 to 19 rad range at 0 to 8 weeks' gestation showed no negative effects. It is possible that exposure during the earliest weeks results in high spontaneous abortion rates of affected fetuses.[130(p 253)]

Attempts to establish a reliable threshold for the teratogenic and mutagenic effects are hampered by the necessity of using enormous population samples to measure the effects of low-level ionizing radiation (defined as one exposure as high as 20 rads).[113] Whereas 1,000 persons are needed to demonstrate the effects of 100 rads, 100,000 persons are needed to demonstrate the effects of 10 rads, and 10 million may be needed to demonstrate conclusively the effects of 1 rad.[128,134]

These problems are further complicated by the fact that the genetic and teratogenic results of radiation exposure are not distinguishable from those brought about by other causes. Moreover, should genetic changes occur, they may be in the form of recessive traits that may not be identified for several generations. Animal research has indicated that the probability of mutation equals the normal spontaneous abortion rate at an exposure of 500 mrads or less per hour.[129] This dosage is considered high for occupational settings and would indicate that most women who work with radiation are unlikely to have an increased risk of genetically induced problems. The Committee on the Biologic Effects of Ionizing Radiation, drawing on research in mice, placed the radiation dose necessary to double the incidence of spontaneous mutations between 50 and 250 rads,[135] but some analysts believe that this range may be far too conservative.[129]

Based on numerous studies, including studies of the Japanese who were exposed to atomic radiation and the early radiologists who worked without precautions, it has been concluded that ionizing radiation causes cancer, especially leukemia, in humans. Estimates of the risk range from below 1% at doses less than 10 rads[136] to 1 in 10,000 for 1 rad of whole body exposure.[129] There is some controversy about whether the fetus has a heightened susceptibility to radiation-induced cancer, but animal studies do not generally support the argument of increased sensitivity.[135]

Electromagnetic Fields

In recent years, controversy has arisen about the reproductive safety of electromagnetic fields (EMFs), particularly as they relate to spontaneous abortion. Three sources of EMFs have been studied: electric blankets and heated water beds, ceiling cable heat, and video display terminals (VDTs). A recent comprehensive review of the literature about the reproductive and developmental toxicity of EMFs concludes that ''laboratory experimental and epidemiological results to date have not yielded conclusive data to support the contention that such fields induce adverse reproductive effects under the test or environmental conditions studied.''[137(p91)]

Video display terminals have become a common fixture in the home and workplace. A VDT emits both extremely low-frequency (approximately 45 to 60 Hz) and very low-frequency (approximately 15 kHz) electromagnetic fields.[138] Concern about the safety of VDTs was fueled by a 1988 study that found an increased risk of spontaneous abortion in exposed women. In this case-control study, Goldhaber and associates[139] found that women who used a VDT more than 20 hours per week had a significantly increased risk of abortion (OR 1.8) when compared with women who were not exposed or were exposed less than 20 hours per week. Although the authors cautioned against over-interpretation of their findings, the study received a great deal of attention in the popular press. A number of methodologic problems have been identified as possible contributors to the findings of this study. The work may have been complicated by an interviewer bias: the elevated odds ratio was found only in women interviewed by telephone as opposed to women who responded to a mailed questionnaire.[137] The amount of time that elapsed between the spontaneous abortions and data collection may have contributed to inaccurate reporting, and, as is true in retrospective studies, recall bias may have confounded the results. One finding of this study is puzzling: the excess abortion risk from VDT exposures of more than 20 hours per week was found to be inconsistent across occupational categories. This observation suggests that other factors, including occupation-specific stress and ergonomic demands, may be significant.

In another case-control study, 628 women known to have experienced a spontaneous abortion by 20 weeks of gestation were compared with 1,308 controls.[140] Information was collected from all women by computer-assisted telephone interviews. Many potential confounders were assessed and analyzed, including prior reproductive outcomes, insurance coverage, month of conception, and exposures to alcohol and tobacco. The researchers found no apparent relationship between abortion and VDT exposure; a marginally increased risk for first trimester abortion (before or at 12 weeks' gestation) was observed, with an odds ratio of 1.5 for moderate exposure (less than 20 hours per week) and 1.4 for heavier use (more than 20 hours per week). The study also found that the risks for low birthweight and intrauterine growth retardation were slightly elevated for women exposed to VDTs more than 20 hours per week, but the findings were not statistically significant.

A Finnish study compared 191 women who had a spontaneous abortion between 1975 and 1985 with 394 controls.[141] The subjects were selected from a cohort of women who were employed by three companies that had introduced VDTs into the workplace before that time and who worked mainly as bank tellers and clerical workers. The odds ratio for spontaneous abortion was generally not increased in women with VDT exposure; however, workers who used VDTs with high levels of extremely low-frequency magnetic fields had an odds ratio of 3.4 compared with workers who used terminals with low levels of these fields.

A recent case-control study offers a number of advantages over previous studies because of the documented comparability of exposed and nonexposed women relative to the demands of their work.[138] In this study, the experiences of women employed as directory assistance operators and general operators at two companies in eight southeastern states were compared. The only documented difference in the work of the two groups was that the former used VDTs whereas the latter did not. Included in the study were 882 women who had been pregnant during a 3-year period. A spontaneous abortion rate of 14.8% in the exposed group and 15.9% in the nonexposed group yielded an odds ratio of 0.93, which was found nonsignificant. When controlling for hours of exposure, no dose-response relationship was found. Operators who used VDTs had higher abdominal exposure to very low-frequency electromagnetic fields (15 kHz), but exposure to extremely low-frequency fields (45-60 Hz) was similar in the two groups, presumably reflecting background levels. Home computer use was similar in the two groups.

Despite the lack of association most studies found between VDT exposure and spontaneous abortion (or other poor pregnancy outcomes), the question has not yet been resolved because the existing epidemiologic research has all been of retrospective design. Currently, a prospective, nationwide study funded by the National Institute of Child Health and Human Development is under way[142]; it is hoped that the results of this study will do much to clarify the reproductive risks associated with VDTs.

An increased risk of abortion with other sources of electromagnetic fields (e.g., heated waterbeds, electric blankets, and ceiling cable heat) has been reported by Wertheimer and Leeper.[143,144] Their two articles represent the only work in the peer-reviewed literature that reports on the reproductive effects of residential EMF.[137] In their first study,[143] an association between electric blankets and heated waterbeds and early fetal loss was observed; in the second study,[144] the authors report a seasonal pattern of fetal loss consistent with increased ceiling cable use. Again, these two studies received considerable coverage in the lay press. Unfortunately, the resultant anxiety was created by studies with numerous methodologic flaws, uncertain logic, and conclusions not supportable by the published data.[137] To date, no convincing evidence exists to support a relationship between residential electromagnetic field exposures and compromised pregnancy outcomes.

Noise Levels

Exposures that could easily be overlooked in a work history may be detrimental to an unborn child. For example, a cross-sectional study that Lalande, Hétu, and Lambert[145] conducted in Canada indicates that a daily prenatal noise level of 85 to 95 dB for 8 hours significantly increases the risk that the child will have a high-frequency hearing loss. The authors note that the study does not provide sufficient data to establish a safe noise level for the fetal auditory system and that further study is warranted.

PRECONCEPTIONAL COUNSELING

The goal of preconceptional counseling on environmental risk is to provide women and their partners with the information necessary to make informed decisions regarding future exposures. Prospective parents should be helped to understand that the process of interpreting animal data is extremely complex, that 3% of newborns have identifiable defects at birth, and that the defect cannot be ascribed to specific causes in most instances. Each woman and her partner should be encouraged to limit unnecessary exposures to maximize their chances of a healthy outcome.

A full reproductive history should be obtained, including any delayed fertility, spontaneous abortions, premature deliveries, previous infants with intrauterine growth retardation or congenital defects, and fetal or neonatal deaths. Workplace, home, and leisure activity exposures should be explored for both the patient and her partner.

Accurate information should be obtained about any possible exposures and specific exposures investigated. Many states have enacted "right-to-know" legislation, which generally requires employers to make available information on any toxic agents used in the workplace, their potential effects, and ways to avoid exposure.[146] Either the patient can request this information, or, with her permission, the preconceptional counselor can contact the physician, nurse, or industrial hygienist at the patient's place of employment to ask about the types and degrees of exposure. Questions should not be limited to exposures specifically mentioned by the patient, because there may be others that she has not yet considered.[147]

After specific exposures have been identified, information about the known reproductive effects of these exposures may be obtained from a number of sources (see Appendix B). It may be helpful to contact a local physician who has expertise in industrial medicine. Because it is unlikely that information on specific exposures and the relevant studies can be reviewed during the patient's initial preconceptional counseling session, specific plans for follow-up should be made. Such plans may include telephone communication, correspondence, or another visit.

Recommendations to the patient should be based on the most complete information available. The preconceptional counselor should not make general statements such as "All chemicals should be avoided," or alarming comments about inadequately tested substances. On the other hand, the counselor should make it clear that a lack of information linking a specific chemical with adverse outcomes is not a guarantee of its safety. In all likelihood, necessary research has not been initiated or completed. Between 1,000[148] and 2,000[117] new chemicals are introduced annually, and research is backlogged for generations of compounds. The counselor should not be hesitant, after a review of the literature, to share the findings with the patient and conclude that it is not possible to determine whether a particular exposure is safe for her and her future baby.

Termination of employment because of pregnancy is a woman's option, but it is rarely a health necessity.[149] If advising the patient to consider the complete avoidance of an exposure, the counselor should explain the basis for this recommendation and should make it clear when such a recommendation is based on subjective judgment.[144] In some instances, work modifications (e.g., transfer to another unit) or extra precautions (e.g., use of gloves and mask) may be advisable.

The woman and her partner should understand that, in general, habits such as maternal alcohol and tobacco use are far more hazardous for an unborn child than are most workplace exposures.[123] Therefore the counselor should emphasize good general principles of health, such as proper diet, smoking cessation, weight and alcohol control, and regular sleep habits. Rubella immunization should be offered when indicated, and education regarding the importance of early prenatal care should be provided.

Exercise

A s a result of American society's interest in physical fitness, growing numbers of people are undertaking increasingly strenuous physical activity. The effects of such activity on reproductive outcomes are not well understood, and the specific risks and benefits of exercise during the periconceptional period have been virtually unexplored. Despite the lack of conclusive data, the preconceptional counselor must regularly answer questions about the relationship of exercise to pregnancy outcomes.

BACKGROUND

It is difficult to estimate the proportion of women of childbearing age who exercise regularly and the level of exertion that they experience. It has been reported that one third to one half of the population at large is involved in physical fitness activities,[150] but in a 1982 survey only 10.8% of California women ages 18 to 34 admitted to leading sedentary lives.[151] Swimming, bicycling, jogging, and bowling lead the list of most popular activities for the American public, followed by golf, tennis, volleyball, and aerobics.[150]

A number of difficulties arise in efforts to determine the effects of exercise on human pregnancy.[152] For example, baseline values relevant to the study of exercise may be inappropriate during pregnancy because of the physiologic changes associated with pregnancy. Because many variables affect both pregnancy and exercise, it is necessary to control data collection and analysis carefully. The responses to fixed exercise regimens vary widely among individuals. Because of ethical and legal considerations, much of the needed research is conducted through animal studies, but animal models may have limited applicability to human responses. Quadrupeds experience less venous pooling than do humans, tend to eliminate heat through panting rather than through sweating, and, unlike humans, cannot be motivated to perform exhaustive exercise unless there are other stressors. Finally, a woman's physiologic status is continually changing throughout pregnancy, which necessitates controlling for gestational age if recommendations regarding exercise are to be meaningful.

Menstrual Dysfunction

The increasing involvement of women in physical fitness and competitive endurance activities has been accompanied by an increasing incidence of menstrual dysfunction. According to Baker,[153(p695)] "disruption of the menstrual cycle, ranging from mild changes in flow to amenorrhea, is a relatively common problem for the female engaged in strenuous endurance sports.'' The literature, most of which has focused on joggers, indicates a causal relationship between athletic activity and menstrual dysfunction.

Exercise-induced amenorrhea appears to have a multifactorial etiology. After a comprehensive review of the literature, Davajan[154] concluded that exercise alters the hypothalamic-pituitary-adrenal-gonadal complex through ill-defined processes, leading some women to become amenorrheic.[154] Risk factors for exercise-induced amenorrhea include the existence of menstrual abnormalities before the initiation of an exercise program, the performance of endurance activities rather than acute exposures to exercise, and weight loss and stress associated with the exercise regimen.[154] It has been reported that at least 17% of body weight must be in fat for menarche to occur and that 22% body fat is needed to maintain menstrual cycles after age 16.[155] These figures may be useful in calculating when a woman may develop amenorrhea or regain menstrual function.[150,156] There is no definitive evidence that menstrual disorders caused by physical activity are permanently harmful to the female athlete's reproductive system.[153]

Hyperthermia

For the woman capable of conception, the most serious potential risk of exercise during the periconceptional period may be hyperthermia. Animal models and predominantly retrospective human studies have related congenital malformations to fever-induced hyperthermia. Edwards[157] established the working definition for fetal hyperthermia in guinea pigs at 1.5°C above the maternal core temperature, which is equivalent to 38.9°C (102°F) for humans.

The fetus must eliminate heat through the mother, although the factors that govern the process are poorly understood. The only routes for the elimination of fetal heat are the fetal surface, via amniotic fluid, and placental circulatory interchange. These mechanisms for diffusion are available because the temperature of the fetus is higher than that of the mother. In studies of pregnant ewes, it was found that, in the absence of maternal hyperthermia, the fetal temperature was 0.61° ± 0.05°C higher than the mother's.[159] A 1°C rise in maternal temperature decreased the temperature differential, but a 2° to 2.5°C rise in maternal temperature results in a marked widening of the difference, with the fetus becoming proportionately more hyperthermic than its mother. Therefore, maternal temperature affects fetal environment, and the degree of fetal hyperthermia is likely to exceed measurable levels of maternal heat.

Vigorous activity for sustained periods of time can increase human core temperature. For instance, it has been reported that 30 to 60 minutes of strenuous activity can elevate a nonpregnant woman's core temperature to 39°C, whereas strenuous exercise for 15 minutes generally does not increase the temperature to more than 38°C.[160] Many studies have indicated temperature elevations, sometimes to more than 40°C, in marathon runners.[161]

For more than 50 years, the relationship between temperature elevation and congenital malformation has been recognized in chicks.[162] More recently, the relationship has been observed in other species, including sheep, rats, mice, rabbits, guinea pigs, and monkeys.[163,164] Defects observed in the animal models differ, however. Exposed guinea pigs are most likely to have facial anomalies and skeletal defects, including arthrogryposis and talipes; monkeys are most likely to have midfacial hypoplasia, talipes, and scoliosis.[163] In addition to congenital anomalies, spontaneous abortions occur in bonnet monkeys after heat exposure.[165]

In the early 1960s, a British report noted that the incidence of human malformation doubled after febrile illness of the mother during the first trimester.[166] In the late 1970s and early 1980s, a number of studies conducted at the University of Washington indicated that hyperthermia at critical points of gestation produces dysmorphogenesis in the human similar to that observed in experimental animals. When Smith and colleagues retrospectively reviewed eight cases in which maternal temperature had been elevated at 4 to 6 weeks of gestation, they found similarities among the offspring, including severe mental deficiency, seizures, hypotonia, microophthalmia, midface hypoplasia, and mild impairment of distal limb development.[167] In five patients exposed to hyperthermia at 7 to 16 weeks of gestation, the observed characteristics among their offspring included hypotonia, neurogenic arthrogryposis, and central nervous system dysgenesis. The cause of hyperthermia in these cases varied; in one case, it was associated with sauna bath exposure.

In a follow-up study, Miller, Smith, and Shepard[168] attempted to correlate anencephaly with maternal hyperthermia. Of 63 anencephalic pregnancies, 11% of the women had a history of hyperthermia at 23 to 26 days of gestation, which is the time of normal anterior neural tube closure. In two cases, the hyperthermia was attributed to sauna bathing. Of the 64 control subjects, none reported an episode of hyperthermia around the time of neural tube closure.

A recent prospective follow-up study of 23,491 women has determined that exposure during the first trimester of pregnancy to heat in the form of hot tub, sauna, or fever is associated with an increased risk for neural tube defects (NTDs).[169] Women reporting any heat exposure during the first trimester had a crude relative risk of 1.6 that their fetuses would develop an NTD. The adjusted relative risks (controlling for maternal age, folic acid supplementation, family history of neural tube defects, and exposure to other heat sources) were as follows: 2.8 for hot tub use (95% confidence interval (CI) 1.2 to 6.5); 1.8 for sauna exposure (95% CI 0.4 to 7.9); 1.8 for fevers higher than or equal to 37.8°C (100°F) (95% CI 0.8 to 4.1), and 1.2 for electric blanket use (95% CI 0.5 to 2.6). The authors speculate that hot tub exposure has the strongest effect because of the efficiency of hot water immersion in raising the body's core temperature. They also interpret the findings relative to electric blankets as not being "materially associated" with an increased risk. The study was not able to quantify core temperatures or precise number, length, or timing of exposures. Nevertheless, the study suggests that women considering conception should be advised to avoid situations in which their core temperature could be raised, after discontinuing their method of birth control.

A study to determine the effect of sauna and hot tub exposure on core temperature indicated that discomfort generally causes healthy nonpregnant women to remove themselves from the sources of heat before their core temperature reaches the 38.9°C temperature previously identified as the teratogenic threshold.[158] The authors concluded in "a decidedly conservative estimate" that a healthy woman of childbearing age can remain in a 39°C hot tub for at least 15 minutes and in a 41.1°C tub for at least 10 minutes before her core temperature reaches a level that may be injurious to the developing embryo or fetus.

Other Effects of Exercise

Beyond hyperthermia, exercise has other physiologic effects on the pregnant woman and her fetus. The woman's connective tissue becomes more lax secondary to hormonal influence during pregnancy, and her center of gravity changes as the pregnancy advances. These occurrences make the pregnant woman more susceptible to injury. Blood volume, heart rate, and cardiac output increase during pregnancy, as does the tendency toward hemoconcentration during exercise. These changes significantly reduce cardiac reserve during increased physical activity.[160] As a result, exercise that was well tolerated during the prepregnancy period may require modification as pregnancy progresses.

Safe levels of exertion are commonly estimated by means of target heart rates. A typical formula for setting this rate for nonpregnant women is $70\% \times (220 - \text{age})$.[170] Some authorities have suggested that this formula is appropriate for pregnant women as well.[171]

Exercise induces a major change in blood flow from the splanchnic and renal tissue to muscles for increased effort and to skin for increased heat dissipation. Although this could result in fetal stress secondary to decreased uterine flow, Speroff indicates that the fetus is protected from this event in three ways.[171] First, placental flow decreases less than does uterine blood flow. Second, the pregnant uterus increases the extraction of available oxygen. Third, the acute decrease in maternal plasma volume during exercise results in hemoconcentration and increased oxygen-carrying capacity.

The effect of maternal exercise on fetal breathing movements and the fetal heart rate is variably reported in the literature, with the majority of studies involving third-trimester gestations.[172,173] There are great differences in the breathing patterns of individual fetuses, even when the mother is at rest, and specific patterns of exercise-induced breathing responses and the potential significance of these responses have yet to be established. In a review of studies of fetal heart rate responses during short-term cycling or graded treadmill testing, Gorski[173] found various effects but concluded that the fetal heart rate in healthy pregnant women does not appear to be significantly affected in any predictable manner. The fetal effects of exercise are more predictable in women with pregnancy complications associated with fetal distress. In these women, the fetal heart rate decreases at the initiation of exercise and then accelerates. In one case, the fetal heart rate acceleration lasted for two hours after maternal exercise.[173]

The most commonly reported negative fetal outcome associated with maternal physical activity is low birthweight.[152] Many of the studies in humans have involved working women, however, which suggests a selection bias or confounding variables that make extrapolation to other forms of physical activity difficult. The findings of animal studies have been inconsistent, with species variation notable. Well-matched prospective studies are needed to determine if and when maternal exercise patterns affect fetal growth.[149]

There is some concern about the possible harmful effects of specific forms of exercise. The official position of the Undersea and Hyperbaric Medical Society, for example, is to discourage women from diving during pregnancy until further studies are undertaken.[174] Current data conflict on the risks of decompression sickness in the fetuses of experimental animals, and the teratogenic effects of hyperoxia, hypercapnia, and the maternal inhalation of breathing gases at increased pressure are unknown.[175] If a woman insists on diving, she should be advised not to dive deeper than 10.06 meters (33 feet) for the period of time extending from the preconceptional period through 6 weeks postpartum.[175] Similarly, water skiing is regarded as a potentially harmful activity for pregnant women, because women skiers traveling more than 30 mph have been noted to experience a vaginal douche effect.[176]

The escalating involvement of pregnant women in aerobic exercise programs has led to several studies of its effect on maternal and fetal well-being. A study of 12 women involved in aerobic exercise and a control group of 8 women involved in no regular exercise demonstrated no differences in labor durations, Apgar scores, or fetal growth, although there was a small but significant rise in the fetal heart rate during exercise.[177] A prospective study of 141 low-risk pregnant women placed at random into control and study groups that differed only in the frequency of aerobic exercise revealed no differences in neonatal morbidity or obstetric complications.[178] In both studies, the target heart rate for the women was less than 80% of the maximum heart rate, and neither study indicated that aerobic training had a beneficial or detrimental effect on the duration of labor.

Swimming may be a particularly appropriate exercise during pregnancy.[179] Immersion results in plasma volume expansion, which appears to compensate for the exercise-induced hemoconcentration seen in pregnant women, thus protecting the mother and fetus from any adverse effects of reduced maternal cardiac reserves. In addition, immersion may ameliorate edema. Because edema plagues as many as 50% of pregnant women, this benefit could significantly decrease the discomforts of pregnancy. Finally, water suspension protects the woman's joints, which are more susceptible to injury during pregnancy.

PRECONCEPTIONAL COUNSELING

In regard to exercise, the goal of preconceptional counseling is to guide the patient toward decisions that are compatible with her lifestyle, with her changing physiologic capabilities during pregnancy, and with normal fetal development. Therefore, the counselor should take into account the type and extent of exercise that the patient enjoys, the climate in which she undertakes it, the physiologic effects of exercise on her, and the psychologic benefits that she gains through the exercise program. The counselor should obtain a baseline of information not only on these considerations but also on her menstrual history, her reproductive history, and her perceptions of the effect of pregnancy on her current exercise regimen.

The onset of menstrual irregularities should be assessed in regard to an exercise program. If previous abnormalities appear to have been aggravated by exercise, decreased activity may reverse the irregularities. The body fat ratios of women with menstrual abnormalities should also be assessed. Women who are very lean may regain menstrual regularity by increasing their percentage of body fat.

Women engaged in vigorous exercise programs should be made aware that hyperthermia may have teratogenic effects and that this potential risk is greatest during the earliest weeks of pregnancy. Because core temperature sensitivities to exercise appear to be individual, it is difficult to offer a generalized prescription for exertion that is appropriate for all women. According to Bullard,[180(p981)] however, "It seems reasonable to advise the patient involved in strenuous activities, such as marathon running, to plan her pregnancy, if at all possible, and to reduce her level of participation in the first six to eight weeks of pregnancy." The counseling of women who live in hot, humid climates requires extra caution. The American College of Obstetricians and Gynecologists has recommended that the maternal core temperature not exceed 38°C and that strenuous activities, following an appropriate warm-up period, not exceed 15 minutes.[160] These guidelines, felt by some to be too restrictive, are currently under debate and discussion.

Generally, unless there is a risk of core temperature elevation, women can continue their preexisting exercise routines into pregnancy. They should understand, however, that the physical encumbrances of an advancing pregnancy may interfere with their levels of performance. Erdelyi found that two thirds of 172 pregnant athletes were able to continue their usual sports activities during the first 3 to 4 months of pregnancy but that decreasing efficiency caused them to discontinue the activity thereafter.[181] This is a particularly important counseling point for those women who are psychologically dependent on a certain level of performance for their sense of self-worth. Women should be advised that certain exercises, such as those that cause a compression of the vena cava, are best avoided during later pregnancy and that the preconceptional recommendations may require modification if unforeseen complications occur in the pregnancy.

A review of the woman's reproductive history may prove helpful in offering appropriate exercise recommendations. The American College of Obstetricians and

Gynecologists has issued a list of relative and absolute contraindications to vigorous exercise during pregnancy.[160] A number of the conditions could be considered preconceptional contraindications if identified in the woman's past pregnancy performance:

- history of three or more spontaneous abortions
- history of premature rupture of the membranes
- history of premature labor
- history of incompetent cervix
- history of placenta previa
- history of intrauterine growth retardation

Possible medical contraindications for exercise as suggested by the college include

- hypertension
- thyroid disease
- diabetes
- cardiac disease
- excessive obesity
- extreme underweight
- sedentary lifestyle

Because physical fitness, practiced in moderation, may have beneficial effects for pregnant women, the woman with an extremely sedentary lifestyle should be encouraged to assume a preconceptional level of activity that can be continued into pregnancy. Swimming or briskly walking at least three times per week are appropriate suggestions. The woman should be taught to gauge her level of exertion by monitoring her cardiac and respiratory effort. A preconceptional target heart rate can be individualized by means of the following formula: $70\% \times (220 - \text{age})$. The American College of Obstetricians and Gynecologists recommends that a pulse rate during pregnancy should not exceed 140 beats per minute.[160] In addition, a level of breathlessness that interferes with conversational ability is most likely too strenuous.[171]

Maternal Age

W omen at both ends of the reproductive continuum have traditionally been assigned high-risk labels in pregnancy because the incidence of poor outcomes is increased for each of these groups. The literature supports the theory that age is the cause of poor outcomes in some instances and refutes it in others. Both physiologic and psychologic variables should be considered in assigning risk and in providing preconceptional counseling relative to age. Adolescents, for example, may not be at increased physiologic risk but may lack psychologic and social readiness for pregnancy and the parenting role. The older patient may be at higher physiologic risk because of the natural aging process but is more likely to enter the childbearing process with psychologic assets that younger women do not have. Although adolescents are extremely unlikely to seek preconceptional services independently, many questions related to the timing of pregnancy and to advanced maternal age surface during preconceptional counseling.

BACKGROUND

In recent years, the birth rate to women over 30 has increased markedly. In 1989, the rate for women ages 30 to 34 was 78.7 per 1,000 women; for women ages 35 to 39 it was 29.7; and for women over 40 it was 5.2.[182(p3)] These rates reflect significant increases over the numbers recorded in the 1970s. The 1989 rate for women ages 30 to 34 was the highest observed in more than 20 years. Similarly, the birth rate for women ages 35 to 39 increased more than 50% during the 1980s.[179] These figures are very modest, however, when compared with rates from the 1960s. At that time, the birth rate for women ages 30 to 34 exceeded 110 births per 1,000 women; for women ages 35 to 39 it was nearly 60; and for women ages 40 to 44 it was about 17.[183(p23)] The birth rate to children ages 10 to 14 has remained fairly constant since 1955 (1.2 per 1,000) and has dropped dramatically for young women ages 15 to 19 (90.4 per 1,000 to 58.1 per 1,000 in 1989).[179(p3),180(p24)] Despite these findings, the birth rate for teenagers is currently the highest recorded in 20 years.[184] However, birth and fertility rates do not provide information on actual conceptions because they are computed on live births. Approximately 25% of all pregnancies and 40% to 50% of adolescent pregnancies end in elective abortion.

In addition to changes in birth rates, the actual number of women over 35 who become pregnant has increased dramatically in recent years. Two phenomena help to explain the increasing numbers. Between 1980 and 1990, the number of women in the United States ages 35 to 44 was forecast to increase by 42% due to aging of the baby boom generation.[185] Second, many women are delaying childbirth; statistics show that between 1970 and 1986 the rate of first births more than doubled in this country among women 30 to 39 years old and increased by 50% for women 40 to 44 years old.[186] It has been postulated that women are delaying childbirth because of career priorities, a desire to further their education, infertility, control over fertility, late and second marriages, and financial concerns.[187]

The Adolescent Mother

In this country, 1 of every 10 adolescents ages 15 to 19 becomes pregnant each year; 84% of these pregnancies are unintended.[188] In 1988, there were approximately 9,000 births to women under the age of 15; 161,000 to women ages 15 to 17; and 293,000 to women ages 18 to 19.[188]

Studies on the physiologic risks of adolescent childbearing present conflicting information. Some reports have indicated that earlier childbearing has biologic advantages, whereas others have indicated that it is associated with increased complications for mother and child. Complications frequently cited include pregnancy-induced hypertension, anemia, prolonged labor, contracted pelvis, and cephalopelvic disproportion. The latter two complications have not been confirmed in recent studies.[189] It is generally believed that biologic risks are significant to perinatal outcomes if the pregnancy occurs earlier than 3 years after the menarche. Mothers under 15 have been reported to have a higher maternal mortality rate than do mothers older than age 20 and an infant mortality rate 2 to 3 times greater.[89,190]

Birthweight has received the most scientific scrutiny of all outcomes associated with adolescent childbearing.[190] The low-birthweight rate for mothers younger than 15 years old is 12.9%; for women ages 15 to 19 it is 9.3%.[191(p24)] Although young maternal age has frequently been associated with low birthweight,[192] age itself is not accepted as the cause.[190] Risk factors associated with adolescence, such as low socioeconomic status, inadequate prenatal care, primiparity, and marginal nutritional status,[189,191] are most likely to be responsible for the birthweight distributions of adolescents' neonates and for the other physiologic outcomes associated with adolescent childbearing. There is general agreement in the literature that adolescent childbearing is associated with long-term social and economic problems that compound the risk for the young adolescent who has not reached biologic maturity. Such problems include lower educational achievement, lower income, higher rates of enrollment on welfare, higher total number of pregnancies, higher rates of divorce, and, in some instances, lower cognitive development in the offspring.[189,190]

The Older Mother

Older pregnant women are not infrequently described in the obstetric literature in unfavorable terms, such as "postmature," "obstetrically senescent," "premenopausal," "geriatric," and "participating in childbearing in the twilight of the reproductive period.''[187] In 1958, the Council of the International Federation of Obstetricians and Gynecologists established the term *elderly primigravida* for women who experience their first pregnancy at age 35 or older.[193] The term is still commonly used, although some feel it is offensive. The term *mature primigravida* has been recommended as a suitable replacement.[162]

Although some dissenting reports appear in the literature, the preponderance of research indicates that women who give birth during and beyond their mid-30s experience more problems than do younger women; their children also have a higher incidence of problems. As early as the eighteenth century, the pregnancies of women of advanced maternal age were designated as high-risk pregnancies.[187,193] The categorization was secondary to maternal rather than fetal or neonatal concerns; presently, the categorization continues, but the primary concern is for the fetus/neonate.[193] The degree of risk is controversial because of study imperfections, sample size limitations, changing obstetric practices, and inconsistencies in terms. Advanced maternal age, for example, is variably defined in the studies; most researchers set the lower limit at age 35, although some use age 40, and a few include only women older than age 44.

After a comprehensive evaluation of existing data on pregnancy outcomes for women of advanced maternal age, Hansen[194(p728)] noted that ''prospective population-based studies are non-existent.'' He puts forth the following conclusions: for those not surgically sterile, the ability to conceive decreases with increasing age; the incidence of problems for those who do conceive is higher than that of the general population. Such problems include hypertension, preeclampsia, diabetes, low birthweight, macrosomia, extended labor, cesarean delivery, placenta previa, abruptio placentae, spontaneous abortion, chromosomal abnormalities, congenital malformation, and neonatal and maternal mortality. Not surprisingly, Hansen found that the incidence of hypertension and diabetes increases with advancing age, a phenomenon explained by the maternal aging processes. It is possible that hypertension, preeclampsia, and diabetes result in higher perinatal mortality rates when they occur in women over age 35.

The Collaborative Perinatal Project of the National Institute of Neurological and Communicative Disorders and Stroke, in which researchers evaluated data from 44,386 deliveries in 12 U.S. hospitals between 1959 and 1966, provides some insight into the cause of increasingly poor outcomes with advancing age.[195] The perinatal mortality rate for the studied births increased progressively from 25 per 1,000 at a maternal age of 17 to 19 to 69 per 1,000 after maternal age 39. Stillbirths accounted for 92% of the increase in the perinatal mortality rate. These figures indicate that the increased mortality rate is due to maternal factors, which are more often responsible for fetal deaths than are fetal factors. Of the increase in perinatal deaths, 14% were attributable to congenital malformations, 50% to problems associated with uteroplacental underperfusion, and 36% to other disorders. Controlling for accepted relationships (such as smoking and placenta previa; low maternal pregravid weight and placental growth retardation) resulted in the conclusion that maternal age itself is a causal factor in the increasing incidences of abruptio placentae, large placental infarcts, placental growth retardation, placenta previa, and premature rupture of the membranes seen in women of advancing age. The study indicates that the aging process compromises uteroplacental blood flow, which is of potential or proved significance to all the conditions mentioned except premature rupture of the membranes. This hypothesis is supported by the finding that the incidence of sclerotic lesions of the myometrial arteries in a sample of 62 nonpregnant, normotensive women examined at autopsy increased from 11% at ages 17 to 19 to 83% after age 39.[195]

A study of nearly 175,000 singleton births to Scandinavian women found that those age 30 and older have a 40% greater risk of experiencing a late fetal death than women ages 20 to 24. The findings held even when other risk factors, such as smoking status, education, and pregnancy complications, were considered.[196] For women age 35 and older, the risk of low birthweight and preterm delivery was nearly twice as high as that for women ages 20 to 29. At least two studies indicate that the higher perinatal mortality rates associated with advanced maternal age may be ameliorated by tertiary-level prenatal and intrapartum care.[187,197]

It is undisputed that the incidence of chromosomal abnormalities increases with age. Although the correlation between age and Down syndrome has received considerable attention in the lay literature, the age-related risks for other chromosomal abnormalities have not received similar coverage. Cytogenic abnormalities other than trisomy 21, however, contribute significantly to the overall rate of chromosomal problems in the offspring of women at all ages, with trisomy 18 (Edwards' syndrome), trisomy 13 (Patau's syndrome), and XXY genotype (Klinefelter's syndrome) all increasing in frequency with advancing maternal age.[195] Women age 36, for example, have an estimated incidence of 6.7 chromosomally anomalous infants per 1,000 births, compared with an estimated incidence of 2.1 for women age 26.[198] The incidences of Down syndrome in the infants of women at these ages are 3.1 and 0.7, respectively.[p14] Information about estimated age-specific risks for chromosomal abnormalities is provided in Appendix C.

Despite increasing risks for chromosomal abnormalities with advancing maternal age, relatively few women avail themselves of amniocentesis. Prenatal testing is either unavailable or unacceptable to many women. Reliable utilization statistics for prenatal diagnosis in the United States are unavailable. Estimates from the mid-1980s indicate that approximately 25% of pregnant women younger than age 35 receive amniocentesis as compared with 50% of women over 35, although 80% of women in the latter group desire testing when informed of its availability.[199] In a 1981 study of 163 women age 33 or older, researchers attempted to identify the reasons for these poor utilization rates.[200] Of the women in the study, all of whom had delivered normal newborns, 68% had heard of amniocentesis for prenatal diagnosis, but only 13% recalled first learning of the procedure from a physician or other health care professional. Despite their general familiarity with amniocentesis, most of the women lacked a clear idea of its specific purpose or associated risks. Of the 38 women over age 35 who were knowledgeable about the procedure, 82% had not been offered amniocentesis by their physicians, and 63% had not requested it themselves for a variety of reasons, including a belief that the procedure was unnecessary or too risky. Eight percent of the knowledgeable women who had not requested the procedure indicated that their rejection of the abortion alternative was an important factor. Seven women who had requested the procedure did not undergo it; in six cases, this was because the physician denied the request.

In another study of 74 women over age 34 who were referred for genetic amniocentesis, eight elected not to undergo the procedure for such reasons as perceived risks, lack of guarantees, difficulty in maintaining a past pregnancy, and moral concerns about abortion.[201] Those who did undergo the procedure expressed several concerns: risk of spontaneous abortion and fetal injury; fear of the unknown; worries about associated pain; and negative attitudes from others, such as spouse, friends, relatives, and physician. Reassurance that the child did not have Down syndrome was the major perceived benefit, followed by sex identification.

Although fetal and neonatal risks are the current major obstetric concerns in the pregnancies of mature women, there is also some maternal risk. An analysis of maternal deaths between 1974 and 1978 indicated that the maternal mortality rate for women age 35 or older was approximately 4 times greater than that for women ages 20 to 34.[202] The leading reported cause of death for the older women was obstetric hemorrhage, followed by embolism and hypertensive disease. Leading causes of death for the younger women were embolism and hypertensive conditions, in that order. Despite the increased risk, women over age 35 can be reassured: 1982 data reveal an overall maternal mortality rate of 7.89 per 100,000 live births compared with 24.2 per 100,000 for women of advanced maternal age.[203]

A potential problem for older women is decreasing fecundity. The mature woman who anticipates pregnancy and seeks preconceptional counseling, as well as the younger woman who seeks advice about the "ideal" time to conceive, is likely to voice fertility-related questions. That age affects the length of time required to achieve pregnancy is well supported in the literature,[194,204] but the reasons are not completely clear. Male fecundity, which may also decrease with age, and coital frequency, which is believed to decline with length of marriage, are possible contributing factors.[204] Female-related causes of age-associated infertility include premature menopause, endometriosis, anovulation, leiomyomas, medical illness, and psychologic factors.[205]

In a French study, Schwartz and Mayaux[206] evaluated fecundity as a function of age in 2,193 women who underwent artificial insemination after their husbands were found to be sterile. This approach made it possible to hold male-related fecundity and the effect of coital frequency constant. As shown in cumulative pregnancy rates over 12 cycles, 74.1% of the women ages 26 to 30 conceived, 61.5% of the women ages 31 to 35 conceived, and 53.6% of the women older than 35 conceived. Such reports have prompted at least one recommendation that, contrary to current trends, women pursue their child-bearing goals in their 20s and postpone career development until their 30s.[204] As a result of a study of 86 couples who had their first child at the ages of 20, 30, or 40, Weingarten and Daniels[207] believe this recommendation to be too stringent. Both men and women in the study population experienced psychologic and economic strain with early parenthood, and women who had their first child at age 30 or older were likely to be employed in positions where they earned higher salaries and had better opportunities for advancement than did younger women. The authors conclude that women and their partners should consider postponing pregnancy until their late 20s rather than their 30s, which would allow both prospective parents to develop a coherent sense of self, a relationship resilient enough to meet the challenges of parenthood, and a meaningful work life without significantly compromising the likelihood of conception.

PRECONCEPTIONAL COUNSELING

In preconceptional counseling related to age, women and their partners need a realistic appraisal of reproductive risks, education and guidance about strategies to reduce risks, and anticipatory guidance on postconceptional care. Translating aggregate population ratios into statistics appropriate to individual counseling requires thoughtful skill, however. Ratios may be unduly alarming and provide little insight into personal risk. For example, while it is true that a 40-year-old woman is 3 times more likely than a 35-year-old woman to give birth to an infant with Down syndrome, she still has a 99% chance for an unaffected child.[208] Similarly, multiparas older than 35 have been reported to have a two-[209] to ten-fold[210] increase in the incidence of diabetes in pregnancy when compared with their younger counterparts. However, even the ten-fold increase translates into a rate of less than 10%.

Because advancing age is associated with an increase in chronic health problems, women over age 35 who seek preconceptional care should be carefully examined for the signs and symptoms of diabetes and hypertension, as well as for those of less commonly occurring problems (e.g., renal disease). If any such condition is uncovered, appropriate recommendations should be offered. These patients should also be aware that they are at increased risk for diabetic and hypertensive complications of pregnancy that, although they will not necessarily compromise their future child's health, may necessitate more rigorous prenatal monitoring and, possibly, increased bedrest. The latter information is especially important to the woman who is unwilling to interrupt her usual professional or domestic routines because of pregnancy.

Following the decision to become pregnant, many mature couples find it difficult to conceive. Anticipatory concerns may be raised by the patients themselves; if not, the counselor should introduce the topic. To prevent disabling anxiety, the counselor should take a hopeful but realistic approach. If the patient is in her 30s, the counselor should advise her and her partner that continued postponement of attempts to conceive could increase fertility problems. It is recommended that the preconceptional counselor be familiar with local infertility programs and with the criteria of those programs for accepting patients at various ages. In general, the older woman with a conception delay warrants an expedited workup.[211]

Individuals or couples who seek preconceptional counseling should understand that the incidence of several chromosomal abnormalities increases with advancing maternal age (see Appendix C). The preconceptional period is an ideal time to educate patients about the purposes and techniques of prenatal diagnosis and the limitations of the procedures. Patients should understand that many conditions cannot be diagnosed prenatally and that the procedures offer probabilities rather than guarantees.

Good general principles of health care, such as proper diet, smoking cessation, weight control, alcohol avoidance, and regular sleep habits, should be discussed in relation to pregnancy outcomes. Rubella immunization should be offered whenever indicated, and the importance of early prenatal care should be emphasized.

References

Alcohol Use

1. National Institute on Drug Abuse, US Department of Health and Human Services. Washington DC: Government Printing Office 1991; Publication No. ADM 91-1732.
2. Johnson SF, McCarter RJ, Ferencz C: Changes in alcohol, cigarette and recreational drug use during pregnancy: Implications for intervention. *Am J Epid* 1987;126:695-702.
3. Serdula M, Williamson DF, Kendrick JS, et al: Trends in alcohol consumption by pregnant women, 1985 through 1988, *JAMA* 1991;265:876-879.
4. Ouellette EM: A report on fetal alcohol syndrome. Presented to the House Select Committee on Children, Youth, and Families, June 1983.
5. Alcohol and the fetus—Is zero the only option? *Lancet* 1983;1:682-683.
6. Streissguth AP, Landesman-Dwyer S, Martin JC, et al: Teratogenic effects of alcohol in humans and laboratory animals. *Science* 1980;209:353-361.
7. Kline J, Stein Z, Shrout P, et al: Drink-ing during pregnancy and spontaneous abortion. *Lancet* 1980;2:176-180
8. Harlap S, Shiono PH: Alcohol, smoking, and incidence of spontaneous abortions in the first and second trimester. *Lancet* 1980;2:173-176.
9. Marbury MC, Linn S, Monson RR, et al: The association of alcohol consumption with outcome of pregnancy. *Am J Public Health* 1983;73:1165-1168.
10. Kaufman MH: Ethanol-induced chromosomal abnormalities at conception. *Nature* 1983;302:258-260.
11. Abel EL: *Fetal Alcohol Syndrome and Fetal Alcohol Effects.* New York, Plenum Press, 1984.
12. Lemoine PH, Harousseau JP, Menuet JC: Les enfants de parents alcooliques: Anomalies observées á propos de 127 cas. *Ouest Médical* 1968;21: 476-482.
13. Jones KL, Smith DW: Recognition of fetal alcohol syndrome in early infancy. *Lancet* 1973;11:999-1001.
14. Rosett HL: A clinical perspective of the fetal alcohol syndrome. *Alcoholism Clin Exp Res* 1980;4:119-122.
15. Streissguth AP, Herman CS, Smith

DW: Intelligence, behavior and dysmorphogenesis in the fetal alcohol syndrome: A report of 20 patients. *Pediatrics* 1978;92:363-367.

16. Sokol RJ, Miller SI, Reed G: Alcohol abuse during pregnancy: An epidemiological study. *Alcoholism Clin Exp Res* 1980;4:135-145.

17. Ouellette EM, Rosett HL, Rosman NP, et al: Adverse effects on offspring of maternal alcohol abuse during pregnancy. *N Engl J Med* 1977;297:528-530.

18. Smith DW: Fetal drug syndromes: Effects of ethanol and hydantoins. *Pediatr Res* 1979;1:165-172.

19. Hanson JW, Streissguth AP, Smith DW: The effects of moderate alcohol consumption during pregnancy on fetal growth and morphogenesis. *Pediatrics* 1978;92:457-460.

20. Halliday HL, Reid M, McClure G: Result of heavy drinking in pregnancy. *Br J Obstet Gynaecol* 1982;89:892-895.

21. Sulik KK, Johnston MC, Webb MA: Fetal alcohol syndrome: Embryogenesis in a mouse model. *Science* 1981; 214:936-938.

22. Rosett HL, Weiner L, Lee A, et al: Patterns of alcohol consumption and fetal development. *Obstet Gynecol* 1983;61: 539-546.

23. Little RE: Moderate alcohol use during pregnancy and decreased infant birth weight. *Am J Public Health* 1977;67: 1154-1156.

24. Clark WB, Midanik L: Alcohol use and alcohol problems among United States adults: Results of 1979 national survey, in *Alcohol Consumption and Related Problems,* US Dept of Health and Human Services publication No. (ADM)82-1190. Rockville, Md, National Institute on Alcohol Abuse and Alcoholism, 1982, pp 3-52.

25. Little RE, Asker RL, Sampson PD, et al: Fetal growth and moderate drinking in early pregnancy. *Am J Epidemiol* 1986;123:270-278.

26. Mills JL, Graubard BI, Harley EE, et al: Maternal alcohol consumption and birthweight: How much drinking during pregnancy is safe? *JAMA* 1984;252: 1875-1879.

27. Landesman-Dwyer S, Ragozin AS, Little RE: Behavioral correlates of prenatal alcohol exposure: A four-year follow-up study. *Neurobehav Toxicol Teratol* 1981;3:187-193.

28. Neugut RH: Fetal alcohol syndrome: How good is the evidence? *Neurobehav Toxicol Teratol* 1982;4:593-594.

29. Spohr H-L, Wilms J, Steinbausen H-C: Prenatal alcohol exposure and longterm developmental consequences. *Lancet* 1993;341:907-910.

30. Streissguth AP, Randels SP, Smith DF: A test-retest study of intelligence in patients with fetal alcohol syndrome: Implications for care. *J Am Acad Child Adolesc Psychiatry* 1991;30:684-587.

31. Henderson GI, Patwardhan RV, Hoyumpa AM, et al: Fetal alcohol syndrome: Overview of pathogenesis. *Neurobehav Toxicol Teratol* 1981;3:73-80.

32. Halmesmaki E, Ylikorkala O: Concentrations of zinc and copper in pregnant problem drinkers and their newborn infants. *Br Med J* 1985;291:1470-1471.

33. Majewski F: Alcohol embryopathy: Some facts and speculations about pathogenesis. *Neurobehav Toxicol Teratol* 1981;3:129-144.

34. Fetal effects of maternal alcohol use. Council Report. *JAMA* 1983;249:2517-2521.

35. FDA Drug Bulletin, vol 11, No. 2, Department of Health and Human Services, Public Health Service, Food and Drug Administration, Rockville, Md, July 1981.

36. Centers for Disease Control: Counseling practices of primary-care physicians—North Carolina, 1991. *MMWR* 1992;41:565-568.

37. Rosett HL: Strategies for prevention of fetal alcohol effects. *Obstet Gynecol* 1981;57:1-7.

38. Rosett HL, Weiner L, Edelin KC: Treatment experience with pregnant problem drinkers. *JAMA* 1983;249: 2029-2033.

39. Selzer ML: The Michigan Alcoholism Screening Test: The quest for a new diagnostic instrument. *Am J Psychiatry* 1971;1127:1653-1658.

40. Ewing JA: Detecting alcoholism: The CAGE questionnaire. *JAMA* 1984;252: 1905-1907.

41. Sokol RJ: Quick prenatal screen for fetal alcohol syndrome. *Med Aspects Hum Sex* 1985;19:92-93.

42. Sokol RJ, Martier SS, Ager JW: The T-ACE questions: Practical prenatal detection of risk-drinking. *Am J Obstet Gynecol* 1989;160:863-870.

43. Rosett HL, Weiner L: Identifying and treating pregnant patients at risk from alcohol. *Calif Med Assoc J* 1981;125: 149-154.

44. Sokol RJ, Miller SI, Martier S: *Identifying the Alcohol Abusing Obstetrical Gynecologic Patient: A Practical Approach,* US Dept of Health and Human Services publication No. (ADM)83-1163. Rockville, Md, National Institute on Alcohol Abuse and Alcoholism, 1981.

Tobacco Use

45. Longo LD: Some health consequences of maternal smoking: Issues without answers, in *Birth Defects, Original Article Series.* White Plains, NY, March of Dimes—Birth Defects Foundation, 1982, vol 18, pp 13-31.

46. Ballantyne JW: *Manual of Antenatal Pathology and Hygiene: The Fetus.* Edinburgh, William Green & Sons, 1902.

47. Simpson WJ: A preliminary report on cigarette smoking and the incidence of prematurity. *Am J Obstet Gynecol* 1957;73:808-815.

48. *The Health Consequences of Smoking for Women: A Report of the Surgeon General,* US Dept of Health and Human Services publication No. HHS396. Government Printing Office, 1980.

49. *MMWR:* Cigarette smoking among adults—United States, 1988. 1991;40: 757-765.

50. U.S. Department of Health and Human Services: The health consequences of smoking for women: A report of the Surgeon General. DHHS, publication No. CDC89-8411, Washington DC: U.S. Department of Health and Human Services, 1989.

51. Fingerhut LA, Kleinman JC, Kendrick JS: Smoking before, during and after pregnancy. *AJPH,* 1990;80:541-544.

52. Floyd RL, Zahniser C, Gunter EP, Kendrick JS: Smoking during pregnancy: Prevalence, effects and intervention strategies. *Birth* 1991;18:48-53.

53. Lincoln R: Smoking and reproduction. *Fam Plann Perspect* 1986;18:79-84.

54. Feldman PR: Smoking and healthy pregnancy: Now is the time to quit. *Md State Med J,* October 1985, pp 982-986.

55. Meyer MB, Jonas BS, Tonascia JA: Perinatal events associated with maternal smoking during pregnancy. *Am J Epidemiol* 1976;103:464-476.

56. Sexton M, Hebel JR: A clinical trial of change in maternal smoking and its effects on birth weight. *JAMA* 1984; 251:911-915.

57. Kline J, Stein Z, Susser M, et al: Environmental influences on early reproductive loss in current New York City study, in Porter IH, Hook EB (eds): *Human Embryonic and Fetal Death.* New York, Academic Press, 1980, pp 225-240.

58. Himmelberger DU, Brown BW, Cohen EN: Cigarette smoking during preg-

nancy and the occurrence of spontaneous abortion and congenital abnormality. *Am J Epidemiol* 1978;108:470-479.

59. Fedrick J, Alberman ED, Goldstein H: Possible teratogenic effect of cigarette smoking. *Nature* 1971;231:529-530.

60. Thompson JD (ed): Women who smoke, in *Bulletin of the Department of Gynecology and Obstetrics of Emory University School of Medicine.* Atlanta, Emory University School of Medicine, 1981, vol 3(1).

61. Christianson RA: Gross differences observed in the placentas of smokers and nonsmokers. *Am J Epidemiol* 1979; 110:178-187.

62. Baird DD, Wilcox AJ: Cigarette smoking associated with delayed conception. *JAMA* 1985;253:2979-2983.

63. Lewak N, van den Berg B, Beckwith JB: Sudden infant death syndrome risk factors. *Clin Pediatr* 1979;18:404-411.

64. Benowitz NL: Smokeless tobacco, nicotine and human disease, in *Health Implications of Smokeless Tobacco Use.* Bethesda, Md, NIH Consensus Development Conference, 1986, pp 91-94.

65. Verma RC, Chansoriya M, Kaul KK: Effect of tobacco chewing by mothers on fetal outcomes. *Indian Pediatr* 1983; 20:105-111.

66. Meyer MB, Tonascia JA: Maternal smoking, pregnancy complications, and perinatal mortality. *Am J Obstet Gynecol* 1977;128:494-502.

67. Longo LD: Carbon monoxide in the pregnant mother and fetus and its exchange across the placenta. *Ann NY Acad Sci* 1970;174:313-341.

68. Longo LD: Carbon monoxide: Effects on oxygenation of the fetus in utero. *Science* 1976;194:523-525.

69. Orleans CT: Understanding and promoting smoking cessation: Overview and guidelines for physical intervention. *Ann Rev Med* 1985;36:51-61.

70. Anda RF, Remington PL, Sienko DG,

et al: Are physicians advising smokers to quit? A patient's perspective. *JAMA* 1987;257:1916-1919.

71. Centers for Disease Control: Counseling practice of primary care physicians—North Carolina, 1991. *MMWR* 1992;41:565-568.

72. Campbell JL, Valente CM, Levine D, et al: Using four simple steps, physicians do influence smoking behavior. *Md State Med J* 1985;34:50-55.

73. Still J, Mannion M: Smoking and pregnancy. *Physician Assist* 1983;7:114-124.

74. Shipley RH: *Quit Smart, a Guide to Freedom from Cigarettes,* ed 2. Durham, NC, JB Press, 1985.

75. Orleans CS, Shipley RH: Take heart, there are ways to quit smoking, in Heyden S (ed): *The Heart Book.* New York, DeLair Publishing Co, 1981, chap 2.

76. American College of Obstetricians and Gynecologists: Smoking and reproductive health. *ACOG Technical Bulletin* 180. Washington, DC, ACOG, 1993.

77. Mullen PD, Quinn VP, Ershoff DH: Maintenance of nonsmoking postpartum by women who stopped smoking during pregnancy. *Public Health Briefs* 1990;80:992-994.

Illicit Drug Use

78. *MMWR:* Statewide prevalence of illicit drug use by pregnant women—Rhode Island. 1990;39:225-227.

79. Chasnoff IJ, Landress HJ, Barrett ME: The prevalence of illicit-drug or alcohol use during pregnancy and discrepancies in mandatory reporting in Pinellas County, Florida. *N Engl J Med* 1990; 322:1202-1206.

80. Neerhof M, MacGregor S, Retzky S, Sullivan T: Cocaine abuse during pregnancy: Prevalence and perinatal outcome. *Am J Obstet Gynecol* 1989;161: 633-638.

81. Frank D, Zuckerman BS, Amaro H, et al: Cocaine use during pregnancy: Prevalence and correlates. *Pediatrics* 1988;82:888-895.

82. Osterloh J, Lee B: Urine drug screening in mothers and newborns. *Am J Dis Child* 1989;143:791-793.

83. National Institute on Drug Abuse, Rockville, MD: National household survey on drug abuse. *Population estimates 1990.* Washington DC: U.S. Government Printing Office, 1991. DHHS, publication No. ADM91-1732.

84. Gomby DS, Shiono PH: Estimating the number of substance exposed infants, in *The future of our children.* Los Angeles: Center for the Future of Children, The David and Lucille Packard Foundation, 1991.

85. Mayes LC, Granger RH, Bornstein MC, Zuckerman B: Commentary: The problem of prenatal cocaine exposure—A rush to judgment. *JAMA* 1992;267:406-408.

86. Fried PA: Marihuana use by pregnant women and effects on offspring: An update. *Neurobehav Toxicol Teratol* 1982;4:451-454.

87. Hingson R, Alpert JJ, Day N, et al: Effects of maternal drinking and marijuana use on fetal growth and development. *Pediatrics* 1982;70:539-546.

88. Qazi QH, Mariano E, Beller E, et al: Is marihuana smoking fetotoxic? *Pediatr Res* 1982;16:272.

89. Linn S, Schoenbaum SC, Monson RR, et al: The association of marijuana use with outcome of pregnancy. *Am J Public Health* 1983;73:1161-1164.

90. Cook PS, Petersen RC, Moore DT: *Alcohol, tobacco and other drugs may harm the unborn.* Washington, DC: Office for Substance Abuse Prevention, U.S. Department of Health and Human Services, 1990 DHHS publication No. ADM90-1711.

91. Zuckerman B, Frank DA, Hingson R, et al: Effects of maternal marijuana and cocaine use on fetal growth. *N Engl J Med* 1989;320:762-768.

92. Parker S, Zuckerman B, Bauchner H, et al: Jitteriness in full-term neonates: Prevalence and correlates. *Pediatrics* 1990;85:17-23.

93. Fried PA, Watkinson B: Twelve- and 24-month neurobehavioral follow-up of children prenatally exposed to marijuana, cigarettes and alcohol. *Neurotoxicol Teratol* 1988;10:305-313.

94. Fried PA, Watkinson B: Thirty-six and 48-month neurobehavioral follow-up of children prenatally exposed to marijuana, cigarettes, and alcohol. *J Dev Behav Pediatr* 1990;11:49-58.

95. Greenland S, Staisch KJ, Brown N, et al: Effects of marijuana on human pregnancy, labor and delivery. *Neurobehav Toxicol Teratol* 1982;4:447-450.

96. Tennes K: Effects of marijuana on pregnancy and fetal development in the human, in Braude MC, Ludford JP (eds): *Marijuana Effects on the Endocrine and Reproductive Systems.* NIDA Research Monograph 44. Rockville, Md, Department of Health and Human Services, Public Health Service and National Institute on Drug Abuse, 1984, pp 115-123.

97. Chasnoff IJ, Burns WJ, Schnoll SH, et al: Cocaine use in pregnancy. *N Engl J Med* 1985;313:666-669.

98. Chasnoff IJ, Chisum G, Kaplan WE: Maternal cocaine use and genitourinary tract malformations. *Teratol* 1988;37:201-204.

99. Slutzker L: Risks associated with cocaine use during pregnancy. *Obstet Gynecol* 1991;79:778-789.

100. American College of Obstetricians and Gynecologists: *Cocaine in pregnancy.* ACOG Committee Opinion 114. Washington, DC, ACOG, 1992.

101. Mayes LC, Granger RH, Bornstein MH, Zuckerman B: Commentary: The

problem of prenatal cocaine exposure—A rush to judgment. *JAMA* 1991; 267:406-408.

102. *The Use of Drugs During Pregnancy.* Hearing Before the Select Committee on Narcotics Abuse and Control, House of Representatives, 96th Congress, Second Session, February 6, 1980.

103. Dwyer J: Substance abuse in pregnancy. *Public Health Currents,* vol 26, No. 2. Columbus, Ohio, Ross Laboratories, 1986.

104. Zuspan FP, Zuspan KJ: Drug addiction in pregnancy, in Rayburn WF, Zuspan FP (eds): *Drug Therapy in Obstetrics and Gynecology,* Norwalk, Conn, Appleton-Century-Crofts, 1982, chap 4.

105. Wilson GS, Desmond MM, Wait RB: Follow-up of methadone-treated and untreated narcotic-dependent women and their infants: Health, developmental and social implications. *J Pediatr* 1981;98:716-722.

106. Pasto ME, Grazian LJ, Tunis SL, et al: Ventricular configuration and cerebral growth in infants born to drug-dependent mothers. *Pediatr Radiol* 1985;15: 77-81.

107. Kolata GB: Behavioral teratology: Birth defects of the mind. *Science* 1978; 202:732-734.

108. Strauss AA, Modanlou HD, Bosu SA: Neonatal manifestations of maternal phencyclidine (PCP) abuse. *Pediatrics* 1981;68:550-552.

109. Chasnoff IJ, Burns WJ, Hatcher RP, et al: Phencyclidine: Effects on the fetus and neonate. *Dev Pharmacol Ther* 1983;6:404-408.

110. Long SY: Does LSD induce chromosomal damage and malformations? A review of the literature. *Teratology* 1972;6:75-90.

111. Dumars KW: Parental drug usage: Effect upon chromosomes of progeny. *Pediatrics* 1971;47:1037-1041.

112. *Drugs and Pregnancy. It's Not Worth the Risk,* publication ISBN 942348-17-6. Rockville, Md, American Council for Drug Education, 1986.

Environmental Exposures at Home and at Work

113. Kurzel RB, Cetrulo CL: Chemical teratogenesis and reproductive failure. *Obstet Gynecol Surv* 1985;40:397-424.

114. Schardein JL: *Chemically Induced Birth Defects.* New York, Marcel Dekker, 1985.

115. Effects of toxic chemicals on the reproductive system. Council Report. *JAMA* 1985;253:3431-3437.

116. Smithells RW: Environmental teratogens of man. *Br Med J* 1976;32:27-33.

117. Kurzel RB, Cetrulo CL: The effect of environmental pollutants on human reproduction, including birth defects. *Environ Science Technol* 1981;15:626-640.

118. Haas JF, Schottenfeld D: Risks to the offspring from parental occupational exposures. *J Occup Med* 1979;21:607-613.

119. Greenberg J: Implications for primary care providers of occupational health hazards on pregnant women and their infants. *J Nurse Midwifery* 1980;25:83-92.

120. *Genetic Predisposition to Chemically Induced Birth Defects.* Reproductive Toxicology, a medical letter on Environmental Hazards to Reproduction, Reproduction Toxicology Center, vol 2, No. 2, March 1983.

121. Brix KA: Environmental and occupational hazards to the fetus. *J Reprod Med* 1982;27:577-583.

122. Warshaw LJ: Employee health services for women workers. *Prev Med* 1978;7: 385-393.

123. Shepard TH: Counseling pregnant women exposed to potentially harmful

agents during pregnancy. *Clin Obstet Gynecol* 1983;26:478-483.

124. Strobino B, Kine J, Stein ZA: Summary of published data and an annotated bibliography on exposure and reproductive function, in Bloom AD (ed): *Guidelines for Studies of Human Populations Exposed to Mutagenic and Reproductive Hazards.* White Plains, NY, March of Dimes—Birth Defect Foundation, 1981.

125. Kalter H, Warkany J: Congenital malformations: Etiologic factors and their role in prevention, Part I. *N Engl J Med* 1983;308:424-431.

126. Wilson JG: *Environment and Birth Defects.* New York, Academic Press, 1973.

127. McCann M: The impact of hazards in art on female workers. *Prev Med* 1978; 7:338-347.

128. White GL, Murdock RT: Ionizing radiation in occupational medicine. *Physician Assist* 1986, 10(2):39-52.

129. Webster EW: The effects of low doses of ionizing radiation. *J Tenn Med Assoc* 1983;76:499-510.

130. Simpson JL, Globus MS: *Genetics in Obstetrics and Gynecology,* ed 2. Philadelphia: WB Saunders Company, 1992.

131. Beebe GW: The atomic bomb survivors and the problem of low-dose radiation effects. *Am J Epidemiol* 1981;114:761-783.

132. Mossman KL, Hill LT: Radiation risks in pregnancy. *Obstet Gynecol* 1982;60:237-242.

133. Yamazaki JN, Schull WJ: Perinatal loss and neurological abnormalities among children of the atomic bomb. *JAMA* 1990;264:605.

134. Land CE: Estimating cancer risks from low doses of ionizing radiation. *Science* 1981;209:1197-1203.

135. Committee on the Biological Effects of Ionizing Radiation. *The Effects on Populations of Exposure to Low Levels of Ionizing Radiation: 1980.* Washington, DC, National Academy Press, 1980, p 220.

136. Swartz HM, Reichling BA: Hazards of radiation exposure for pregnant women. *JAMA* 1978;239:1907-1909.

137. Chernoff N, Rogers JM, Kavet R: A review of the literature on potential reproductive and developmental toxicity of electric and magnet fields. *Toxicol* 1992;74:91-126.

138. Schnorr TM, Grajewski BA, Hornung RW, et al: Video display terminals and the risk of spontaneous abortion. *N Engl J Med* 1991;324:727-733.

139. Goldhaber MK, Polen MR, Hiatt RA: The risk of miscarriage and birth defects among women who use video display terminals during pregnancy. *Am J Ind Med* 1988;13:695-706.

140. Windham GC, Fenster L, Swan SH, Neutra RR: Use of video display terminals during pregnancy and the risk of spontaneous abortion, low birthweight, or intrauterine growth retardation. *Am J Ind Med* 1990;18:7675-7688.

141. Lindbohm M-L, Hietanen M, Kyyronen P, et al: Magnetic fields of video display terminals and spontaneous abortion. *Am J Epidemiol* 1992;136:1041-1051.

142. McConough PG: Editorial comment. *Fertil Steril* 1990;53:185.

143. Wertheimer N, Leeper E: Possible effects of electric blankets and heated waterbeds on fetal development. *Bioelectromagnetics* 1986;7:13-22.

144. Wertheimer N, Leeper E: Fetal loss associated with two seasonal sources of electromagnetic field exposure. *Am J Epidemiol* 1989;129:220-224.

145. Lalande NM, Hétu R, Lambert J: Is occupational noise exposure during pregnancy a risk factor of damage to the auditory system of the fetus? *Am J Ind Med* 1986;10:427-435.

146. Frank-Stromberg M, Krafka B, Gale D, et al: Carcinogens: Are some risks acceptable? *Am J Nurs* 1986;86:813-817.
147. Bond MB: Reproductive hazards in the workplace. *Contemp Ob Gyn,* September 1986, pp 57-66.
148. Rosenberg MJ, Kuller LH: Reproductive epidemiology, in Seabrook EC, Parkinson DK (eds): *Reproductive Health Policies in the Workplace.* Symposium Proceedings, May 1982. Pittsburgh, Pa, Family Health Council of Western Pennsylvania, 1983, pp 202.
149. Pries CN: Reproductive effects of occupational exposure. *Am Fam Physician* 1981; 24:161-165.

Exercise

150. Hastings AW, Bankhead CD, Frye JP: The fitness boom. Must staying in shape extract a price? *Med World News,* July 23, 1984, pp 44-56.
151. Centers for Disease Control: Annual Summary: 1982. *MMWR* 1983;31:128.
152. Lotgering FK, Gilbert RD, Longo LD: The interactions of exercise and pregnancy: A review. *Am J Obstet Gynecol* 1984;149:560-568.
153. Baker ER: Menstrual dysfunction and hormonal status in athletic women: A review. *Fertil Steril* 1981;36:691-696.
154. Davajan V: The effect of exercise on the menstrual cycle, in Artal R, Wiswell RA (eds): *Exercise in Pregnancy.* Baltimore, Williams & Wilkins, 1986, chap 4.
155. Frisch RE, McArthur JW: Menstrual cycles: Fatness as a determinant of minimal weight for height necessary for their maintenance or onset. *Science* 1974;185:949-951.
156. Trussell J, Frisch RE: Menarche and fatness: Re-examination of the critical body composition hypothesis. *Science* 1978;200:1506-1509.

157. Edwards MJ: Congenital defects in guinea pigs following induced hyperthermia during gestation. *Arch Pathol* 1967;84:42-48.
158. Harvey MAS, McRorie MM, Smith DW: Suggested limits to the use of the hot tub and sauna by pregnant women. *Can Med Assoc J* 1981;125:50-53.
159. Cefalo RC, Hellegers AE: The effects of maternal hyperthermia on maternal and fetal cardiovascular and respiratory function. *Am J Obstet Gynecol* 1978; 131:687-694.
160. American College of Obstetricians and Gynecologists: *Exercise during Pregnancy and the Postnatal Period.* Washington, DC, ACOG, 1985.
161. Maron MB, Wagner JA, Horvath SM: Thermoregulatory responses during competitive marathon running. *J Appl Physiol* 1977;42:909-914.
162. Alsop FM: The effect of abnormal temperatures upon the developing nervous system in chick embryos. *Anat Rec* 1919;15:307-332.
163. Brix KA: Environmental and occupational hazards to the fetus. *J Reprod Med* 1982; 27:577-583.
164. Edwards MJ: The effects of hyperthermia on pregnancy and prenatal development. *Exp Embryol Teratol* 1974;1: 91-133.
165. Hendrickx AG, Stone GW, Hendrickson RV, et al: Teratogenic effects of hyperthermia in the bonnet monkey *(Macaca radiata). Teratology* 1979;19: 177-182.
166. McDonald AD: Maternal health in early pregnancy and congenital defect. Final report on a prospective inquiry. *Br J Prev Soc Med* 1961;15:154-166.
167. Smith DW, Clarren SK, Harvey MAS: Hyperthermia as a possible teratogenic agent. *J Pediatr* 1978;92:878-883.
168. Miller P, Smith DW, Shepard TH: Maternal hyperthermia as a possible cause of anencephaly. *Lancet* 1978;1: 519-521.

169. Milunsky A, Ulcickas M, Rothman KJ, et al: Maternal heat exposure and neural tube defects. *JAMA* 1991;268:882-885.

170. Thomas GS, Lee PR, Franks P, et al: *Exercise and Health—The Evidence and the Implications.* Cambridge, Mass, Oelgeschlager Gun & Hain Publishers, 1981, pp 82-83.

171. Speroff L: Exercise during pregnancy. *Contemp Ob/Gyn,* June 1984, pp 25-29.

172. Artal R, Yitzhak R: Fetal responses to maternal exercise, in Artal R, Wiswell RA (eds): *Exercise in Pregnancy.* Baltimore, Williams & Wilkins, 1986, chap 14.

173. Gorski J: Exercise during pregnancy: Maternal and fetal responses: A brief review. *Med Sci Sports Exerc* 1985;17:407-416.

174. Bolton ME: Scuba diving and fetal well-being: A survey of 208 women. *Undersea Biomed Res* 1980;7:183-189.

175. Kizer KW: Women and diving. *Physician Sportsmed* 1981;9:85-92.

176. Noelle G: Water skiing hazards: Nature and prevention. *J Sports Med* 1974; 11: 212-216.

177. Collings CA, Curet LB, Mullin JP: Maternal and fetal responses to a maternal aerobic exercise program. *Am J Obstet Gynecol* 1983;145:702-707.

178. Kulpa PJ, Bridget MW, Visscher R: Aerobic exercise in pregnancy. *Am J Obstet Gynecol* 1987;156:1395-1403.

179. Katz VL, McMurray R, Cefalo RC: Aquatic exercise during pregnancy, in Mittelmark RA, Wiswell RA, Drinkwater BL, (eds): *Exercise in Pregnancy,* ed 2. Baltimore: Williams & Wilkins, 1991.

180. Bullard JA: Exercise and pregnancy. *Can Fam Physician* 1981;27:977-982.

181. Erdelyi GJ: Gynecological survey of female athletes. *J Sports Med Phys Fitness* 1962;2:174-179.

Maternal Age

182. Horton JA, (ed): *The Women's Health Data Book.* Washington, DC, The Jacobs Institute of Women's Health, 1991.

183. Taeuber C, (ed): *Statistical Handbook on Women in America.* Phoenix, Arizona, The Oryx Press, 1991.

184. National Center for Health Statistics. Advance report of final natality statistics, 1989. *Monthly Vital Statistics Report* Hyattsville, Maryland, NCHS, 1991;40(8)(suppl).

185. Adams MM, Oakely GP, Marks JS: Maternal age and births in the 1980s. *JAMA* 1982;247:493-494.

186. National Center for Health Statistics: Trends and variations in first births to older women, 1970-86. *Vital and Health Statistics* Series 21, no 47, Washington, DC, Government Printing Office, 1989. DHHS publication, No DHS89-1925.

187. Kirz DS, Dorchester W, Freeman RK: Advanced maternal age: The mature gravida. *Am J Obstet Gynecol* 1985; 152:7-12.

188. Trussell, J: Teenage pregnancy in the United States. *Fam Plann Perspect* 1988;20:262-272.

189. McAnarney ER, Hendee WR. Adolescent Pregnancy & Its Consequences. JAMA 1989;262:74-77.

190. Capitulo KL, Maffia AJ: *Adolescent pregnancy.* Series 4, Nursing issues for the 21st century; module 2. White Plains, New York, March of Dimes Birth Defects Foundation, 1992.

191. Strobino DM: The health and medical consequences of adolescent sexuality and pregnancy: A review of the literature, in Hofferth SL, Hayes CD (eds): *Risking the Future: Adolescent Sexuality, Pregnancy and Childbearing,* vol 2. Washington, DC, National Academy Press, 1987, chap 5, pp 111-119.

192. Committee to Study the Prevention of Low Birthweight, Division of Health Promotion and Disease Prevention, Institute of Medicine. *Preventing Low Birthweight.* Washington, DC, National Academy Press, 1985, pp 100-102.

193. Morrison I: The elderly primigravida. *Am J Obstet Gynecol* 1975;121:465-470.

194. Hansen JP: Older maternal age and pregnancy outcome: A review of the literature. *Obstet Gynecol Surv* 1986; 41(suppl):726-742.

195. Naeye RL: Maternal age, obstetric complications, and the outcome of pregnancy. *Obstet Gynecol* 1983;61:210-216.

196. Cnattingius S, Forman MR, Berendes HW, Isotalo MD: Delayed child-bearing and risk of adverse perinatal outcome: A population-based study. *JAMA* 1992;268:886-890.

197. Berkowitz GS, Skovron ML, Lapinski RH, Berkowitz RL: Delayed childbearing and the outcome of pregnancy. *N Engl J Med* 1990;322:659-664.

198. Hook EB: Rate of chromosome abnormalities at different maternal ages. *Obstet Gynecol* 1981;58:282-285.

199. Fletcher JC, Wertz DC: Ethical aspects of prenatal diagnosis: Views of U.S. medical geneticists. *Clin Perinatol* 1987;14(2):293-311.

200. Lippman-Hand A, Piper M: Prenatal diagnosis for the detection of Down syndrome: Why are so few eligible women tested? *Prenat Diagn* 1981;1:249-257.

201. Davies BL, Doran TA: Factors in a woman's decision to undergo genetic amniocentesis for advanced maternal age. *Nurs Res* 1982;31:56-59.

202. Buehler JW, Kaunitz AM, Hogue CJ, et al: Maternal mortality in women aged 35 years or older: United States. *JAMA* 1986;255:53-57.

203. Fonteyn VJ, Isada NB: Nongenetic implication of childbearing after age thirty-five. *Obstet Gynecol Surv* 1988; 43:709-719.

204. DeCherney AH, Berkowitz GS: Female fecundity and age, editorial. *N Engl J Med* 1982;306:424-426.

205. Dorfman SF: Age as a factor in pregnancy. *Contemp Ob/Gyn,* February 1986, pp 68-77.

206. Schwartz D, Mayaux MJ: Female fecundity as a function of age: Results of artificial insemination in 2193 nulliparous women with azoospermic husbands. *N Engl J Med* 1982;306:404-406.

207. Weingarten K, Daniels P: When to have children, editorial. *N Engl J Med* 1982; 307:372.

208. Hook EB, Lindsjo A: Down's syndrome in livebirths by single year maternal age interval in a Swedish study: Comparison with results from a New York State study. *Am J Hum Genet* 1978;30:19.

209. Tysoe FW: Effect of age on the outcome of pregnancy. *Trans Pac Coast Obstet Gynecol Soc* 1970;38:8-15.

210. Grimes DA, Gross GK: Pregnancy outcomes in black women aged 35 and older. *Obstet Gynecol* 1981;58:614-620.

211. Gindoff PR, Jewelewicz R: Reproductive potential in the older woman. *Fertil Steril* 1986;46:989-999.

3

Nutrition History

E nsuring optimal nutrition throughout the childbearing years may prove a critical step toward improving reproductive outcomes. Studies have been conducted, books have been written, and protocols have been designed to emphasize the importance of adequate maternal nutrition. Yet many women continue to have nutritional imbalances, either as the direct result of poor dietary intake or as the indirect result of the ingestion of vitamins in excessive amounts, the use of certain drugs, smoking, or alcohol abuse. Unfortunately, many women receive information about the importance of optimal nutrition during pregnancy only when it is too late for them to change their habits in a timely manner.

In most instances, it cannot be proved that impaired nutritional status is the cause of a poor pregnancy outcome. Rather, maternal nutritional status interacts with a host of other factors to determine outcome. However, identifying patients with nutritional deficiencies preconceptionally and helping them to achieve optimal nutrition may reduce the number of reproductive problems.

All patients who seek preconceptional health counseling should be screened for nutritional risks. At a minimum, the counselor should ask whether the patient
- practices vegetarianism
- practices pica
- has a history of bulimia or anorexia
- follows a special diet or had a special diet prescribed as a child
- supplements her diet with vitamins
- uses medications that affect nutrient balance
- has an intolerance for milk

In addition, the counselor should determine the appropriateness of weight for height and the hematocrit for every patient.

Other components of the preconceptional history may also uncover risks for nutritional imbalances. Examples include tobacco use, drug and alcohol abuse (see Chapter 2, Social History), and the presence of chronic diseases, such as phenylketonuria and diabetes mellitus.

BACKGROUND

Intuition indicates that good nutrition during pregnancy is important to keep pace with maternal physiologic changes and fetal development. Scientific research into the effect of nutrition on human reproductive outcomes, however, has appeared on the scene relatively recently.

In animals and humans, nutritional deficiencies and excessive amounts of isolated nutrients, vitamins, and minerals have been shown to result in pregnancy loss, low birthweight, or congenital malformation. Animal studies have shown that offspring may be congenitally malformed when specific nutrients are removed from the diet.[1,2] In humans, extreme periconceptional malnutrition may cause covert spontaneous abortion of severely malformed embryos, resulting in undetected pregnancies.

Data from the Pregnancy Nutrition Surveillance System reveal that women who are underweight at the time of conception are 50% more likely to have a low-birthweight infant than their counterparts who are of average periconceptional weight.[3] The nutritional status of the mother in the preconceptional period and during pregnancy appears to affect not only her offspring but also succeeding generations; women who were themselves low-birthweight infants are more likely to give birth to low-birthweight infants, thus carrying on the intergenerational process.[4,5]

Adequate fetal growth and development depend on a steady supply of nutrients from the mother. In the human, the nutritional requirements of the embryo and fetus are met by three mechanisms:

1. During the prenidation phase, the blastocyst absorbs nutrients from the fallopian tube and uterine fluids.
2. During the implantation phase, a sinusoidal space (lacuna) forms in the decidua, and the fetus receives nutrients directly from the maternal blood.
3. For most of the pregnancy, the fetus receives nutrients across the placental membrane.

The mother must undergo considerable physiologic adaptation during pregnancy to meet her own changing metabolic needs and to supply the fetus with essential nutrients. Additional calories are required for the adaptation of maternal tissue, the development of the placenta, and the growth of the fetus. The total energy cost attributed to pregnancy is approximately 75,000 kcal, or 300 additional kcal/day. When the mother's total caloric intake is insufficient, her own tissue does not provide the necessary nutrients to any great extent; consequently, nutrients to support fetal growth may be inadequate. Maternal malnutrition also prevents the expected increase in blood volume. As a result, cardiac output and blood flow to the uterus fail to increase, which may affect placental development and fetal growth.[6]

Animal research indicates that nutritional deficiencies immediately before and at the time of mating have adverse effects on pregnancy, whereas nutritional deprivation during the latter part of pregnancy has little effect on the offspring.[7] Giroud's extensive review[8] of the literature on animal nutrition during pregnancy clearly demonstrates that the levels of nutrients and minerals during the embryonic period are critical for favorable reproductive outcome.

Unlike animal investigations, human studies are not abundant; moreover, human studies cannot be scientifically regulated and controlled. However, human epidemiologic studies have linked maternal malnutrition in times of famine to adverse pregnancy outcome. Severe dietary restriction before and during pregnancy appears to increase the risk of low birthweight and congenital abnormalities in the off-spring.[9-11] If the malnutrition is limited to early pregnancy, the major effect is an increased perinatal mortality rate secondary to congenital malformation, particularly of the central nervous system. Severe congenital malformation related to nutritional deficiencies is not observed if the malnutrition occurs only late in pregnancy,[12] but birthweight is decreased by 300 to 400 g.[11]

The human reproductive effects of malnutrition were observed during the famine in Holland during World War II.[12,13] Each Dutch citizen was allotted 900 to 1,200 calories per day during the 8-month period from October 1944 to May 1945. This experience resulted in amenorrhea in 50% of the women; a 30% reduction in the birth rate; increased rates of stillbirth, neonatal death, and malformation in infants *conceived* during the famine; and a decrease in the average infant's birthweight of 300 to 400 g, with a proportional decrease in placental weight. The decreases in birthweight and placental weight were correlated both with famine in the third tri-mester and with famine in the earlier stages of pregnancy. Lethal malformations of the central nervous system increased by 170% in babies conceived during the food shortage, while other malformations increased by 30%. The highest stillbirth rate (42 per 1,000), neonatal mortality rate (23 per 1,000), and perinatal mortality rate (65 per 1,000) were recorded during December 1945, 8 to 9 months after the most severe food shortage.

A review of the reproductive effects of poor maternal nutrition in Berlin as a result of World War II revealed similar findings.[12,13] The incidence of neural tube defects and other malformations did not increase in this population during the war, when the food supplies were deemed adequate, but the food shortages that followed the defeat of the German army were associated with an increase in the rate of con-genital malformation. The findings of a Guatemalan study also indicate that poor maternal nutrition has an adverse effect on pregnancy outcomes; an average reduc-tion in birthweight of 400 g was observed after restriction of the mother's caloric intake.[14] The placental weight was proportionally reduced. Diet supplementation with protein and calories restored the normal birth and placental weights for the population.

It appears from these studies that the fetus is not immune to the effects of mater-nal nutrition, even if the pregnant woman has previously been well nourished. Fur-thermore, it seems that the mother protects her nutrient reserves at the expense of the fetus and that the fetus is not a perfect parasite.[12-14] In addition, the studies suggest that a nutritionally deficient diet periconceptionally may be an important cause of congenital malformation.

The Significance of Nutrients, Vitamins, and Minerals

Few authors on maternal nutrition address the influence of preconceptional nutri-tional status on pregnancy outcomes or the specific role of various nutrients in successful organogenesis. Worthington-Roberts and colleagues,[15] however, describe the physiologic basis of nutritional needs at length, including the significance of many nutrients during organogenesis. They note that the "central place that protein occupies in the synthesis of new tissue sometimes obscures the emphasis that should be placed on other nutrients."[15(p92)] Worthington-Roberts[16] has also observed that maternal health, including nutritional status, begins before conception.

Protein and Amino Acids

A positive nitrogen balance exists during gestation to meet the needs secondary to the physiologic and metabolic changes of pregnancy and the growth and development of the fetus. Animal proteins contain the eight essential amino acids that the human body cannot synthesize. During pregnancy, these amino acids should make up approximately 10% of total calories,[8(p214)] because optimal fetal growth and development require that at least 50% of all amino acids be made up of these eight essential amino acids (leucine, isoleucine, phenylalanine, valine, lysine, methionine, threonine, and tryptophan).[17]

The recommended daily allowance (RDA) for protein during pregnancy is 60 g, or approximately 15 g more than the prepregnancy amount. This additional protein can be obtained through 3 oz. of tuna (23 g of protein) and two medium-size eggs (12 g of protein). Strict vegetarians must ingest a variety of plant proteins to maintain an adequate intake of essential amino acids. (Examples of nonmeat protein sources are listed in Appendix D.) Experimental animal studies indicate that protein-restricted diets started 30 days before pregnancy and maintained throughout gestation result in decreased fetal weight and, importantly, decreased DNA content in fetal brain cells.[18-20]

Although an adequate intake of amino acids is necessary, excessive amounts of amino acids may have adverse effects on the fetus. Aspartame (Nutrasweet or Equal) is a food additive that contains two commercially produced amino acids and has a sweetening power 180 to 200 times that of sucrose. Aspartame is found in many foods and beverages, and questions have been raised about the potential toxic effects of the methyl ester amino acids, l-aspartate, and l-phenylalanine. The administration of extremely large doses of aspartame to infant mice has resulted in hypothalamic neuronal necrosis.[21]

The plasma concentration of phenylalanine in the normal adult is less than 2 mg/dl; toxic levels in normal adults and children are 19 to 20 mg/dl. A maternal level as low as 10 mg/dl may be toxic for the fetus, however, because phenylalanine concentrates in the fetus. Although the administration of aspartame in a 200-mg/kg dose to normal adult subjects increases the plasma concentration of phenylalanine to this 10-mg/dl level, this dose is equivalent to ingesting 24 L of aspartame-sweetened beverage.[21,22] Even so, because elevated plasma phenylalanine levels result in mental retardation in children with classic phenylketonuria (PKU), there is some question about the fetal safety of aspartame ingestion by pregnant patients who have atypical or mild hyperphenylalanemia or are heterozygous for PKU.

Aspartame has three principal components: aspartate, phenylalanine, and methanol. There seems to be little concern about the safety of aspartate during pregnancy, because the amino acid does not cross the primate placental membrane, even at maternal levels 100 times the normal level.[23(p581)] As mentioned earlier, phenylalanine, the second metabolite of aspartame, not only crosses the placenta but also concentrates in the fetus. It seems highly unlikely, however, that the ordinary intakes of phenylalanine during pregnancy could raise fetal levels to the 20-mg/dl neurotoxic levels. The placental transfer of methanol and its potential effects on the fetus are not known, but the projected amount of methanol ingested from aspartame-containing products appears to be less than that received from 12 oz. of unsweetened fruit juice.[24]

The American Medical Association recently reviewed the effects of aspartame on pregnancy and determined that the food additive does not appear to be teratogenic.[25] Despite the large number of animal studies, the lack of human data on the effect of aspartame during organogenesis warrants the recommendation that women who are considering pregnancy or who are pregnant use aspartame in moderation (i.e., two to three servings of food or beverages that contain added aspartame per day).

Carbohydrates

Throughout human pregnancy, glucose is the main energy source for the developing embryo and fetus. At term, 20 mg of glucose per minute are transferred across the placenta. During pregnancy, carbohydrate intake should average 200 to 300 g per day, representing an increase over nonpregnancy intake. This increase can be obtained from ordinary foodstuffs. For example, milk supplies 12 g of carbohydrates per 8 oz.; bread, approximately 15 g per slice; and fruit, 15 g per average serving.

Abnormally high blood glucose levels just before and during the first 7 to 8 weeks of gestation have been implicated in the increased rate of congenital malformation observed in the offspring of diabetes mellitus patients. On the other hand, prolonged carbohydrate deficiency causes the placenta and fetus to utilize amino acids for energy, thus adversely affecting fetal growth. Clearly, it is critical to maintain normal blood glucose levels during the immediate prepregnancy period and during organogenesis for normal fetal growth and development.

Lipids

Fatty acids are the main energy source for the pregnant woman. These acids are broken down into their component parts and transferred across the placental membrane. Linoleic acid, an essential unsaturated fatty acid, is necessary for normal fetal and infant growth and development both before and after birth.[26] Although no congenital anomalies have been reported as a result of specific dietary lipid deficiencies or excesses, the increased incidence of congenital malformation in infants of diabetic mothers may be related in part to abnormal metabolism of lipids secondary to maternal hyperinsulinemia.[27]

Vitamins

For the most part, vitamins are not produced in the body and must be supplied by the diet. The dosage of vitamins in prenatal supplements reflects increases in the RDA for pregnancy and cannot replace a diet that contains adequate amounts of protein, fats, and carbohydrates. In the United States, vitamin deficiencies are usually not a problem; most commonly used foods are either fortified or enriched (e.g., vitamins A and D in milk, iodine in table salt, and B vitamins and iron in bread and breakfast cereals). Appendix E lists vitamin and mineral requirements and recommended food sources.

Between 39% and 47% of women of childbearing age supplement their diets with vitamin or mineral preparations.[28] These findings were derived from a telephone survey of nearly 3,000 persons regarding their doses of supplementation for 21 nutrients. The median intake for those identifying themselves as supplementers ranged from levels consistent with the RDA to levels more than 6 times the recommended intake. In some instances, women reported supplementation at greater than 60 times the RDA. Persons whose supplementation meets or exceeds 10 times the RDA are considered to be ingesting megadoses. Such amounts for some nutrients, especially the fat-soluble vitamins, may prove harmful to fetal development.

Fat-soluble vitamins. The vitamins A, D, E, and K are fat soluble. Vitamins A and D are essential to normal reproduction. Except for vitamin K, which is synthesized by microorganisms normally present in the gastrointestinal tract, all fat-soluble vitamins are stored in the body.

Vitamin A is readily available as a nonprescription vitamin. During pregnancy, the RDA for vitamin A is unchanged from the prepregnancy requirement of 4,000 IU. This amount is easily obtained by eating a varied diet that includes deep yellow, orange, and green vegetables. Supplementation with this nutrient, while common, is not recommended in women of reproductive age because of the risk of fetal teratogenicity.[29] Isotretinoin (Accutane) is a synthetic relative of vitamin A used to treat cystic acne. The drug has proved highly teratogenic in humans. Accumulating evidence indicates that several of the naturally occurring compounds that are included under the vitamin A label may result in similar malformations. Most reports suggest that an intake of 20,000 to 50,000 IU is required for teratogenicity[29]; however, one report associated the phenotypic isotretinoin syndrome with first-trimester supplementation of 2,000 IU of vitamin A.[30] Unfortunately, vitamin A tablets that contain 25,000 IU or more are readily available.

The prepregnancy requirement of 200 IU of vitamin D per day increases to 400 IU/day during pregnancy. Because vitamin D is endogenously produced in the skin through the action of the sun's ultraviolet rays on the vitamin's precursor, dihydrocholesterol, deficiencies of vitamin D are rare. Vitamin D regulates calcium metabolism and, as such, is needed for the proper development of the fetal bones and teeth. Not only is vitamin D in liver, eggs, and cod but also almost all commercially available milk in the United States is fortified with 400 IU of vitamin D per quart. Like megadoses of vitamin A, megadoses of vitamin D may have adverse fetal effects; for example, 4,000 IU of vitamin D may lead to severe infantile hypercalcemia and a syndrome of an elfin face, pulmonic or supravalvular aortic stenosis, and growth retardation of the fetus.[31,32] Pregnant women may unknowingly ingest excessive amounts of vitamin D from a combination of several sources (e.g., natural foods rich in vitamin D, fortified foods, overzealous supplementation, and ultraviolet light exposure). Unfortunately, the margin of safety with vitamin D is not as great as that with other vitamins.[33]

Vitamin E (α-tocopherol) has a variety of roles in human metabolism, but it was considered nutritionally unnecessary for animals until recently. Now, however, it appears that there is a high incidence of central nervous system and skeletal defects, as well as habitual abortion, in rats that have a vitamin E deficiency.[15] Nonpregnant and pregnant women require 15 IU of vitamin E daily. Vitamin E is present in almost all food in the American diet, and deficiencies are rare. Megadoses of vitamin E have been recommended for the treatment of many conditions, ranging from heart disease and thrombophlebitis to sterility, and for the prevention of aging. In addition, megadoses of 400 IU have been recommended for the treatment and prevention of cystic mastitis.[34] Such megadoses during human pregnancy have not been associated with birth defects.[35]

Produced by the intestinal flora, vitamin K is essential for blood clotting factors. There is no RDA for vitamin K, however. In the human, vitamin K deficiency may be exogenously induced by the use of anti-vitamin K drugs, such as phenobarbital, diphenylhydantoin, and warfarin. Such a deficiency may lead to fetal or neonatal hemorrhage.[36] It is not clear whether either the diphenylhydantoin syndrome or the warfarin syndrome is a direct result of fetal drug exposure or whether fetal effects result from a vitamin K deficiency secondary to maternal drug ingestion.[37] There are no known adverse effects of megadoses in humans, although rats fed high doses of vitamin K are reported to have an increase in the spontaneous fetal resorption rate and in skeletal abnormalities.[38]

Water-soluble vitamins. Because the water-soluble vitamins are not stored in the body, they must be routinely replenished by a typical diet, which contains adequate quantities of these vitamins. These vitamins include vitamin B_1 (thiamine), vitamin B_6 (pyridoxine), vitamin C (ascorbic acid), folic acid, vitamin B_{12} (cyanocobalamin), vitamin B_2 (riboflavin), and niacin.

The RDA for vitamin B_1 increases during pregnancy by 36% over the prepregnancy level to 1.5 mg. A diet severely deficient in vitamin B_1 during pregnancy may not adversely affect the mother, but the infant may have beriberi.[39] In neither humans nor animals have any detrimental effects been reported secondary to excessive vitamin B_1 intake during pregnancy.

The prepregnancy RDA for pyridoxine is increased by 40% to 2.2 mg. Hypoplasia of the thymus and spleen, as well as diminished neonatal immunocompetence, has been observed in animals with preconceptional and antenatal deficiencies in pyridoxine.[40] In humans, a prenatal vitamin B_6 deficiency has been asso-

ciated with mental retardation.[41] The treatment of pulmonary tuberculosis with isoniazid may lead to an increased excretion of vitamin B_6 and, thus, a deficiency.
Excessive doses of vitamin B_6 do not appear to be detrimental to humans or animals.

A woman's daily requirement for vitamin C increases during pregnancy by 17%
to 70 mg. Vitamin C deficiency in humans has been associated with an increased
incidence of spontaneous abortion and premature birth.[15,42] Megadoses of more than
600 mg/day have not been associated with any adverse effects in humans.[43]

Folic acid is one of the nutrients most likely to be deficient in a pregnant woman's diet. Found in foods such as liver, spinach, asparagus, broccoli, and most grains,
folic acid is needed for the rapid division of cells, normal protein metabolism, and
erythropoiesis. Multiple fetal malformations have been observed in the offspring of
folate-deficient rats and humans.[44,45] In humans, induced folate deficiency secondary
to the administration of anti-folic acid medication (e.g., methotrexate and aminopterin) during pregnancy is associated with an increased rate of abortion and severe
fetal anomalies.[2,45] The recommended daily requirement for folic acid in pregnant
women is 400 μg, compared with an RDA of 180 μg in nonpregnant women. Recent
research documenting preventive advantages of higher folic acid intake in women
during the periconceptional period has prompted the Centers for Disease Control to
recommend that all women of reproductive potential have a daily intake of 400 μg.

Neural tube defects (NTDs) occur in approximately 0.5 to 1.0 per 1,000 births
in the United States and affect an estimated 2,500 newborns annually.[46] The likelihood of recurrence in a subsequent pregnancy is estimated at 10 times the background risk.[47] Observations that indicate a link between maternal folate deficiency
and central nervous system abnormalities in the offspring have given rise to a number
of studies intended to determine whether manipulation of maternal folate ingestion
offers protection to the fetus.[48-55]

Laurence and colleagues[48] undertook a randomized controlled trial in South
Wales to prevent recurrence of neural tube defects through maternal supplementation
with 4 mg of folic acid daily. Supplementation was begun at the time contraception
was discontinued. Of the 44 women who took supplements preconceptionally, none
had a recurrence; of the 67 women who did not receive supplementation, six had
recurrences, resulting in a statistically significant difference. The researchers concluded that folic acid supplementation might prove an effective and efficient method
of primary prevention of neural tube defects and called for a large multicenter trial.
An interesting observation regarding their study is the difficulty the researchers had
in recruiting and retaining subjects: they note that "as a trial of the methodology of
preventing neural tube defects by giving prophylactic folate the trial was
unsuccessful."[48]

A large case-control study reported by Milunsky and colleagues[53] generated
enthusiasm for the protective advantages of folic acid. The study involved assessment of dietary intake of folic acid as well as supplementation of the nutrient in
23,491 women undergoing maternal serum α-fetoprotein screening or amniocentesis

around 16 weeks of gestation. Supplementation was defined as ingestion of a multivitamin supplement at least once a week (although 87% of the users took a multivitamin pill daily). The study found a substantially reduced risk of NTDs among women who took multivitamins that contained folic acid during the first 6 weeks of gestation. The prevalence of neural tube defects was 3.5 per 1,000 in the population who did not use vitamins before or during the early weeks of pregnancy combined with those who supplemented only before conception; the rate for women who initiated vitamins beyond the seventh week of gestation was 3.2, and the prevalence for women who took multivitamins during the first 6 weeks of pregnancy was 1.1. The independent or interrelated effects of other nutrients in the multivitamin preparations on neural tube development could not be assessed. The authors conclude that their data, combined with the findings of other studies, provide evidence that use of multivitamin preparations containing folic acid during the first 6 weeks of pregnancy will reduce by more than 50% the rate of occurrence of NTDs. At approximately the same time, a study published by Mills and colleagues[56] concluded that "the periconceptional use of multivitamins or folate-containing supplements by American women does not decrease the risk of having an infant with a neural tube defect." Mills' study focused on self-prescribed vitamin intake by querying women after delivery about their periconceptional use.

In 1991, the Medical Research Council Vitamin Study Research Group published the results of their multicenter trial, which investigated whether supplementation with folic acid or a mixture of seven other vitamins around the time of conception affected the rate of occurrence of neural tube defects.[52] In seven countries other than the United States, 1,817 women at risk for giving birth to infants with NTDs because of a previously affected pregnancy were randomly assigned to one of four groups: supplementation with folic acid, supplementation with other vitamins, supplementation with a multivitamin that contained folic acid, and no supplementation. The study demonstrated a 72% protective effect of folic acid supplementation (4 mg daily) around the time of conception; supplementation with other vitamins resulted in no significant protective effect. The dramatic findings resulted in the trial's being prematurely discontinued. The CDC subsequently recommended that women who have had a prior pregnancy affected by a NTD and who are planning conception should consume 4 mg of folic acid daily beginning at least 1 month before conception and continuing through the first 3 months of pregnancy.[57]

The question of whether folic acid also offers protection against the first occurrence of neural tube defects was the focus of a Hungarian study published in 1992.[55] The study determined that periconceptional supplementation with 12 vitamins, including 0.8 mg of folic acid, four minerals, and three trace elements, significantly reduced the incidence of neural tube defects when compared with a similar population supplemented only with trace minerals. A case-control study published in 1993[54] found a 60% reduction in neural tube defects among women who used daily multivitamins containing folic acid during the periconceptional period; the study documented a significant protective effect for supplements containing 0.4 mg of folic acid. The study also demonstrated a significant trend of decreasing risk with increasing dietary intake of folate.

Accumulating evidence on the protective effects of folic acid has led the United States Public Health Service (USPHS) to issue a landmark recommendation: ''All women of childbearing age in the United States who are capable of becoming pregnant should consume 0.4 mg of folic acid per day for the purpose of reducing their risk of having a pregnancy affected with spina bifida or other NTDs.''[58] The agency offered a warning, however, that total folate consumption should be maintained at less than 1 mg per day, except under the supervision of a physician, because high intakes may complicate the diagnosis of vitamin B_{12} deficiency and could have other, as yet unknown, ramifications. The CDC notes three potential approaches to ensuring adequate intake by all fertile women: improvement of dietary habits (the recommended intake can be achieved by making careful food choices that are consistent with the U.S.D.A. dietary pyramid), fortification of the U.S. food supply, and use of dietary supplements (the recommended dose is available in over-the-counter vitamin preparations). The Food and Drug Administration (FDA) is currently examining these options to determine the best method of achieving the USPHS goal without risking overconsumption of the nutrient. The CDC believes that compliance with the recommendation could result in a 50% reduction in the rate of neural tube defects in this country. The American College of Obstetricians and Gynecologists has not endorsed the recommendation, however, citing conflicting evidence and the lack of prospective, randomized, controlled studies.[59]

Pregnancy increases a woman's RDA for vitamin B_{12} by 10% to 2.2 μg. In rats, multiple congenital anomalies have been associated with vitamin B_{12} deficiency. In humans, deficiencies are rare except among strict vegetarians who do not supplement their diets with vitamin B_{12}. When deficiencies do occur, they are associated with pernicious anemia and, usually, infertility. Neither a deficiency nor an excessive intake of vitamin B_{12} appears to have a teratogenic effect in humans.

No human toxic or teratogenic effects have been associated with deficiencies or excesses in riboflavin or niacin (nicotinic acid). The RDAs for riboflavin and niacin are 1.6 mg and 17 mg NE, respectively, which are slightly higher than nonpregnant requirements.

Minerals

Information about the role of minerals in human reproductive outcome has generally been gleaned from small studies or case reports. It has long been known, however, that the correct balance of minerals is important for good reproductive outcome in animals. Extrapolation from animal data to humans is difficult but deserves further study and attention.

Iron. The increased blood volume and red blood cell mass during pregnancy increase the pregnant woman's need for iron. It has been estimated, however, that 40% of all adult women and 56% of all pregnant women are deficient in iron stores, and it is difficult to make up this deficiency by diet alone. It may, for example, take a woman as long as 2 years to replace the iron requirements lost during a term pregnancy.

Appendix F contains a list of excellent food sources of iron. Approximately 10% to 15% of the iron in food is absorbed under normal conditions; during pregnancy, absorption increases 30% to 40% or a maximum of 6 mg/day. There are two types of iron in various foodstuffs, the heme and the nonheme type, and these types have different rates of bioavailability. Iron from vegetable and grain foods (nonheme iron) is poorly absorbed by the body, whereas iron in meat, fish, and poultry (heme iron) is absorbed more efficiently. Certain foods, drinks, minerals, and nutrients (e.g., tea, milk, cereal, eggs, calcium, and food additives) may alter the amount of iron absorbed.

The RDA for iron is 15 mg for nonpregnant women. However, the average menstruating woman has a dietary intake of only 10 to 12 mg of iron per day; furthermore, she loses 1 to 2 mg through menstruation. Because only 10% to 15% of her iron intake is absorbed, she can easily become deficient. Pregnancy increases iron loss by an additional 2.5 mg/day because of the requirements of the fetus and bleeding at the time of delivery. Therefore, most women need iron supplementation in addition to an optimal diet to meet the iron requirements of pregnancy. For patients who are not iron deficient before pregnancy, the administration of a prenatal supplement that provides 30 mg of elemental iron per day should be sufficient (Appendix G). When greater amounts of iron are prescribed to treat iron-deficiency anemia, supplementation with approximately 15 mg of zinc and 2 mg of copper is recommended, because the iron may interfere with the absorption and utilization of these trace elements.[60] Although anemic women have a greater incidence of premature delivery and increased perinatal mortality,[61,62] there is no evidence that iron deficiency is associated with an increased incidence of congenital malformation.

Calcium. Calcium needs during pregnancy have been determined to be 1,200 mg/day. Depending on maternal age, this represents an increase of 0% to 50% over nonpregnant requirements. The total fetal calcium requirement is about 30 g. Approximately 300 mg/day is required during the third trimester for mineralization of the fetal skeleton. A dietary balance of calcium and phosphorus is necessary for the optimal action of both minerals. The RDA for calcium and phosphorus during pregnancy can be met by drinking 1 quart of whole or lowfat cow's milk. Other dairy products that are high in calcium, such as cheese, yogurt, and ice cream, may be substituted (Appendix H).

Many black, Asian, Hispanic, and native American women are lactose-intolerant. An effort should be made to identify these women and to ensure that they receive adequate amounts of calcium, either by increasing their intake of nondairy calcium-containing foods or by taking supplements. Many of these women can tolerate chocolate milk, milk in cooked foods (e.g., custard and cheeses), and fermented dairy products (e.g., yogurt). Calcium absorption from fermented dairy products is equal to that from milk.

Calcium supplementation is unnecessary except for women who cannot or will not eat dairy products. If supplementation is needed, calcium carbonate offers the best absorption; good sources of calcium carbonate are inexpensively available as over-the-counter drugs (Appendix I). Supplementation with "natural" calcium supplements, such as those made from bonemeal, oyster shell, and dolomite, are not recommended, because they may contain high concentrations of lead.[63]

Decreased levels of maternal calcium have been associated with neonatal hypocalcemia and, if the deficiency is severe or prolonged, abnormal fetal bone development and mineralization.[64] It has been suggested that there is also an association between calcium deficiency and preeclampsia. There is some evidence that, in populations with low calcium intake, the incidence of preeclampsia is higher and that calcium supplementation reduces the incidence of preeclampsia.[65]

Iodine. The RDA for iodine for the pregnant and the nonpregnant woman is 175 μg. Severe maternal iodine deficiency may cause cretinism in the offspring. Most people in the United States consume acceptable amounts of iodine, although the "goiter belt" of the Great Lakes region is known to have a low iodine content in its drinking water.

Excessive iodine intake during pregnancy (e.g., through the use of certain prescription and over-the-counter drugs with high iodine concentrations) may have adverse fetal effects. Patients treated for asthma and chronic bronchitis with iodine-containing medication (e.g., Combid and Quadrinal) have delivered offspring with congenital goiter, hypothyroidism, and mental retardation.[66] The amount of iodine provided by such medication may equal 500 to 1,000 times the RDA for pregnancy. X-ray contrast media also contain large amounts of iodine. In addition, repeated use of vaginal douches that contain iodine could be hazardous. Kelp tablets found in health food stores typically contain 0.15 to 0.2 mg of iodine, and the ingestion of 10 to 20 such tablets daily, combined with heavy use of iodized salt and a prenatal vitamin-mineral supplement, could result in a toxic level of iodine; this combination should be avoided.

Zinc. Considerable interest has developed in the significance of zinc deficiency in adverse pregnancy outcomes. An essential nutrient, zinc is a constituent of a number of metalloenzymes and a necessary cofactor for other enzymes. Because zinc is essential for RNA and DNA synthesis, it is essential for the growth of all tissues. An extra margin of safety of zinc is needed because of its small body pool and rapid rate of turnover. The RDA for zinc during pregnancy is increased by 3 mg to 15 mg.

Plasma zinc levels decrease throughout pregnancy. It has been hypothesized that this decrease is secondary to fetal demand for maternal zinc, an increased zinc requirement, or inadequate zinc intake during pregnancy.[67,68]

Like folic acid and iron, zinc must be supplied daily by the diet. Zinc is lost through the kidneys and through sweat glands, and those who participate in strenuous exercise (e.g., marathon running) may be deficient in zinc. Zinc intake is closely related to the amount of protein in the diet. Because it is difficult to meet the RDA for zinc unless the diet contains some animal protein foods, vegetarians may be deficient in this mineral.[69] Red meat, liver, eggs, and seafood, especially clams, oysters, and mussels, are good sources of zinc. [70,71]

A zinc deficiency is highly teratogenic in rats and nonhuman primates,[70,71] and epidemiologic studies indicate that the rate of congenital malformation is high in a human population with a zinc deficiency.[72] In Scandinavia, women with low serum levels of zinc had a high incidence of offspring with congenital malformation.[73] Soltan and Jenkins[74] found low plasma zinc concentrations in 54 women who gave birth to malformed offspring. Epidemiologic studies in countries such as Iran, Egypt, and India, where zinc deficiencies are common because of vegetarian practices, have revealed high rates of congenital malformations of the central nervous system.[75,76] Ruth and Goldsmith[77] have suggested that zinc deficiency may be related to the fetal alcohol syndrome, as transient dietary zinc deficiency increases the manifestation of fetal alcohol effects in rats.

It appears that maternal zinc status may have a direct effect on pregnancy outcome and that information concerning dietary zinc intake should be an important part of a nutritional history.[78] Hambridge and colleagues[79] reported that the routine administration of iron supplements (such as ferrous sulfate, 300 mg/day) during pregnancy correlated with a decline in the plasma concentration of zinc. The significance of this study is difficult to interpret, but it does point to the need to recommend good zinc sources for patients on indicated supplemental iron therapy.

In rats, the intake of zinc in excessive amounts has been associated with fetal loss and growth retardation.[80] The human effects of excessive zinc levels have not been established.

Fluoride. There is no RDA for fluoride specific to pregnancy, and it is not contained in prenatal vitamin preparations. In one study, Horowitz and Keifetz[81] found that the incidence of caries in the offspring of women who drank fluoridated water during pregnancy was the same as that in controls. When Glenn and colleagues[82] examined the 5- to 9-year-old children of nearly 500 women who had been exposed to different levels of fluoride supplementation during the second and third trimesters of pregnancy, however, they found that the children of those women who had received fluoridated water were 99% caries-free. The children who had not been exposed to supplemental prenatal fluoride were 15% caries-free.

Excessive fetal fluoride exposure in rats has been associated with significant mottling of deciduous teeth.[83,84] The use of fluoride during pregnancy remains controversial, and there has been no standard recommendation for routine prenatal fluoride supplementation.

Copper. According to experimental animal studies, a deficiency of copper may have a teratogenic effect.[85] For example, the rate of congenital malformation was increased in pregnant rats with a copper deficiency induced by D-penicillamine.[86] Patients on D-penicillamine have been reported to give birth to offspring with congenital abnormalities similar to those observed in animals with copper deficiencies.[87] Copper supplementation before conception and during pregnancy is advisable for those with diseases that require medication associated with copper deficiency.

Weight and Pregnancy Outcome

Malnutrition may take the form of overweight or underweight, or it may be discernible in eating habits or addictions that prevent proper absorption or intake of nutrients. The relative importance of preconceptional weight status and diet compared with prenatal weight gain and nutrition on fetal growth is unknown.[88] However, it is becoming increasingly clear that the mother's preconceptional weight status is an important determinant. A study that examined more than 2,700 term births documented that a combination of pregravid weight and weight gain during pregnancy related to birthweight for all women except those identified as morbidly obese.[89]

It has been estimated that 85,000 kcal are required to meet the energy needs of pregnancy in an average-size woman. Younger patients and those who are underweight need additional calories. To ensure a properly distributed caloric intake, 15% to 20% should be provided by protein, 20% to 30% by fats, and 55% to 60% by carbohydrates. A gradual increase in weight of 25 to 35 lbs (11.5 to 16 kg) is recommended for a pregnant woman of normal prepregnancy weight.

A woman is underweight if she is 10% or more below the ideal weight for her height and age. Any woman who weighs less than 100 lbs automatically falls into this category. The primary obstetric risk for the underweight woman is the delivery of a growth-retarded infant with the attendant increased risk of perinatal mortality.[90-92] When a poor maternal weight gain is added to a low pregravid weight, the incidence of growth retardation becomes more than 40%, compared with 2% in the general population.[93]

The recommended pregnancy weight gain for women identified to be underweight in the preconceptional period is 28 to 40 lbs (12.5-18 kg).

Comparing the obstetric performance and pregnancy outcomes of 3,534 underweight patients with those of patients whose prepregnancy weight was normal, Edwards and colleagues[94] found that the underweight women had significantly higher rates of cardiorespiratory problems, anemia, premature rupture of the membranes, preterm birth, and offspring with low birthweight and low Apgar scores. It appears that maternal metabolic needs take preference over fetal requirements when prepregnancy weight is low.[95]

In general, women who are overweight at conception have increased obstetric risks. Because obesity usually results from the ingestion of an excessive number of calories rather than nutrients, the obese patient may be more malnourished than the underweight woman. A woman is described as moderately overweight if her weight is 120% to 135% of her ideal body weight for her age and height. Very overweight patients (i.e., those whose weight is greater than 135% of their ideal body weight) are at increased risk for chronic hypertension, preeclampsia, diabetes mellitus, and thromboembolic complications.[96] Furthermore, obese patients are more likely than are other patients to have macrosomic infants, which may lead to birth trauma, dysfunctional labor, and cesarean delivery. The risks associated with surgery are increased in obese patients, because cardiovascular, respiratory, and anesthetic complications and postoperative wound infections occur more frequently.[97] The ideal weight gain during pregnancy for women who conceive at greater than 120% and 135% of the ideal weight for height is 15 to 25 lbs (7-11.5 kg) and 15 lbs (6.8 kg), respectively.

Obese patients should reduce their weight before pregnancy, since weight reduction during pregnancy is not recommended. Because a rapid prepregnancy weight loss may deplete the body of essential nutrients, the patient should stabilize her weight for 2 to 3 months before conception. At the time of conception, the patient should be on a diet of 1,800 to 2,000 kcal/day in combination with an exercise program.

Pica

Pregnant and nonpregnant women can be subject to pica, the compulsive ingestion of substances that have little or no nutritional value. Craved substances commonly reported include dirt, clay, and starch. Less frequently, patients report cravings for burned matches, charcoal, cigarette ashes, baking soda, coffee grounds, and tire inner tubes. The causes of pica are varied, ranging from psychological to cultural phenomena. Pica is not limited to any one geographic area, race, or status within a culture.

The adverse effects of pica may be secondary to the patient's substitution of the craved substance for other foods, resulting in calorie or nutrient malnourishment, or to the ingestion of excessive calories, resulting in undesirable weight gain. The ingested substances may be directly toxic to the bowel, may contain material that the body does not tolerate, or may inhibit absorption of essential nutrients. Anemia should be corrected, because anemia may be a contributing factor in pica. Nutritional counseling should include suggestions of foods that may substitute for craved substances, such as nonfat dry milk for laundry starch. Psychiatric consultation may be necessary.

Anorexia and Bulimia

Anorexia nervosa is characterized by low self-esteem, unrealistic goals, and a delusional denial of the appearance of thinness. Like extreme fasting, anorexia nervosa is usually associated with amenorrhea. If an anorectic patient should become pregnant, her risks are similar to those of a woman who conceives under famine conditions. Bulimia, or food gorging and emesis, may occur independent of a diagnosis of anorexia nervosa. As in hyperemesis gravidarum, the primary risk during pregnancy is the possibility of depletion of the nutrients essential for maternal adaptations and fetal development.

The prevalence of anorexia nervosa and bulimia, both observed primarily in adolescents and young adults, is difficult to assess. Bulimia is believed to be far more common, with reports ranging from 3.2% to 13% in college women. Other populations identified to be at risk are gymnasts, ballet dancers, and jockeys.[98] Bulimia and anorexia nervosa are chronic conditions whose identification and interventions are best undertaken in the preconceptional period.

Vegetarianism

Ovo-lactovegetarians include dairy products, eggs, and plants in their diets. Those who consume milk and milk products but no eggs are termed lactovegetarians. Vegans eat only plant food, omitting meat, fish, eggs, and dairy products. The ingestion of excessive quantities of plant food may lead to early satiation and thereby prevent the patient from increasing her caloric intake during pregnancy, as recommended. Furthermore, because some plant proteins contain only a few of the essential amino acids, a vegan diet places the woman at a particularly high risk for amino acid deficiencies. In addition, the amounts of vitamin B_{12}, zinc, calcium, vitamin D, and iron in the diet may be inadequate during pregnancy. Identified deficiencies can be addressed through careful food selection and, in some instances, supplementation.

Drug-Alcohol-Nutrition-Mineral Interactions

Alcohol's direct toxic effects upon the gastrointestinal tract may result in maldigestion, malabsorption, and poor utilization of amino acids and vitamins.[99] It has been demonstrated that the urinary excretion of zinc and folic acid is increased after alcohol ingestion.[77,100] Vitamin supplementation, particularly with vitamin B_1 and folic acid, is common in the treatment of alcoholism.

The reproductive effects of alcohol appear to be long-lasting and may be evident in neonates long after their mothers have ceased to consume alcohol. Little and colleagues[101] studied 50 infants of mothers who did not drink alcohol and 100 infants of mothers who had a history of alcoholism. Of the infants in the latter group, 50 were born to women who reported total abstinence during pregnancy but who had a history of alcoholism before conception; the other 50 infants were born to alcoholic women who reported drinking heavily during pregnancy. The mean birthweight of the infants born to the abstinent alcoholics was 258 g less than that of the control infants. The infants of the other alcoholics weighed 493 g less at birth than the control infants. These findings suggest that even a history of maternal alcoholism may pose a risk to fetal growth because of a depletion of the mother's nutritional stores, regardless of her alcohol use during pregnancy (see Chapter 2).

Like alcohol, prescription and nonprescription drugs may affect the patient's nutritional status. Patients on long-term isoniazid therapy for tuberculosis, for example, can develop a peripheral neuropathy secondary to deficiencies in vitamin B_6 and niacin. The action of mineral oil, which patients may self-prescribe for the treatment of constipation, can impair the absorption of fat-soluble vitamins (i.e., A, D, E, and K). Long-term use of broad-spectrum antibiotics can change the flora in the gastro-intestinal tract and interfere with the synthesis of vitamin K, which requires the presence of certain microorganisms. The levels of vitamins A and D are reduced in patients on cholestyramine for certain hyperlipidemic states.[102] Chronic use of aspirin has been shown to decrease vitamin C uptake in leukocytes and impair the protein binding of folate.[103] Appendix J outlines some common drug and vitamin interactions.

Caffeine and Pregnancy

Annually, 28 gallons of coffee with caffeine are consumed per individual in the United States; one of three Americans consumes an average of 200 mg of caffeine per day. It is not unusual for consumption to reach the level of 10 to 12 mg/kg of body weight, which may equal 800 mg/day.[104]

Caffeine is a 1,3,7-trimethylxanthine that is in approximately 63 species of plants, including coffee beans, cocoa beans, cola nuts, and tea leaves. Commercially, it is ubiquitous. It is found in soft drinks, cocoa, tea, coffee, chocolate, prescription drugs, and certain over-the-counter drugs used as stimulants and diuretics (Appendixes K and L). The amount of caffeine in coffee and tea depends on the type of grind and the length of brewing. The caffeine content of drip coffee, for instance, is higher than that of percolated coffee. Soft drinks are a common source of caffeine; nearly 34 gallons per person are consumed annually in the United States. Approximately 95% of the caffeine in a typical cola drink and 100% of the caffeine in citrus drinks have been added by the manufacturer.

The time required for the body to eliminate one half of the caffeine introduced varies; it takes less than 3 hours in children and smokers, approximately 3 to 7 hours in nonsmokers, up to 13 hours in women on birth control pills, and 10 to 20 hours in pregnant women in the third trimester. In general, moderate amounts of caffeine are not harmful to the average healthy adult. Although individuals vary in their reactions, the consumption of 6 to 10 cups of coffee per day, or 600 to 1,000 mg of caffeine, may lead to anxiety, restlessness, delayed onset of sleep and frequent awakening, and heart palpitations.

Caffeine is structurally similar to the purine DNA-based pairs, adenine and guanine. Because of this association, extensive mutagenic and teratogenic testing has been done in a variety of animal species. It has been found that caffeine increases the level of adenosine 3^1-,5^1-cyclic monophosphate, which may impair fetal cellular growth. In sheep, caffeine increases the blood level of catecholamines and decreases uterine blood flow.[105] In general, however, studies of the teratogenic effects of caffeine in humans and animals have produced contradictory results.

In 1980, the FDA advised pregnant women to avoid caffeine during pregnancy. The action was based on studies of pregnant rats who had offspring with skeletal defects following forced feeding of caffeine by stomach tube.[106] The dosage was equivalent to the human intake of 56 to 87 cups of brewed coffee per day. At lower dosages, equivalent to 4, 8, and 28 cups per day, no birth defects were seen. The FDA questioned the method of forced feeding and sponsored a set of "sipping studies" in which the rats received caffeine in their drinking water at a total dosage consistent with the forced feeding studies. The offspring of these rats did not have the malformations seen in the offspring of the force-fed rats.[107]

Human studies have yielded inconsistent results. In a survey of 800 pregnant women, Weathersbee, Olsen, and Lodge[108] identified 16 women who consumed more than 600 mg of caffeine daily; of these women, 15 had spontaneous abortion, fetal death, or premature delivery. The authors postulate that caffeine caused these adverse effects by increasing the circulating levels of catecholamines, thus altering uterine and placental blood flow. Linn and colleagues[109] interviewed 12,205 "normal" women during the first trimester; after controlling for smoking and other variables, no relationship was found between low birthweight, prematurity, or congenital anomalies and coffee or tea consumption of 4 or more cups. A study reported in 1991 found a relationship between daily caffeine consumption of greater than 300 mg and intrauterine growth retardation and low birthweight. This level of consumption did not affect the incidence of preterm delivery.[110] The study suffered from methodologic problems common to this type of research: data collection occurred up to 9 months after birth; sources of caffeine other than tea, coffee, and soft drinks were not included; and the method of coffee preparation, which affects caffeine concentration, was not reported. In addition, gestational age was calculated from the mother's report of the last menstrual period. Mills and colleagues[111] studied a cohort of 431 women identified within 21 days of conception and prospectively monitored their caffeine intake during pregnancy to determine its relationship to spontaneous abortion and fetal growth. This carefully designed study detected no evidence that "moderate" (<300 mg/day) caffeine use increased the risk of spontaneous abortion, intrauterine growth retardation, or microcephaly. This lack of association was also noted for women consuming at least 300 mg caffeine, after adjusting for other risk factors, most notably smoking. The latter group consisted of only 24 women, however, and the upper limit of caffeine intake for this group is unknown.

The possibility that caffeine exposure affects conception has particular preconceptional significance. A study by Wilcox, Weinberg, and Baird[112] found that women who consumed more than the equivalent of 1 cup of coffee per day were half as likely to achieve conception than women who drank less. Because the study was retrospective and other maternal characteristics that may affect fertility were not equally represented in the cases and controls or were not assessed, the preconceptional counselor should not rely heavily on the findings in making recommendations.

PRECONCEPTIONAL COUNSELING

The goals of preconceptional counseling regarding nutrition are (1) to identify and address nutrient excesses and deficiencies and (2) to inform the patient about nutritional needs during pregnancy. Eating is not just a matter of physical requirements; it is closely related to a patient's social activities, her feelings about her appearance, her independence, and her acceptance.[113] Therefore, nutritional counseling must be individualized to meet not only the physical but also the psychological needs of the patient. It is not easy to change eating habits, but it may be easier when the rationale for changes or modifications in habits is clear.[114] A woman may be more likely to change her habits preconceptionally if she understands the long-term implications of her current nutritional status on her own health and, particularly, on reproductive outcomes.

Ideally, the preconceptional counselor should obtain a nutrition history, including a 24-hour recall. A daily diet usually meets the RDAs for all nutrients if it includes a variety of foods in the amounts recommended by the U.S.D.A food guide pyramid:

- 2 to 3 servings of milk, yogurt, and cheese
- 2 to 3 servings of meat, poultry, fish, dry beans, eggs, and nuts
- 3 to 5 servings of vegetables
- 2 to 4 servings of fruit
- 6 to 11 servings of bread, cereal, rice, and pasta
- sparing use of fats, oils, and sweets

A patient who eats such a diet does not need a vitamin or mineral supplement. The current recommendation is that all women of reproductive potential consume 0.4 mg of folic acid daily to reduce the risk of neural tube defects in their offspring. This amount can be achieved through food selection or through supplementation with an over-the-counter multivitamin; use of prenatal prescription vitamins is unnecessary. In addition to being expensive, their use could result in daily intake of more than 1 mg per day, which exceeds the USPHS recommendation. Women who have previously had a pregnancy complicated by a neural tube defect are the exception; these women should be prescribed folic acid supplementation in the amount of 4 mg daily beginning at least 1 month before conception and continuing through the first 3 months of pregnancy. The preconceptional counselor is advised, however, to keep abreast of changing recommendations, because many believe that future research will reveal that lower doses have the same protective effect while decreasing the risk of toxicity.

Supplementation should also be provided to women who have an iron-deficiency anemia. The counselor should review the food intake of the anemic woman and, when appropriate, advise her of appropriate iron-rich food choices (see Appendix F). She should also receive an iron supplement that contains 60 mg of elemental iron (Appendix G) three times a day for a sufficient period, usually 3 to 6 months, to correct the anemia and rebuild iron stores. Therapeutic supplementation with iron should include consideration of additional zinc and copper intake, because iron can interfere with the physiologic availability of these two important elements.

If there are no dairy products in the diet recall, the counselor should question the patient about her usual intake. If she can tolerate milk and milk products, the counselor should prescribe their inclusion in her daily diet, explaining that adequate calcium intake is necessary for her own long-term health needs and for those of her prospective child. If the patient is unwilling to introduce dairy products into her diet or is unable to tolerate them, the counselor should try to introduce other foods high in calcium (see Appendix H) and should consider supplementation (see Appendix I). Care must be taken to avoid prescribing calcium supplements in forms that are high in lead content.

The 24-hour diet recall should be reviewed for vitamin and other drug ingestions. If the woman has a potentially harmful drug-nutrient interaction (see Appendix J), the counselor should attempt to correct it through alterations in medication, through diet, or through appropriate vitamin or nutrient supplementation before conception. The counselor should ask a patient who takes more than one multivitamin per day to bring in her vitamins so that total dosage can be evaluated and megadose exposure avoided. After asking about the reasons for supplementation, the counselor should tactfully advise the patient on the actual versus the perceived benefits of supplemental vitamins.

The most likely drug-nutrient interaction is associated with alcohol use. Alcohol abuse has been associated with decreased levels of zinc and folic acid, as well as with general malnutrition. Every effort should be made to identify the alcohol-abusing patient and to address not only her addiction but also its nutritional effects (see Chapter 2). The preconceptional use of a multivitamin that contains zinc and folic acid may be appropriate for these patients.

The patient's weight indicates the general reliability of the diet recall. When there is a marked discrepancy, referral to a nutritionist or registered dietitian for a more detailed history may be appropriate. Markedly underweight women who indicate good caloric intake through their food recall may be practicing deviant eating behaviors, such as bulimia. It may take considerable time in such cases for the preconceptional counselor to establish a nonthreatening rapport. Eventually, referral to a psychologist or to a special eating disorders clinic is likely to be necessary.

The preconceptional counselor should have a chart readily available to determine accurately the appropriateness of the patient's weight for her height (Appendix M). If the patient is underweight or overweight, the counselor should try to help her more closely approach the ideal. The patient needs to understand and accept the rationale for the counselor's recommendations regarding her weight before she is likely to change her eating behavior. If the chronically under- or overweight patient indicates a desire to change her weight, a nutritionist should be consulted to design an appropriate diet. Both groups of patients deserve frequent visits to acknowledge progress and reinforce motivation.

Both underweight and overweight women should be aware of the recommended weight gain specific to their situations during pregnancy. Preconceptional counseling may facilitate the thin woman's effort to reach 120% of her ideal weight during pregnancy, while it helps the obese woman to disavow commonly held beliefs that pregnancy will result in a net weight loss.

If a woman is a vegetarian, her essential amino acid intake may be marginal or below normal. Ovo-lactovegetarian diets, incorporating the principles of complementary proteins, are usually adequate in protein and all other nutrients; therefore, they pose no risk to a pregnant woman[114] or developing fetus. However, a nutritionist or registered dietitian should assess such a diet for completeness. If a woman is a vegan, eating only foods of plant origin, she may be consuming a low-energy, low-protein, mineral-poor diet. The major risks of such a diet are that it may result in low mineral and vitamin levels preconceptionally, a low prepregnancy weight, and, if continued during pregnancy, an inadequate weight gain. The vegan who is considering pregnancy should be encouraged to expand her food intake to include milk and eggs and to use mineral and vitamin supplements.

Pica is difficult to identify and difficult to change. Patients generally recognize that their craving is unusual and may be less than candid because of the associated embarrassment. The counselor must make nonjudgmental efforts, however, to identify any current craving or any cravings associated with past pregnancies, as some of the craved substances may be dangerous. Substituting nutritious foods of similar consistency may prove useful.

References

1. Hurley LS: Teratogenic aspects of manganese, zinc, and copper nutrition. *Physiol Rev* 1981;61:249-295.
2. Hurley LS: Nutritional deficiencies and excesses, in Wilson JG, Fraser FC (eds): *Handbook of Teratology.* New York, Plenum Press, 1977, vol 1, pp 261-308.
3. Kim I, Hungerford DW, Yip R, et al: Pregnancy Nutrition Surveillance System—United States, 1979-1990. *MMWR* 1992;41 (SS-7):25-71.
4. Ounsted M, Scott A, Ounsted C: Transmission through the female line of a mechanism constraining human fetal growth. *Ann Hum Biol* 1986;13:143-151.
5. Hackman E, Emanuel I, vanBelle G, et al: Maternal birth weight and subsequent pregnancy outcome. *JAMA* 1983; 250:2016-2019.
6. Winick M: Maternal nutrition and fetal growth. *Perinatol Neonatal* 1986;10: 28-34.
7. Wynn M, Wynn A: Effects of nutrition on reproductive capability. *Nutr Health* 1983;1:165-178.
8. Giroud A: Nutritional requirements of the embryo. *World Rev Nutr Diet* 1973; 18:195-262.
9. Osofsky HJ: Relationships between nutrition during pregnancy and subsequent infant and child development. *Obstet Gynecol Surv* 1975;30:227-241.
10. Philips C, Johnson NE: The impact of quality of diet and other factors on birth weight of infants. *Am J Clin Nutr* 1977; 30:215-225.
11. Falkner F: Maternal nutrition and fetal growth. *Am J Clin Nutr* 1981;34:769-774.

12. Stein Z, Susser M, Saenger G, et al: *Famine and Human Development: The Dutch Hunger Winter of 1944/45.* New York, Oxford University Press, 1975.

13. Smith C: Effects of maternal undernutrition upon the newborn infant in Holland (1944-45). *J Pediatr* 1947;30:229.

14. Lechtig H, Habicht JP, Delgado H, et al: Effect of food supplementation during pregnancy on birthweight. *Pediatrics* 1975;56:508-520.

15. Worthington-Roberts BS, Vermeersch J, Williams SR: Physiological basis of nutritional needs, in *Nutrition in Pregnancy and Lactation,* ed 3. St. Louis, Times Mirror/Mosby College Publishing, 1985, pp 77-131.

16. Worthington-Roberts B: Nutrition and maternal health. *Nutr Today* 1984;19:6-19.

17. Goldsmith GA: The new dietary allowances. *Nutr Today* 1968;3:16-19.

18. Platt BS, Stewart RJC: Reversible and irreversible effects of protein-calorie deficiency on the central nervous system of animals and man. *World Rev Nutr Diet* 1971;13:43-85.

19. Stewart RJC, Platt BS: Nervous system damage in experimental protein-calorie deficiency, in Scrimshaw R, Gordon L (eds): *Malnutrition, Learning and Behavior.* Cambridge, Mass, MIT Press, 1968, pp 168-180.

20. Zamenhof S, VanMarthens E, Margolis FL: DNA (cell number) and protein in neonatal brain: Alteration by maternal dietary protein restriction. *Science* 1968;160:322-323.

21. Aspartame and other sweeteners. *Med Lett Drugs Ther* 1982;24:1-2.

22. *Decision of the Public Board of Inquiry, Aspartame,* (FDA) docket 75F-0335. US Dept of Health and Human Services, 1980.

23. Pitkin RM: Aspartame ingestion during pregnancy, in Stegink LD, Filer LJ (eds): *Aspartame: Physiology and Biochemistry.* New York, Marcel Dekker, 1984, pp 555-563.

24. Tenbrink MS, Stroud KW: Normal infant born to mother with PKU. *JAMA* 1982;247:2239-2240.

25. Aspartame: Review of safety issues. Council Report. *JAMA* 1985;254:400-402.

26. Deuel HJ, Martin CR, Alfin-Slater RB: The effect of fat level of the diet on general nutrition: XII. The requirement of essential fatty acids for pregnancy and lactation. *J Nutr* 1954;54:193-204.

27. Randle PJ, Garland PB, Hales CH, et al: The glucose fatty acid cycle: Its role in insulin sensitivity and the metabolic disturbances of diabetes mellitus. *Lancet* 1963;1:785-789.

28. Stewart ML, McDonald JT, Levy AS, et al: Vitamin/mineral supplement use: A telephone survey of adults in the United States. *J Am Diet Assoc* 1985; 85:1585-1590.

29. Institute of Medicine: *Nutrition during Pregnancy.* Washington, DC, National Academy Press, 1990.

30. Lungarotti MS, Marinelli TM, Calabro A: Multiple congenital anomalies associated with apparently normal intake of vitamin A; a phenocopy of isotretinoin syndrome? *Am J Med Genet* 1987;27:245-248.

31. Pitkin RM: Megadose nutrients during pregnancy, in *Alternative Dietary Practices and Nutritional Abuses in Pregnancy.* Washington, DC, National Academy Press, 1982, pp 203-211.

32. Committee on Nutrition, American Academy of Pediatrics: The relationship between infantile hypercalcemia and vitamin D: Public health implications in North America. *Pediatrics* 1967;40:1050.

33. Seeling MS: Vitamin D and cardiovascular, renal and brain damage in infancy and childhood. *Ann NY Acad Sci* 1969;147:539-582.

34. Abrams AA: Use of vitamin E in chronic cystic mastitis. *N Engl J Med* 1965;272:1080-1085.

35. Roberts HJ: Perspectives on vitamin E as therapy. *JAMA* 1981;246:129-131.

36. Kaminetzky HA, Baker H: Micronutrients in pregnancy. *Clin Obstet Gynecol* 1977;20:363-380.

37. Hurley LS: *Developmental Nutrition.* Englewood Cliffs, NJ, Prentice-Hall, 1980.

38. Kousige Y: Study of developmental pharmacology on vitamin K. *Folia Pharmacol* 1973;69:285.

39. Van Gelder DW, Darby FV: Congenital and infantile beriberi. *J Pediatr* 1944; 25:226-235.

40. Vitamin B$_6$ deficiency and immune responses. *Nutr Rev* 1976;34:188-189.

41. Frimpter GW, Andelman RJ, George WF: Vitamin B$_6$-dependency syndromes: New horizons in nutrition. *Am J Clin Nutr* 1969;22:794-803.

42. Martin MP, Bridgforth E, MacGanity WJ, et al: The Vanderbilt Cooperative. Study of maternal and infant nutrition: V. Ascorbic acid. *J Nutr* 1957;62:201-224.

43. Cochrane WA: Overnutrition in prenatal and neonatal life: A problem? *Can Med Assoc J* 1975;93:893-899.

44. Armstrong RC, Monie IW: Congenital eye defects in rats following maternal folic acid deficiency during pregnancy. *J Embryol Exp Morphol* 1966;16:531.

45. Kitay DZ: Folic acid and reproduction. *Clin Obstet Gynecol* 1979;22:809-817.

46. Centers for Disease Control: Recommendations for the use of folic acid to reduce the number of cases of spina bifida and other neural tube defects. *MMWR* 1992;41:1-7.

47. Elwood JM, Elwood JH: *Epidemiology of Anencephalus and Spina Bifida.* Oxford University Press, 1980.

48. Laurence KM, James N, Miller MH, et al: Double-blind randomized control of folate treatment before conception to prevent recurrence of neural tube defects. *Br Med J* 1980;282:1509-1511.

49. Smithells RW, Seller MJ, Harris R, et al: Further experiences of vitamin supplementation for prevention of neural tube defect recurrences. *Lancet* 1983;1: 1027-1931.

50. Mulinare J, Cordero JF, Erickson JD, et al: Periconceptional use of multivitamins and the occurrence of neural tube defects. *JAMA* 1988;260:3141-3145.

51. Bowen C, Stanley FJ: Dietary folate as a risk factor for neural tube defects: evidence from a case control study in Western Australia. *Med J Aust* 1989; 150:613-619.

52. MRC Vitamin Study Research Group: Prevention of neural tube defects: Results of the Medical Research Council Vitamin Study. *Lancet* 1991;338: 131-137.

53. Milunsky A, Jick H, Jick S, et al: Multivitamin/folic acid supplementation in early pregnancy reduces the prevalence of neural tube defects. *JAMA* 1989;262: 2847-2852.

54. Werler MM, Shapiro S, Mitchell AA: Periconceptional folic acid exposure and risk of occurrence of neural tube defects. *JAMA* 1993;269:1257-1261.

55. Czeizel AE, Dudas I: Prevention of the first occurrence of neural-tube defects by periconceptional vitamin supplementation. *N Engl J Med* 1992;327: 1832-1835.

56. Mills JL, Rhoads GG, Simpson JL, et al: The absence of a relation between the periconceptional use of vitamins and neural-tube defects. *N Engl J Med* 1989;321:430-435.

57. Centers for Disease Control: Use of folic acid for prevention of spina bifida and other neural tube defects 1983-1991. *MMWR* 1991;40:513-516.

58. Centers for Disease Control: Recommendations for the use of folic acid to

reduce the number of cases of spina bifida and other neural tube defects. *MMWR* 1992;41:1-7.

59. American College of Obstetricians and Gynecologists: *Nutrition in Pregnancy.* ACOG Technical Bulletin 179, Washington, DC, 1993.

60. Institute of Medicine. *Nutrition during Pregnancy.* Washington, DC, National Academy Press, 1990.

61. Luke B: *Maternal Nutrition.* Boston, Little Brown & Co, 1979.

62. Kitay DZ, Habort RA: Iron and folic acid deficiency in pregnancy. *Clin Perinatol* 1975;2:255.

63. Lead in "natural" calcium pills still causes concern. *Tufts University Diet and Nutrition Letter.* November 1987.

64. Bowden JW, Osborne JW: Tracer study on the effect of dietary calcium deficiency during pregnancy. *J Dent Res* 1962;41:1349.

65. Belizan JM, Villar J: The relationship between calcium intake and edema-, and proteinuria- and hypertension-gestosis: A hypothesis. *Am J Clin Nutr* 1980;33:2202.

66. Carswell F, Kerr MM, Hutchinson JH: Congenital goiter and hypothyroidism produced by maternal ingestion of iodides. *Lancet* 1970;1:1241.

67. Prasad AS: Clinical, biochemical, and pharmacological role of zinc. *Annu Rev Pharmacol Taxicol* 1979;19:393-426.

68. Kynast G, Saling E: The relevance of zinc in pregnancy. *J Perinat Med* 1980; 8:171-182.

69. Swanson CA, King JC: Human zinc nutrition. *J Nutr Educ* 1979;11:181-183.

70. Hurley LS: Trace metals in mammalian development. *Johns Hopkins Med J* 1981;148:1.

71. Sandstead HH, Fosmire GS, Halas ES, et al: Zinc deficiency effects on brain and behavior of rats and Rhesus monkeys. *Teratology* 1977;16:229.

72. Bergman NKE, Makosch G, Tewas KH: Abnormalities of hair zinc concentration in mothers of newborn infants with spina bifida. *Am J Clin Nutr* 1980; 33:2145.

73. Jameson S: Effects of zinc deficiency in human reproduction. *Acta Med Scand* 1976; 1(suppl):593.

74. Soltan MH, Jenkins MH: Maternal and fetal plasma zinc concentration and fetal abnormalities. *Br J Obstet Gynaecol* 1982;89:56.

75. Caudar AO, Bacacan E, Arcasoy A, et al: Effect of nutrition on serum zinc concentration during pregnancy in Turkish women. *Am J Clin Nutr* 1980; 33:542.

76. Sever L, Emanuel J: Is there a connection between maternal zinc deficiency and congenital malformations of the nervous system in man? *Teratology* 1973;7:117.

77. Ruth RE, Goldsmith SK: Interaction between zinc deprivation and acute ethanol intoxication during pregnancy in rats. *J Nutr* 1981;111:2034.

78. Hambridge KM, Casey CE, Krebs NF: Zinc, in Mertz M (ed): *Trace Elements in Human and Animal Nutrition,* ed 5. Orlando, Fla, Academic Press, 1986, vol 2, pp 1-137.

79. Hambridge KM, Krebs NF, Sibley L, et al: Acute effects of iron therapy on zinc status during pregnancy. *Obstet Gynecol* 1987;70:593-596.

80. Schlicker SA, Cox DH: Maternal dietary zinc and development. *J Nutr* 1968;95:287-294.

81. Horowitz HS, Keifetz SB: Effects of prenatal exposure to fluoridation on dental caries. *Public Health Rep* 1967; 82:297-304.

82. Glenn FB, Glenn WD, Duncan RC: Fluoride tablet supplementation during pregnancy for caries immunity: A study of offspring produced. *Am J Obstet Gynecol* 1982;143:560.

83. Schour J, Smith MC: Mottled teeth: Experimental and histological analysis. *J Am Dent Assoc* 1935:22:796.

84. Smith CM, Smith HV: The occurrence of mottled enamel on temporary teeth. *J Am Dent Assoc* 1935;22:814.

85. Hurley LS, Keen CL: Teratogenic effects of copper, in Nriagu J (ed): *Copper in the Environment: II. Health Effects.* New York, John Wiley & Sons, 1979, pp 33-56.

86. Keen CL, Mark-Savage P, Lonnerdal B, et al: Low tissue copper and teratogenesis in rats resulting from D-penicillamine. *Fed Proc* 1981;40:917.

87. Solomon L, Abrams G, Dinner M, et al: Neonatal abnormalities associated with D-penicillamine treatment during pregnancy. *N Engl J Med* 1977;296:54-55.

88. Worthington-Roberts BS, Klerman LV: Maternal nutrition, in Merkatz IR, Thompson JE (eds): *New Perspective on Prenatal Care.* New York, Elsevier, 1990;237.

89. Abrams BF, Laros RK: Prepregnancy weight, weight gain, and birth weight. *Am J Obstet Gynecol* 1986;154:503-509.

90. Gordon AM: *Nutritional Management of High Risk Patient.* Berkeley, Calif, Society for Nutrition Education, 1981.

91. Anderson GD: Nutrition in Pregnancy. *South Med J* 1979;72:1304-1314.

92. Jacobson HH: Diet in pregnancy. *N Engl J Med* 1977;297:1051-1053.

93. Brown JE, Jacobson HH, Askue LH, et al: Influence of pregnancy weight gains on the size of infants born to underweight women. *Obstet Gynecol* 1981; 57:13-17.

94. Edwards LE, Alton IR, Barrada MI, et al: Pregnancy in the underweight woman: Course, outcome and growth patterns of the infant. *Am J Obstet Gynecol* 1979;135:297-302.

95. Naeye RL: Nutritional/nonnutritional interactions that affect the outcome of pregnancy. *Am J Clin Nutr* 1981;34: 727-731.

96. Calandra C, Abell DA, Beischer NA: Maternal obesity in pregnancy. *Obstet Gynecol* 1981;57:8-12.

97. Strauss RJ, Wise L: Operative risks of obesity. *Surg Gynecol Obstet* 1978; 146:286-291.

98. Committee on Diet and Health, Food and Nutrition Board, Commission on Life Sciences, National Research Council: *Diet and Health: Implications for Reducing Chronic Disease Risk.* Washington, DC, National Academy Press, 1989;584-585.

99. Lieber CS: *Medical Disorders of Alcoholism: Pathogenesis and Treatment.* Philadelphia, WB Saunders Co, 1982.

100. Russel RM, Rosenberg IH, Wilson PD, et al: Increased urinary excretion and prolonged turnover time of folic acid during ethanol ingestion. *Am J Clin Nutr* 1983;38:64-70.

101. Little RE, Streissguth AP, Barr HM, et al: Decreased birth weight in infants of alcoholic women who abstained during pregnancy. *J Pediatr* 1980;96:974-977.

102. Roe DA: Diet-drug interactions and incompatibilities, in Hathcock JH, Coon J (eds): *Nutrition and Drug Interactions.* New York, Academic Press, 1978, chap 11.

103. Ovesen L: Drugs and vitamin deficiency. *Drugs* 1979;18:278-298.

104. Graham DM: Caffeine—Its identity, dietary sources, intake and biologic effects. *Nutr Rev* 1978;36:97-102.

105. Srisuphan W, Bracken MB: Caffeine consumption during pregnancy and association with late spontaneous abortion. *Am J Obstet Gynecol* 1986;154: 14-20.

106. Spiller J (ed): *The Methylxanthine Beverages and Foods; Chemistry, Consumption and Health Effects.* New York, Alan Liss, 1984, p. 393.

107. Collins TF, Welsh JJ, Black TN, et al:

A study of the teratogenic potential of caffeine ingested in drinking water. *Food Chem Toxicol* 1983;21(6):763-777.

108. Weathersbee PS, Olsen LK, Lodge JR: Caffeine and pregnancy: A retrospective survey. *Postgrad Med* 1977;62:64-69.

109. Linn S, Schoenbaum SC, Monson RR, et al: No association between coffee consumption and adverse outcome in pregnancy. *N Engl J Med* 1982;306:141-145.

110. Fenster L, Eskenazi B, Windham GC, et al: Caffeine consumption during pregnancy and fetal growth. *Am J Public Health,* 1991;81:458-461.

111. Mills JL, Holmes LB, Aarons JH, et al: Moderate caffeine use and the risk of spontaneous abortion and intrauterine growth retardation. *JAMA* 1993;269:593-597.

112. Wilcox A, Weinberg C, Baird D: Caffeinated beverages and decreased fertility. Epidemiology Branch, National Institute of Environmental Health Sciences, Research Triangle Park, NC. *Lancet* 1988;2:1453-1456.

113. Ritchey SJ, Taper LJ: Nutritional health of the adult female, in Henry F, Kamlani B (eds): *Maternal and Child Nutrition.* New York, Harper & Row, 1983, chap 1.

114. Hinton SM, Kerwin DR: Nutritional concerns of women, in Hinton SM (ed) *Maternal, Infant and Child Nutrition— A Resource Book for Health Professionals.* Chapel Hill, NC, Health Sciences Consortium, 1981, chap 5.

4

Medical History

A though disorders of the endocrine, metabolic, pulmonary, cardiovascular, renal, neurologic, and hemopoietic systems may affect pregnant women, they do not necessarily alter the outcome of pregnancy. The preconceptional approach to the woman with a significant medical problem, including cancer, must take into account the effect that the disease and its current or past therapeutic regimens may have on the intrauterine environment and fetal development, as well as the effect that pregnancy may have on the woman's disease process.

The preconceptional counselor begins the evaluation of the medical risk status of a patient by asking whether she has or has ever had

- diabetes mellitus
- a thyroid disorder
- hyperphenylalaninemia (may be identified by inquiring about special diets in childhood)
- asthma
- heart disease
- chronic hypertension
- deep venous thrombosis
- kidney disease
- systemic lupus erythematosus
- epilepsy
- a hemoglobinopathy
- cancer

Any positive response should prompt further investigation into therapy regimens and past medical records. If a patient is being treated for a chronic disease, the preconceptional counselor must coordinate his or her recommendations with those of other medical care providers. This ensures that all providers appreciate the patient's total plan of care and spares the patient the anxiety of sorting through conflicting recommendations.

Diabetes Mellitus

C arbohydrate intolerance affects approximately 1.5 million women of repro-ductive age in the United States, and diabetes mellitus is the most common serious disease to affect the maternal-fetal dyad. Advances in antenatal and intra-partum maternal-fetal surveillance, ultrasonography, and neonatal care, together with a clearer understanding of the pathophysiology of diabetes mellitus, have dramati-cally reduced the maternal and perinatal mortality associated with this disease. Despite these reductions, the 6% to 10% incidence of congenital malformation in the infants of diabetic mothers remains 2 to 3 times that of the infants of nondiabetic mothers, and malformation associated with diabetes mellitus is the leading cause of perinatal death.[1] The most common types of abnormalities seen in infants of diabetic mothers, including ventricular septal defects, neural tube defects, and caudal regres-sion syndrome, involve organs that are formed within the first 7 to 8 weeks of gestation, which indicates that preventive strategies must be placed in the precon-ceptional period.[2-4]

BACKGROUND

Approximately 90% of patients with diabetes have type II disease, which is usually diet-controlled and is not ketosis-prone; 10% have insulin-dependent type I diabetes, which is ketosis-prone and has more serious vascular involvement.

Blood Glucose Levels Associated with Congenital Malformation

Many of the problems seen in the infants of insulin-dependent diabetic mothers are the direct result of high maternal blood glucose levels. In animal models, the apparent teratogenic effect of diabetes mellitus is correlated with the degree of glucose control during organogenesis.[5] In 1973, Pedersen and Møolsted-Pedersen[4] reported a 5.6% rate of major congenital malformation among the offspring of diabetic mothers who attended a specialized prepregnancy program for glucose control, whereas the rate among the offspring of diabetic mothers who did not participate in the prepregnancy clinic was 12.2%. These findings prompted Pedersen[6(p196)] to hypothesize that the congenital malformations were associated with ''incomplete metabolic compensa-tion'' in the first trimester and to advocate that ''a diabetic woman should contem-plate pregnancy only after advice and a full compensation of her metabolism.''

To determine the metabolic control of glucose over a period of time, measure-ment of a glycosylated hemoglobin level has been used. A normal, minor hemoglobin in adults, glycosylated hemoglobin is distinguished from hemoglobin A in the red blood cell by the nonenzymatic, irreversible addition of a glucose moiety to the terminal valine of the β chain. This binding occurs after the red blood cells leave the marrow and is proportional to the plasma glucose concentrations to which the red blood cells have been exposed. Once the hemoglobin has been combined with glucose, it forms hemoglobin A_{1c}, A_{1a1}, A_{1a2}, and A_{1b}. The majority (80%) of glycosylated hemoglobin is hemoglobin A_{1c}. Therefore, measurement of hemoglobin A_{1c} provides a retrospective and integrated index of glucose control over the previous 4 to 8 weeks.[7]

The normal hemoglobin A_{1c} levels in nondiabetic women are 4% to 8%. Care must be taken in interpreting hemoglobin A_{1c} values, however, because the techniques used to determine these values differ greatly from one laboratory to another. During pregnancy, there is an additional difficulty: the increased erythrocyte production during pregnancy may decrease the mean age of circulating red blood cells and falsely decrease the level of hemoglobin A_{1c}. On the other hand, fetal hemoglobin in the maternal circulation may falsely elevate the measured level of hemoglobin A_{1c}.

Miller and colleagues[8] retrospectively correlated elevated maternal levels of hemoglobin A_{1c} with major congenital anomalies in infants of diabetic mothers. On the basis of hemoglobin A_{1c} levels drawn before 13 weeks of gestation, they divided the women into two groups. The infants born to the diabetic mothers in the better-controlled group, as indicated by a near-normal level of hemoglobin A_{1c} ($\leq 8.5\%$), had a severe congenital anomaly rate of 3%, remarkably close to the rate for the general population. Those born to the diabetic mothers in the more poorly controlled group (hemoglobin A_{1c} level $\geq 8.5\%$) had a congenital malformation rate of 22%.[8]

The work of Ylinen and colleagues[9] supports the association between maternal hyperglycemia during organogenesis and congenital malformation. These researchers measured the level of hemoglobin A_{1c} in 142 insulin-dependent diabetic women before the end of the fifteenth week of gestation. Those who gave birth to malformed infants had mean hemoglobin A_{1c} values of 9.5% (± 1.8); those who gave birth to infants without congenital malformation had hemoglobin A_{1c} values of 8% (± 1.4). When the level of hemoglobin A_{1c} was equal to or more than 10% during the first 15 weeks of pregnancy, 35% of the infants had major anomalies.

Fuhrmann and associates,[10] in a report on 420 pregnancies of insulin-dependent diabetic women, emphasized the importance of preconceptional glucose control in reducing the incidence of congenital malformation. Twenty-three (5.5%) of the offspring had congenital malformations. The malformation rate was 1.4% in the infants of 420 comparable nondiabetic women. Of the 420 insulin-dependent diabetic women, strict metabolic control began after 8 weeks of gestation in 292. As this group delivered 22 of the 23 malformed infants, the incidence of congenital malformation in the group was 7.5%. Intensive metabolic control began before conception in 128 of the diabetic women; only one malformed infant (0.8%) was among the offspring of this group.

As reported in a subsequent study on the management of 200 pregnant diabetic patients, 56 patients whose blood glucose levels were normal in 87% or more of their readings before conception and in the early weeks of gestation gave birth to 57 infants, only one of whom had a fatal congenital malformation.[11] The remaining 144 patients did not participate in preconceptional metabolic control programs and did not begin glucose control efforts until an average of 8 weeks of gestation. This group gave birth to 145 children. Nine of the children had congenital malformations: three were fatal, three were severe, and three were minor. These studies by Fuhrmann, as well as studies by others,[12,14] demonstrate that strict metabolic control for the insulin-dependent diabetic woman before conception and during the first trimester significantly reduces the incidence of congenital malformation.

Vascular, genetic, immunologic, and other metabolic factors may also play a role in the incidence of congenital anomalies in the infants of diabetic women. Determinations of hemoglobin A_{1c} levels indicate only blood glucose control for the 4 to 8 weeks preceding the test; they reveal nothing about other metabolic products that may be altered when blood glucose levels are not controlled. For example, hyperglycemia may induce a myoinositol deficiency in neural tissue that interferes with the mobilization of the arachidonic acid necessary for fusion of the neural tube.[5] Because insulin has a direct effect on amino acid and fat metabolism, it may disturb the relationship of the metabolic or "ambient" fuels available to the developing embryo.

Risks of Pregnancy for the Diabetic Woman

The fetus of the pregnant diabetic woman is likely to be larger than the average fetus. The cause of this macrosomia is still controversial, but it may be due to fetal hyperglycemia and fetal hyperinsulinemia caused by maternal hyperglycemia. Elevated levels of fetal insulin and multiple nutrients stimulate fetal growth.[6,15] Macrosomia may lead to increased maternal morbidity because of the more frequent need for cesarean delivery and to increased perinatal morbidity because of birth trauma. Optimal maternal glucose control with insulin may decrease the incidence of macrosomia.[16]

Pregnant diabetic women have a higher incidence of preeclampsia. This may be associated with a large placenta or may be secondary to vascular disease in the mother that decreases renal function or uterine blood flow.

Because of the pH changes in the urinary tract and the presence of glycosuria, pregnant diabetic women are more susceptible to urinary tract infections. Screening for significant bacteriuria and tests of kidney function are recommended during the prepregnancy period.

Pregnancy does not accelerate the natural course of diabetic nephropathy.[17] However, the complications of pregnancy in the presence of renal disease and hypertension are serious and potentially life-threatening. Pregnancy is inadvisable, therefore, in a diabetic patient who has a creatinine clearance rate equal to or less than 30 ml/min, a blood urea nitrogen value equal to or greater than 30 ml/dl, and hypertension.

Until recently, pregnancy in a patient with proliferative diabetic retinopathy was thought to present a very serious hazard to maternal vision. Today, the course and treatment of ophthalmologic changes in the pregnant diabetic woman are better understood. Diabetic retinopathy may progress or regress during pregnancy, but no controlled prospective studies have suggested that pregnancy either permanently accelerates or retards the disease process. Pregnancy does not interfere with the use of laser photocoagulation treatment; therefore, there is no medical indication for avoidance or termination of pregnancy in the presence of proliferative retinopathy with preretinal or intraocular hemorrhages or vascularization.[18]

The number of reports of diabetes with ischemic heart disease during pregnancy is small, but the maternal mortality rate is high. Therefore, pregnancy is not recommended for a patient with diabetes mellitus and angina pectoris, a prior myocardial infarction, or coronary artery disease.

The genetic factors of diabetes mellitus are not entirely understood. The risk that a mother who has insulin-dependent diabetes mellitus will have a diabetic child is approximately 1%; if both parents are diabetic, this risk increases to approximately 6%.[19] The offspring of a diabetic is approximately 3 times more likely to develop the disease at some time than is the general population. Typing of human leukocyte antigens (HLAs) may permit a more accurate estimation of the risk to an individual fetus. Studies over the past decade have indicated that insulin-dependent (type I) diabetes is genetically on the major histocompatibility complex markers on chromosome 6 linked to specific HLA alleles.[20] The risk for type I diabetes mellitus, for example, may be estimated by analyzing amniotic fluid to determine the fetal HLA type and comparing it with that of the parents or siblings with type I diabetes. The absence of any HLA alleles in common with a diabetic parent or sibling is reassuring, whereas the presence of HLA alleles in common implies that the fetus has an increased risk of later developing type I diabetes.

PRECONCEPTIONAL COUNSELING

The goal of preconceptional counseling for insulin-dependent diabetic women is to reduce the occurrence of obstetric and diabetic complications and to decrease the incidence of congenital abnormalities. To accomplish this, the patient must have optimal diabetic control before and throughout her pregnancy. The patient's fasting blood plasma glucose level should be maintained between 60 and 100 mg/dl; the 2-hour postprandial plasma glucose level, between 100 and 120 mg/dl. These levels can be assessed by self-monitoring blood glucose with a reflectance meter or by frequent blood analyses in a laboratory. The preconceptional goal is to affect blood sugar levels so that the hemoglobin A_{1c} level is within normal limits for the specific laboratory. The preconceptional counselor should coordinate all efforts to achieve these results with the patient's usual health care provider.

The individual patient's general medical condition should be evaluated by means of a complete history, a thorough physical examination, and careful laboratory assessments. Particular attention should be given to the presence or absence of retinopathy, nephropathy, and hypertension, as well as to the degree of metabolic control. A known type I or type II diabetic woman should undergo the following workup preconceptionally:

- determination of glycosylated hemoglobin blood level
- lipid profile
- analysis of 24-hour urine specimen for creatinine clearance and total protein concentration
- ophthalmologic examination with pupillary dilation
- electrocardiogram if the duration of the diabetes has been longer than 10 years

Abnormal findings on any of these studies necessitate appropriate endocrine, ophthalmologic, renal, and cardiac consultations. It is also advisable to consult a nutritionist. The patient should be informed that many of these studies will be repeated throughout pregnancy and that serial ultrasound examinations and fetal evaluation tests will also be needed. Because the incidence of neural tube defects is increased in the offspring of diabetic mothers,[19] patients should be made aware preconceptionally of the availability of maternal serum α-fetoprotein screening and should be counseled about the protective effects of folic acid intake during the periconceptional period (see Chapter 3).[21]

After the initial evaluation, the preconceptional counselor should explain the potential short- and long-term effects of pregnancy on diabetes mellitus, as well as the effects of diabetes mellitus on pregnancy and offspring. The diabetic woman and her partner should be encouraged to discuss their concerns about pregnancy and the offspring openly, because they may have hidden fears or unrealistic expectations. They need the most current scientific information available. In providing such information, the counselor can assist the patient and her partner in arriving at realistic, informed decisions. The couple should understand the theory and practice of diabetic care before and during pregnancy and should be aware that the extensive glucose monitoring and control strategies during the prepregnancy period and during the pregnancy itself may be burdensome.

All diabetic patients should be advised to adhere strictly to the recommended diet and insulin regimen. In addition to a good diet and exercise regimen, the counselor should recommend for the prepregnancy period a standard prenatal vitamin that contains 15 to 25 mg of zinc. Because optimal control may result in episodes of hypoglycemia, the counselor must teach patients to recognize and treat this state. Mild hypoglycemia is easily treated by the patient and is of no serious consequence, but severe and prolonged hypoglycemia is potentially dangerous. Therefore, patients on strict caloric and insulin regimens need to be especially careful to eat regularly and to learn to recognize and treat incipient symptoms of hypoglycemia. Patient education, including the use of injectable glucagon and diet management, requires a coordinated team approach. For most diabetic patients, the educational program and glucose control can be managed on an outpatient basis.

A model preconceptional program for diabetes is functioning in a number of perinatal centers that are part of the State of California Diabetes and Pregnancy Program.[22] During the prepregnancy assessment, patients are asked to use barrier methods of contraception and to keep an accurate menstrual calendar. Once attempted, pregnancy is documented as early as possible. Good general principles of health, such as proper diet, smoking cessation, weight control, avoidance of alcohol, and the early detection and treatment of infections, are encouraged. Rubella immunization is offered if appropriate, and the importance of early prenatal care is stressed.

The diabetic patient and her partner should understand that it is impossible to reduce the incidence of congenital malformation to zero, because there remains a 2% to 3% incidence of severe congenital malformation in the general, nondiabetic population.

Thyroid Disorders

A s many as 5% of women of reproductive age may have thyroid disorders. With appropriate surveillance and therapy, maternal and fetal thyroid function can remain normal throughout pregnancy and not impair pregnancy outcome.

BACKGROUND
Hypothyroidism

An enlargement of the thyroid may indicate hyperplasia secondary to compensation for hypothyroidism. Usually a primary condition in young women, hypothyroidism is diagnosed clinically by the classic signs and symptoms of the disease and is confirmed by a decreased free thyroxine (T_4) index and an elevated serum concentration of thyroid-stimulating hormone (TSH). Untreated maternal hypothyroidism has been associated with impaired fertility, an increased spontaneous abortion rate, and impaired fetal growth and development.[23-25] Studies indicate that the growth and development of infants born to mothers with hypothyroidism who have received appropriate replacement therapy are normal and that there is no increase in the incidence of congenital malformation.[23,26] The fetal hypothalamic-pituitary axis develops and functions independently of the maternal thyroid, allowing safe maternal replacement therapy during gestation.

Hyperthyroidism

Generally diagnosed as Graves' disease, hyperthyroidism occurs in 2 per 1,000 pregnancies. A diagnosis of hyperthyroidism is confirmed by an elevated free thyroxine (T_4) or free triiodothyronine (T_3) index, although other causes of an elevated free thyroxine level (e.g., chronic thyroiditis and subacute viral thyroiditis) should be considered. The symptoms of hyperthyroidism usually antedate pregnancy, and the patient has already received medical or ablative surgical therapy. Fertility is not impaired, and pregnancy does not appear to exacerbate the disease if the thyroid function is well controlled by antithyroid medication. If diagnosis and treatment occurred just before pregnancy, however, symptoms may recur during the first trimester.

In recent years, the administration of antithyroid drugs has largely supplanted surgery as the treatment of choice for hyperthyroidism. Propylthiouracil and methimazole are small molecules that cross the placenta. However, propylthiouracil crosses the placental membrane in concentration approximately one-fourth as often as does methimazole. Cheron and colleagues,[27] reporting on 11 patients treated with propylthiouracil during pregnancy, noted that there was no clinical evidence of thyroid disease in any of the neonates. Their serum thyroxine levels were initially reduced and thyrotropin levels elevated, but both levels quickly reverted to normal. Burrow and associates[28] followed 28 infants exposed to propylthiouracil during their mothers' pregnancies. The children studied ranged from age 2 to age 24, and none demonstrated any impairment of developmental status. Methimazole, on the other hand, not only has a greater potential for decreasing fetal thyroid function but also has been associated with scalp abnormalities in the fetus. No specific congenital malformations have been observed with propylthiouracil.

In the nonpregnant woman, the administration of radioactive iodine is a common therapy for hyperthyroidism. If a woman becomes pregnant within 12 months of radioactive iodine treatment, it is theoretically possible for the radioactivity to affect the developing fetal thyroid adversely.[29,30]

Fetal thyrotoxicosis is a potential problem in pregnancies complicated by a maternal history of Graves' disease. Even if the mother has been asymptomatic and medication-free for a number of years, a persistent maternal thyroid-stimulating immunoglobulin may cross the placenta and cause fetal thyrotoxicosis. A high index of suspicion and close intrauterine monitoring of fetal well-being, including serial ultrasound examinations to identify fetal hydrops and enlargement of the fetal thyroid gland, are appropriate.

Thyroid Cancer

Approximately 1.5% of women of reproductive age have thyroid nodules. Most of these women have multiple thyroid nodules, which are usually benign; the incidence of thyroid cancer is quite low. The most common thyroid neoplasm that develops during the reproductive years is a well-differentiated papillary carcinoma that is associated with an extremely good prognosis if diagnosed early and surgically removed. A history of carcinoma of the thyroid is not a contraindication to pregnancy, nor does pregnancy affect the natural course of the disease.[31-33] After surgery, thyroxine therapy is usually indicated. Because thyroxine is a naturally occurring hormone that is produced by both the mother and fetus, and because there is negligible transplacental transport, it is considered safe during pregnancy.[34]

PRECONCEPTIONAL COUNSELING

The preconceptional counselor's goal is to help patients with all types of thyroid disorders achieve or maintain thyroid function within a normal range with the least amount of medication. It is necessary to determine the specific diagnosis, treatment, and current symptoms of hyperthyroid or hypothyroid function for all patients with a history of thyroid disease. A thyroid function panel should be ordered, even for patients who are currently asymptomatic. It is helpful for the counselor to communicate with the patient's endocrinologist about treatment goals and possible changes in medication.

Patients who are receiving medication for a thyroid condition should understand the importance of continuing their medication before and throughout pregnancy, unless specifically advised to alter the course of therapy. They should be aware that it will be necessary for them to have serial thyroid function studies during pregnancy and that ultrasound examinations of the fetus may be indicated. Each patient should be informed that the signs and symptoms of normal pregnancy may be similar to those associated with her thyroid disorder. However, she should be encouraged to report these signs and symptoms to her physician.

Patients who have been treated with radioactive iodine 131 before pregnancy should be advised that, although there are no proved fetal effects, the safest choice is to use a reliable form of contraception for 1 full year after completion of the treatment.

Blood levels of thyroid-stimulating immunoglobulins should be determined pre-conceptionally on patients with a history of Graves' disease, because these antibodies may cross the placenta. If this immunoglobulin is identified, the patient should be informed that, should she become pregnant, her fetus would be at risk for thyrotoxicosis. This condition cannot be averted by reinstitution of maternal antithyroid medication. Awareness of this potential problem, however, allows for antenatal fetal surveillance and timely neonatal intervention. The preconceptional counselor should reassure patients that the condition is treatable and transient.

Good general principles of health, such as proper diet, smoking cessation, weight control, and avoidance of alcohol, should be emphasized in preconceptional counseling. Rubella immunization should be offered when appropriate, and education regarding the importance of early prenatal care should be provided.

Hyperphenylalaninemia

The precise number of women with phenylketonuria (PKU) who are of childbearing age is unknown. A 1988 report indicated that there were at least 2,800 women in the United States between the ages of 16 and 26 with PKU.[35] Another estimate, made in 1990, indicates that more than 5,500 fecund women in this country have hyperphenylalaninemia[36]; many of them are unknown because they were born before neonatal screening was routine, have been lost to follow-up, or have emigrated to this country. Pregnancy outcomes for women with PKU are traditionally poor; their offspring have high incidences of microcephaly, mental retardation, and congenital heart defects. In addition, increased rates of spontaneous abortion, stillbirth, and intrauterine and postnatal growth retardation have been reported.[37] Research indicates that adherence to a restricted phenylalanine diet beginning in the preconceptional period improves pregnancy outcome.

BACKGROUND

Phenylalanine and tyrosine are essential amino acids found naturally in protein-containing food. Impaired metabolism of phenylalanine to tyrosine results in hyperphenylalaninemia or PKU. Because patients with PKU lack phenylalanine hydroxylase, the level of phenylalanine in their blood and tissue increases with the ingestion of a normal diet. Inherited as an autosomal recessive trait, hyperphenylalaninemia is one of the most frequent inborn defects of amino acid metabolism; it occurs in approximately 1 in 10,000 live births.

The normal phenylalanine level in the blood is less than 2 mg/dl. In classic PKU, the blood phenylalanine level is greater than 20 mg/dl. There are also mild and atypical hyperphenylalaninemias in which the blood level ranges from 3 to 20 mg/dl. The patient with classic PKU lacks the converting hepatic enzyme phenylalanine hydroxylase, whereas a small amount of enzyme activity occurs in mild forms of the disease.

An elevated blood phenylalanine level in infants and young children impairs the myelinization of brain tissue and the growth of the central nervous system. If the condition is untreated, a child with PKU becomes severely mentally retarded. During the last 25 years, all states in the United States and many foreign countries have established programs for the detection and treatment of PKU in neonates. The primary treatment, which is instituted at birth, involves restricting the protein in the diet and substituting an artificial amino acid mixture that is low in phenylalanine.

Until recently, dietary therapy was commonly discontinued when the child was 5 to 8 years of age. In a national collaborative study, Acosta and Wenz[38] determined that the children who remained on the diet were much more like their unaffected siblings in terms of IQ than were those who discontinued the diet. Today, most of the PKU treatment centers in the United States advocate indefinite continuation of the diet, although the issue is still controversial.

As a result of successful treatment, many female neonates with PKU have become normal adult women who are now in their childbearing years. Their offspring are at risk for the maternal PKU syndrome if the women do not adhere to a low phenylalanine diet. In this syndrome, the child does not inherit the autosomal recessive disorder of the mother, but rather is affected in utero by high circulating levels of maternal phenylalanine. The result is a neonate with microcephaly, mental retardation, and serious congenital heart disease.

In their survey and review of 524 pregnancies in 155 women with classic PKU, Lenke and Levy[37] found that when the mother had an untreated blood phenylalanine level of 20 mg/dl or more the frequency of mental retardation among the offspring was 92%; the frequency of microcephaly in the offspring was 73%.[34] In addition, there was an increased incidence of congenital heart disease, spontaneous abortion, and intrauterine growth retardation. Lenke and Levy[37 (p1202)] concluded that

> among untreated pregnancy the frequencies of mental retardation, microcephaly and congenital heart disease were greatly increased over those of the normal population and these increases correlated with the mothers' levels of phenylalanine.

Patients with atypical PKU or mild degrees of hyperphenylalaninemia appear to be less likely to give birth to an affected fetus, although the specific risks for a woman with maternal phenylalanine levels between 3 and 15 mg/dl are not known at this time.[39]

Although the problems associated with maternal PKU were first identified more than 30 years ago, many questions remain about its pathophysiology and treatment.[40]

In the human, phenylalanine crosses the placenta easily, and fetal concentrations are approximately 50% higher than those found in maternal serum. The mechanism of fetal damage in the maternal PKU syndrome is unknown. No convincing explanation has been offered for the pathophysiology and the pathogenesis of the maternal PKU syndrome, and there is no natural animal model that makes it possible to study PKU in a laboratory setting. Hyperphenylalaninemia induced by the administration of phenylalanine to pregnant animals, however, has produced low birthweight and learning defects in the offspring.[41]

Experience with the preconceptional and prenatal treatment of 54 women with PKU indicated that dietary treatment is effective in improving the outcome of these pregnancies but that such treatment does not prevent all the potential adverse fetal effects of maternal PKU.[42] In 13 patients who were treated before pregnancy, there was a significant drop in the phenylalanine levels. Birthweights of the offspring were normal, and there was no evidence of microcephaly or congenital heart disease; in follow-up, however, one of the infants demonstrated a lower-than-average IQ.[42] The outcome of the remaining 41 offspring varied depending on the pretreatment blood level of phenylalanine and the trimester in which treatment started. Even with a significant drop in phenylalanine levels, the outcome varied from mentally normal offspring to neonatal death due to congenital heart disease.[43]

Koch and colleagues[41] attempted to determine (1) the safe levels of maternal blood phenylalanine before conception, at the time of conception, and during pregnancy; (2) the amount of phenylalanine dietary restriction necessary during pregnancy; and (3) the effect of supplemental tyrosine, zinc, and other trace elements on the outcome of pregnancy. They studied five patients, beginning in the prepregnancy period. Each patient had emotional support, close dietary supervision, frequent monitoring of phenylalanine levels, and, once pregnant, serial measurements of blood phenylalanine levels. The authors concluded that blood phenylalanine levels should be kept at less than 5 mg/dl; that emotional support is essential in meeting this goal; and that attention should be given to dietary requirements for tyrosine, vitamins, zinc, and other metals.

In 1987, Farquhar and colleagues[45] followed two patients with borderline IQ, hyperphenylalaninemia, and dietary control of their phenylalanine levels before conception and during pregnancy. To maintain the normal phenylalanine level in the plasma, these patients required intensive intermittent inpatient instruction and outpatient care for months before conception. Both children appeared normal at birth and are achieving normal developmental milestones.

To investigate further the issues surrounding maternal PKU, the National Institute of Child Health and Human Development initiated in 1984 the National Maternal Phenylketonuria Collaborative Study. A preliminary report published in 1992 indicates that preconceptional counseling and early entrance into prenatal care are essential to achieving optimal fetal outcome in women with PKU.[40] The report was based on 237 pregnancies of women with hyperphenylalaninemia. The prospective study enrolled women and initiated indicated treatment before the conception of planned pregnancies or as soon as unplanned pregnancies were made known. Treatment involved providing a diet restricted in phenylalanine to women who had blood phenylalanine concentrations greater than or equal to 10 mg/dl, maintaining blood phenylalanine concentrations between 2 and 10 mg/dl, and supplementing the diet with tyrosine and trace elements as medically indicated. Two different control groups were included in the study design. Results showed that no children born to women who maintained the lowest phenylalanine levels throughout pregnancy ($\leq$ 10 mg/dl) had microcephaly, intrauterine growth retardation, or cardiac defects; 49% of the children born to mothers with intermediate levels (10.1 to 19.9 mg/dl) had microcephaly, as did 90% of the children born to mothers with the highest phenylalanine levels ($\geq$ 20 mg/dl). The incidence of intrauterine growth retardation in the intermediate- and high-level groups was 10% and 90%, respectively. The greatest incidence of cardiac defects was 13% for children born to mothers in the intermediate group. An interesting and disturbing finding is that facial dysmorphism was observed in 97% of the infants born to women with the highest phenylalanine levels, 92% of the infants born to women with intermediate levels, and 88% of the infants born to women with the lowest levels.

PRECONCEPTIONAL COUNSELING

In regard to PKU, the goals of preconceptional counseling are to identify women with elevated levels of serum phenylalanine and to initiate diet therapy when indicated. A careful history is necessary. All women should be asked whether they were on a special diet as children. Because in the past diet therapy was discontinued in early childhood, patients may not readily remember. If there is any question, previous medical records should be obtained.

Education of the patient and her partner about the documented fetal hazards of elevated maternal phenylalanine levels during pregnancy is most important. Appropriate educational materials and directions can be obtained from national collaborative PKU treatment centers (Appendix N).

The patient and her partner should be informed that, even with optimal preconceptional and prenatal care, there is no guarantee that their baby will be normal and that their risk appears to be greater than that for the general population. Research indicates, however, that taking certain steps will maximize their chances for a healthy outcome. The following preconceptional recommendations are based on the recommendations of Acosta and colleagues[46] for pregnant patients:

- Levels of serum phenylalanine, tyrosine, and other plasma amino acids should be determined before the institution of diet therapy.
- The tests should be accompanied by a 3-day diet record to evaluate the natural intake of the amino acids.
- Blood phenylalanine levels should be in the range of 4 to 8 mg/dl, and blood tyrosine levels should be greater than 1 mg/dl before conception. If tyrosine falls below 1 mg/dl, tyrosine supplementation should be given.
- A diet that combines low-protein foods (e.g., fruits and vegetables) with a formula that contains all amino acids except phenylalanine (e.g., Maxamum x^P, Milupa PKU3, and Phenyl-free) should be prescribed. The protein and energy needs of pregnancy, as well as the vitamin and mineral needs, can be met by this diet.
- The patient should be advised that plasma and urine amino acid profiles will be performed monthly and that blood levels of vitamins and minerals will be assessed in each trimester of pregnancy. She should also be aware that serial ultrasound measurements will be made to evaluate fetal growth and development.
- Preconceptional and prenatal vitamin supplementation is not recommended. A PKU patient who ingests 300 g of a phenyl-free formula daily needs only

supplemental folic acid during pregnancy, because the formula contains sufficient vitamins and minerals. If regular prenatal vitamins are taken in addition to the formula, the levels of vitamins A, B_2, B_6, C, D, and niacin become higher than the level recommended during pregnancy.

The implementation of a phenyl-free diet requires the utmost support of family and friends. Because the diet is restrictive and expensive, it imposes social and economic hardships. The support of professionals in PKU treatment programs may help reinforce the patient's resolve.

Good general principles of health, such as proper diet, smoking cessation, weight control, and avoidance of alcohol, should be emphasized in preconceptional counseling. Rubella immunization should be offered when appropriate, and education regarding the importance of early prenatal care should be provided.

Asthma

A sthma is encountered in approximately 1% of pregnant women.[47] Its effects on individual patients and their future offspring are unpredictable, but acute attacks of asthma or chronic lung disease can change maternal pulmonary mechanics, oxygenation of the blood, or uterine blood flow and thus prove harmful. If asthma is stable before pregnancy and remains under control throughout gestation, however, maternal and fetal risks are minimized.

BACKGROUND

The elevated levels of progesterone that accompany pregnancy relax the smooth muscle of the bronchial tree, decrease airway resistance, increase respiratory rate, and increase tidal volume. Maternal arterial oxygen tension and vital capacity remain essentially unchanged, but there is a 40% increase in minute ventilation over non-pregnant levels.[48] Maternal arterial carbon dioxide tension decreases to 30 torr, while the pH rises to 7.44. By term, the patient's initial functional residual volume and capacity have fallen by 20%. These changes may result from the elevation of the diaphragm by the enlarging uterus.[49]

Because oxygen is supplied to the fetus by diffusion across the placental membrane, the amount of oxygen received by the fetus is dependent on maternal and fetal blood flow. The fetus sustains normal growth and development with an umbilical vein oxygen tension of 27 to 30 torr. The three compensatory mechanisms that allow normal growth and development in the presence of a low PO_2 are (1) a greater oxygen affinity and binding capacity in fetal hemoglobin; (2) the flow through the ductus venosus and ductus arteriosus, directing blood to vital areas; and (3) an increased blood flow rate from the fetus to the placenta and peripheral tissue.

A number of studies, most of which are retrospective, have compared outcomes of pregnancies complicated by asthma with those of control populations. There is general but not total agreement that prematurity and low birthweight are more frequently associated with maternal asthma.

Although the level of unbound plasma cortisol is increased during pregnancy, the incidence of asthmatic attacks and the need for corticosteroid therapy do not necessarily decrease. One reason is that the levels of prostaglandins, including the level of prostaglandin $F_{2\alpha}$ ($PGF_{2\alpha}$), a bronchoconstrictor, are increased in blood and amniotic fluid during pregnancy. The increase in the circulating levels of $PGF_{2\alpha}$ during pregnancy, particularly during labor, when the level increases tenfold to thirtyfold, may precipitate bronchospasm in asthmatic patients; however, the action of this prostaglandin appears blunted during pregnancy.

Turner and colleagues[56] reviewed many studies of pregnancy in asthmatic women. Of the 1,114 women in the studies, 235 (22%) experienced an increase in the severity of asthma, 300 (30%) experienced a reduction in the severity of asthma, and 579 (49%) experienced no substantial change during pregnancy. If a first pregnancy exacerbated the asthma, future pregnancies were likely to have the same effect. Usually, these patients had severe asthma and experienced frequent or recurrent attacks when they were not pregnant, despite corticosteroid therapy.[57,58]

A recent study indicates that one third of asthmatic patients decrease their prescribed drug regimens from daily to PRN use, independent of medical advice.[53] These actions may relate to patients' concerns about fetal safety of the drugs. Among the drugs currently used for the treatment of asthma during pregnancy are theophylline, aminophylline, epinephrine, prednisone, beclomethasone dipropionate (inhalation), and terbutaline.[47] For acute attacks of wheezing, terbutaline or epinephrine may be administered without any apparent acute effects on the fetus. Theophylline is used chronically to maintain bronchial dilation and appears free of fetal complications. The usual maintenance dosage of theophylline is 800 to 1,200 mg/day, which sustains a therapeutic blood level of 10 to 20 μg/ml. Aminophylline may be administered intravenously during acute asthmatic attacks.

The use of prednisone is indicated when asthma is unresponsive to bronchodilators. It should be administered initially at a dosage of 30 to 60 mg/day; the dosage should then be reduced every other day until the minimum effective dosage has been determined. When the patient's condition has stabilized, inhaled steroid preparations (e.g., beclomethasone dipropionate) are recommended. If effective, the use of the inhaled steroid allows a reduced dosage of oral steroids or an every-other-day treatment regimen. Beclomethasone dipropionate can be used preconceptionally or during the first trimester.[58]

Tetracyclines should be avoided during pregnancy, because they may lead to staining of the teeth in the offspring. Many commercial asthma preparations contain iodine at dosages that may be safe for the mother but can have detrimental effects on the fetus. These drugs may block fetal binding of elemental iodine and lead to congenital hypothyroidism and goiter.[59]

PRECONCEPTIONAL COUNSELING

For the asthmatic patient, the goal of preconceptional counseling is to stabilize her disease by using the least amount of medication that proves effective. The patient should be advised that clinical studies of pregnancy outcomes in asthmatic patients indicate somewhat higher rates of maternal and fetal morbidity than those of the general population. However, these observations generally apply to asthmatic patients who had active disease at the time of pregnancy and had recurrent episodes during pregnancy. Patients should also be aware that the course of the disease is difficult to predict during pregnancy but that the majority of women either have a decrease in the severity of symptoms or no change. Women whose symptoms worsened during a previous pregnancy should be informed of the possibility of recurrence.

Antiasthmatic drugs can be used safely during the prepregnancy and pregnancy periods. The preconceptional counselor should review the woman's drug regimen with her, discuss the purposes and safety of specific medications, and caution her against changing her regimen without medical consultation. The counselor also should caution patients specifically against the use of tetracyclines and expectorants containing iodine. An oral/inhaler type of glucocorticoid may be used. The counselor should review situations and environmental conditions known to precipitate attacks and suggest ways to reduce such exposures. Patients should be encouraged to seek treatment of all respiratory infections and assured that careful and early treatment will pose less harm to the developing fetus than will maternal respiratory distress. Depending on the time of the year, the administration of the influenza vaccine may be advisable.

Good general principles of health, such as proper diet, smoking cessation, weight control, and avoidance of alcohol, should be emphasized. Rubella immunization should be offered when appropriate, and education regarding the importance of early prenatal care should be provided.

Heart Disease

aternal heart disease may represent a significant life-threatening risk for the prospective mother and conceptus. Because the interruption of pregnancy in women with compromised cardiac status may also pose significant risks, the safest course of action is to evaluate cardiac lesions thoroughly before pregnancy and to discuss the potential ramifications of conception fully before it occurs.

BACKGROUND

The cardiovascular changes associated with normal pregnancy may pose a significant threat to women with impaired cardiac function. The antenatal changes include
- a 40% to 45% increase in blood volume
- a 10% to 20% increase in heart rate above prepregnancy rates (a 30% to 50% increase in cardiac output)
- widening of the pulse pressure
- a decrease in systemic vascular resistance
- a decrease in mean aortic pressure[60]

The labor and delivery process requires further increases in the patient's cardiac output, heart rate, and stroke volume.

It has been estimated that 300 to 500 ml of blood is intermittently squeezed from the uterus and autotransfused into the maternal circulation during each labor contraction. This results in a transient 15% to 20% increase in cardiac output and a 10% increase in mean arterial pressure over prelabor values. Maternal pain and anxiety may result in increased sympathetic stimulation, causing blood pressure and heart rate to rise, especially during the second stage of labor. In the immediate postpartum stage, the redistribution of blood from the uterus to the general circulation creates another temporary increase in blood volume. A temporary increase in cardiac output occurs secondary to a decrease in the size of the uterus and the relief of inferior vena caval compression. The inability of the pregnant woman with cardiac disease to tolerate these demands on her cardiovascular system increases the risk of maternal and fetal morbidity and mortality.

The outcome of pregnancy in association with heart disease depends on the mother's functional impairment, as expressed by the New York Heart Association classification adopted by the American Heart Association[61]:
- class I, asymptomatic
- class II, symptomatic with heavy exercise

- class III, symptomatic with light exercise
- class IV, symptomatic at rest

Pregnancy poses the greatest risk to patients with class III and IV disease, and the clinical functional status of these patients and the cause of the underlying cardiac lesion must be fully evaluated before recommendations regarding conception can be made.

When the mother is asymptomatic (class I) or mildly symptomatic (class II), the perinatal mortality rate among the offspring shows only a slight increase. When the mother has class III disease, however, the perinatal mortality rate increases dramatically to 12%; with class IV disease, the perinatal mortality rate rises to 31%.[60,62]

The incidence of pregnancy in conjunction with heart disease has been at 0.5% to 1.5% for the last 25 years. As a result of advances in cardiovascular surgery, increasing numbers of women with congenital heart disease are experiencing pregnancy; however, much of the heart disease seen in pregnancy is rheumatic or acquired.

Acquired Heart Disease

For women with rheumatic heart disease, the cardiovascular changes of pregnancy may precipitate acute pulmonary edema, atrial fibrillation, or atrial embolic episodes. Usually, these can be treated medically with bedrest, digitalis, diuretics, and anti-arrhythmic drugs, antibiotics, and anticoagulants. When medical treatment fails to resolve these problems, surgical correction by closed mitral valvotomy or even valve replacement may be required.

Hemodynamically, mitral stenosis is the most significant acquired valvular heart lesion encountered during pregnancy.[63] The basic defect is a partial obstruction of blood flow from the left atrium to the left ventricle, with a decrease in cardiac output and an increase in the oxygen concentration of mixed venous blood. The cardiovascular changes of pregnancy may adversely affect the mechanisms by which the patient has been compensating for the defect. As the cardiac output and heart rate increase during pregnancy, the diastolic pressure gradient across the mitral valve further increases, which, in turn, increases left atrial, pulmonary venous, and pulmonary capillary pressures. These changes are usually well tolerated; should atrial fibrillation occur, however, the resulting decrease in left ventricular filling increases the chance of cardiac failure.

Prepregnancy surgery should be considered for the patient with severe mitral stenosis. Otherwise, surgery may become necessary during pregnancy, which not only greatly increases the maternal morbidity and mortality rates, but also threatens the fetus.[64]

The pregnancy-induced expansion of blood volume, together with the decrease in systemic vascular resistance, decreases the risk of pulmonary edema associated with mitral and aortic regurgitation and may decrease the severity of the lesion.

However, the cause of mitral and aortic regurgitation, as well as the cause of associated lesions, must be assessed.

Severe valvular aortic stenosis associated with fixed cardiac output and decreased preload may result in cardiac and cerebral ischemia or compromised uterine blood flow during pregnancy. This critical change may be associated with an increased maternal mortality rate and a high fetal mortality rate.[65] Prepregnancy surgical correction of severe aortic stenosis is recommended.[60]

A patient with ischemic heart disease and a history of recent myocardial infarction, cardiac failure, or significant angina is at high risk during pregnancy.[66] The patient who has a history of ischemic disease but who is asymptomatic and has a negative workup may consider pregnancy. The workup has prognostic limitations, however, and there is a risk of irreversible cardiac failure.

Mitral valve prolapse, which usually occurs as an isolated abnormality, has a greater incidence in women and tends to occur in families.[67] Most women with mitral valve prolapse are asymptomatic and do well during pregnancy, although they may experience palpitations and chest pain. Bedrest and activity restriction may be necessary if cardiac arrhythmia develops. Pregnancy does not appear to increase the risk of complications.

Congenital Heart Disease

The incidence of spontaneous abortion and intrauterine growth retardation is increased in the offspring of women with cyanotic heart disease who are symptomatic and have a high hematocrit secondary to hypoxemia.[68] Surgical correction before pregnancy improves the likelihood of a good pregnancy outcome.[69] However, according to a series of 500 patients studied by Neill and Swanson,[68] the incidence of a congenital heart anomaly is 1.8% in children born to a parent who has congenital heart disease, which is six times the incidence in the general population.

In patients with Eisenmenger syndrome, blood flow from the right ventricle is obstructed and arterial oxygenation is decreased. As a result, pregnancy is associated with markedly increased maternal and fetal mortality and morbidity rates[70]; in view of the 30% to 70% maternal mortality rate, pregnancy is a very high risk. Although the patient may be asymptomatic when not pregnant, the cardiovascular changes during pregnancy are not well tolerated, and the patient becomes symptomatic. Even if the mother survives, the fetal death rate approaches 30%.[71]

Similarly, primary pulmonary hypertension has a maternal mortality rate that approaches 50% and a fetal mortality rate that exceeds 40% if the mother survives. Pregnancy is not advisable for a patient known to have primary pulmonary hypertension,[72] but the disease may not be detected until pregnancy is under way. Investigators at Stanford University have documented the pregnancy-related deterioration of patients with primary pulmonary hypertension.[72] In one patient, they performed a successful heart and lung transplant, and the patient subsequently completed a successful pregnancy. She had a normal exercise tolerance 18 months after the transplant operation and before pregnancy.

Tetralogy of Fallot is a complex of lesions that results in right-to-left shunt and cyanosis. The mortality and morbidity rates for both the mother and the fetus are increased if the following conditions are present:

- a hematocrit greater than 60%
- peripheral arterial oxygen saturation of less than 80%
- an increased right ventricular pressure
- recurrent syncopal episodes

In general, pregnancy should not be attempted until the cardiac defects have been surgically corrected. If surgery is successful and the patient is acyanotic, pregnancy may be uncomplicated.[62-64]

One of the most common congenital heart defects in women is an atrial septal defect. The defect usually has been repaired by the time patients reach adulthood, and they do well during pregnancy.[60] If the lesion has not been repaired, there is an increased incidence of cardiac failure in these patients during pregnancy.

Ventricular septal defects occur less frequently than do atrial septal defects. A large defect is associated with a left-to-right shunt and pulmonary hypertension, which may result in nonremedial cardiac failure. A small defect is compatible with pregnancy.[64,73] Surgical correction, if indicated, should be performed during the prepregnancy period.

Coarctation of the aorta is a serious congenital cardiac defect that may increase the risk of a dissecting aneurysm secondary to the collagen tissue changes of late pregnancy, thus leading to maternal death. Most patients with this condition require prolonged bedrest and strict limitation of physical activity throughout pregnancy and the postpartum period.[74]

Medical and Surgical Therapies
Prosthetic Valves

Although prosthetic cardiac valves improve the quality of life of the cardiac patient, pregnancy in patients who have prosthetic valves poses unique problems.[75] The degree of risk in a pregnant patient with a prosthetic valve depends on the specific valve replaced, the type of valve prosthesis, and the need for anticoagulant therapy. To prevent a systemic embolism, most patients with nonbiosynthetic prosthetic heart valves are treated with oral anticoagulant drugs for life. Because coumarin derivatives have a strong teratogenic potential, heparin is the recommended anticoagulant just before and during pregnancy.[76] In addition, it may be necessary to restrict the physical activity of patients with an artificial mitral valve if there is any evidence of cardiac decompensation secondary to an impaired ability to increase cardiac output during pregnancy.

In a study of 106 pregnancies in 90 patients with valve prostheses, there were no maternal deaths in the antenatal period; however, there were three deaths in the immediate postpartum period and three additional deaths 3 months to 1 year after delivery.[75] Five of the six maternal deaths were related to an episode of cerebral embolus. Of the 106 pregnancies, 80 (75%) yielded healthy, viable infants; there were 13 spontaneous abortions, 5 stillbirths, 4 neonatal deaths, and 4 infants who lived but who had significant anomalies.

The development of nonthrombogenic cardiac valve prosthesis biografts (e.g., porcine xenograft) has been particularly helpful during pregnancy, because the patient with such a graft does not require anticoagulation therapy.[77]

Women with heart disease may be medicated with β-blockers for chronic hypertension or atrial arrythmia; those with mitral stenosis may use them to block heartrate response to exercise. β-blockers should be used judiciously during pregnancy,[78] and fetal and neonatal well-being must be carefully monitored. There is concern that prolonged exposure to these drugs may mask the usual signs of fetal distress, may be associated with increased uterine tone leading to diminished uterine blood flow and intrauterine growth retardation, and may produce transient neonatal hypoglycemia, bradycardia, and respiratory depression.[78,79]

Little information is available on the use of the newer antiarrhythmic agents during pregnancy. Quinidine, however, has been used extensively without adverse fetal effects.[80,81] Both digoxin and digitoxin freely cross the placenta, but they have no negative effect on the fetus.

Coumarin and its derivatives, which cross the placenta easily, have been associated with the warfarin embryopathy. The syndrome consists of facial dysmorphism (e.g., saddle nose, hypoplasia of the nose and ear passages), stippled epiphyses, and short stature. The administration of coumarin derivatives during the third trimester has been associated with fetal intracranial hemorrhage and stillbirth. Because heparin does not cross the placenta and is not teratogenic, a woman who is taking a coumarin derivative should change to heparin before conception or within the earliest weeks of gestation. The risk of warfarin embryopathy may be as high as 25% to 30% if fetal exposure occurs between 6 and 12 weeks of gestation and may be substantially less for exposure confined to earlier in pregnancy.[82] The assurance of fetal protection against warfarin embryopathy that is afforded by switching women to heparin therapy in the preconceptional period may, however, pose maternal risks. Prolonged use of heparin has been associated with the development of osteoporosis in laboratory animals and humans. In a British study of 70 women treated with subcutaneous heparin during pregnancy, immediate postpartum x-rays revealed 12 women with osteopenia and 2 with multiple fractures of the spine. At 6 to 12 months postpartum, the x-ray findings had generally reversed.[83] Based on existing evidence, one reviewer concludes that, although the risk of symptomatic fractures is low, a subclinical reduction in bone density is a potential consequence of long-term heparin use during pregnancy.[82]

The length of maternal heparin exposure can be minimized by reintroducing warfarin in the postpartum period. This action is appropriate even for breast-feeding women, because warfarin has not been detected in breast milk nor associated with anticoagulant effects in breast-feeding infants.[84,85]

PRECONCEPTIONAL COUNSELING

The goals of preconceptional counseling for the woman with heart disease arc to assess her cardiac status and to inform her of the risks of pregnancy specific to her condition. Should the woman choose to attempt pregnancy, steps should be taken to minimize the risks both to her and to her future offspring.

To advise the woman with heart disease appropriately, the counselor needs a knowledge of the type of cardiac defect, its severity, the current clinical status of the patient, and the presence or absence of complicating factors. The patient should be fully aware of her prognosis both with and without pregnancy. She should understand the cardiovascular changes that occur during pregnancy and the specific strain that pregnancy may place on her heart. It may be helpful for the counselor to ask about the course of prior pregnancies, but it is more important to determine the patient's cardiac functional status in the current prepregnancy period.

The patient and her partner should understand that a workup, including a chest roentgenogram, electrocardiogram, or cardiac catheterization, may be necessary to assess her risk. Before initiating any workup or recommendations, however, the counselor should contact the patient's cardiologist regarding previously administered diagnostic tests, existing therapeutic regimens, and the possible significance of the transient cardiovascular changes of pregnancy on the patient's specific cardiac disease. A conference that includes the cardiologist, the preconceptional counselor, the patient, and her partner may prove helpful, particularly if the prognosis for pregnancy is guarded.

Patients with mitral stenosis, mitral regurgitation, and valve prostheses are candidates for endocarditis prophylaxis at delivery. Antenatal antibiotic prophylaxis may be necessary for dental procedures or minor surgical procedures. The importance of this prophylactic therapy should be emphasized during the prepregnancy period.

The patient who requires anticoagulation therapy should receive parenterally administered heparin, rather than oral anticoagulant medication, beginning in the immediate preconceptional period. The patient should accept the need for parenteral therapy when the teratogenicity of coumarin is explained. Patients should be aware, however, that although heparin therapy is protective of the fetus, it may cause reduced bone density in the woman; the effect of this occurrence on the risk of postmenopausal fractures is unknown.

The patient with congenital heart disease and her partner should be aware that their offspring may have an increased risk of cardiac defects but that the risk is small.

In general, women with cardiac disease that is not life-threatening when complicated by pregnancy should be advised not to postpone desired childbearing. Cardiovascular functioning may become increasingly compromised with advancing years. The patient and her partner must understand that, should pregnancy occur, intensive surveillance will be necessary, physical activity may be restricted, and prolonged bedrest may be prescribed. They should also be aware that the postpartum stage, both in the hospital and at home, is an extremely critical time and that additional household assistance may be necessary after the patient is discharged.

Good general principles of health, such as proper diet, smoking cessation, weight control, and avoidance of alcohol, should be emphasized. Rubella immunization should be offered when appropriate. Education regarding the importance of early prenatal care should be provided.

Chronic Hypertension

The potential risks for cerebral hemorrhage, kidney failure, and cardiac failure are well recognized in patients with chronic hypertension. A pregnant woman with chronic hypertension has, in addition, an increased risk of abruptio placentae, preeclampsia, and fetal growth retardation. Good prepregnancy health habits and the control of preconceptional blood pressure may decrease the likelihood of maternal and fetal morbidity from pregnancies complicated by preexisting hypertension.

BACKGROUND

The severity of hypertension correlates directly with maternal morbidity and perinatal mortality rates.[86–88] Chronically hypertensive women have high incidences of superimposed preeclampsia, premature delivery, and intrauterine growth retardation.[89]

If the patient's diastolic blood pressure is equal to or less than 100 torr and she requires little or no antihypertensive medication during the prepregnancy period, the chance of severe exacerbation of hypertension during pregnancy or the development of preeclampsia is not significantly increased. If antihypertensive therapy is needed but diastolic blood pressure is controlled at a level equal to or less than 105 torr, the incidence of maternal and fetal complications associated with hypertension during pregnancy is minimized. A patient whose diastolic pressure is consistently more than 105 torr or who requires high-dose or multiple antihypertensive medications, however, has a 20% or 30% risk of superimposed preeclampsia and an increased risk of abruptio placentae and cardiac failure.[90]

Although contemporary management of the nonpregnant essential hypertensive patient continues to evolve, the generally accepted goal is maintenance of blood pressure at less than or equal to 140/90.[79] Depending on baseline readings and responsiveness, successful interventions may include weight reduction, stress reduction, avoidance of alcohol and tobacco, and single or combination pharmacologic therapy. When pregnancy is contemplated, pharmacologic therapy may require adjustment. Some of the newer therapies have demonstrated fetal risk or have posed theoretical concerns. For instance, angiotensin-converting enzyme (ACE) inhibitors have been associated with a 30% incidence of fetopathy, including irreversible fetal-neonatal renal disease after second- and third-trimester exposure.[91,92] Theoretical concerns exist regarding diminished uteroplacental blood flow with administration of calcium-channel blockers[79] and regarding the ability of the fetus to repond to distress after exposure to β-blockers.[93(p16)] The use of thiazide diuretics, frequently a first-line therapy for nonpregnant hypertensive patients, remains controversial during gestation. These agents negatively affect plasma volume expansion.[93(p17),94] The antihypertensive drug most commonly used during pregnancy and about which the most is known is methyldopa. A follow-up study of children exposed to methyldopa in utero demonstrated no adverse effects by age 7.5 years.[95] Other drugs that appear relatively safe and efficacious when used to treat chronic hypertension during pregnancy are atenolol, clonidine, and hydralazine.[79(p489)]

Some researchers believe that mild chronic hypertension may not require any drug therapy during pregnancy. Sibai and colleagues[96] studied 211 women with this diagnosis throughout pregnancy and found that the majority required no pharmaceutical treatment.

PRECONCEPTIONAL COUNSELING

The goal of preconceptional counseling for the hypertensive woman is to achieve and maintain blood pressure levels within a range compatible with good maternal and neonatal outcomes with as little medication as possible.

When a patient with a diagnosis of chronic hypertension seeks preconceptional counseling, the status of her cardiovascular and kidney function should be assessed and the need for antihypertensive medications evaluated. Ideally, the cardiac and kidney function tests demonstrate no evidence of compromise, and the diastolic blood pressure can be controlled at or below 100 torr with or without medication. A blood urea nitrogen value greater than 30 mg/dl or a serum creatinine concentration equal to or more than 3 mg/dl, together with poorly controlled hypertension, markedly increase both maternal and fetal morbidity and mortality.[97]

A thorough evaluation of the functional cardiac status of the patient, based on electrocardiogram findings, roentgenogram evidence of cardiac size, and results of heart and kidney function tests, is appropriate before the preconceptional counselor offers recommendations concerning the prognosis of pregnancy. If the workup reveals poor cardiac reserves, evidence of ventricular enlargement, or signs of kidney failure, the outlook for a healthy pregnancy may be poor for the patient and the fetus.

For patients who require medication for blood pressure control, the preconceptional counselor should focus on finding a successful therapeutic regimen. Once effective control has been achieved, the medications should be continued throughout pregnancy—provided that the drugs are safe to the developing fetus. The continuation of a drug throughout pregnancy is likely to enhance the postpregnancy compliance rate and potentially decrease the long-term consequences of hypertension.

During the preconceptional period, the patient should be informed about the potential for a good reproductive outcome, the possible complications, and the importance of drug compliance. She should be advised to sleep 8 to 10 hours each night and to take rest periods during the day. Finally, she should understand that she may need to curtail her work as the pregnancy progresses.

The patient should be aware that she may be required to visit her health care provider frequently during pregnancy and that repeated monitoring for creatinine clearance, 24-hour protein excretion, and fetal well-being (by ultrasound examinations and other techniques) will be necessary. The preconceptional counselor should explain that labor may be induced at term if there are signs of fetal distress or earlier if superimposed preeclampsia develops. Evidence of uncontrollable hypertension or renal failure may also precipitate the decision to induce labor.

Good general principles of health, such as proper diet, smoking cessation, weight control, and avoidance of alcohol, should be emphasized. Rubella immunization should be offered when appropriate. Education regarding the importance of early prenatal care should be provided.

Deep Venous Thrombosis

A serious vascular condition, deep venous thrombosis can occur during pregnancy and in the postpartum period. Pulmonary embolism resulting from deep venous thrombosis is a life-threatening situation; it accounts for 150,000 deaths per year in the United States. The incidence of deep venous thrombosis during pregnancy varies between 2 and 5 per 1,000 deliveries. Approximately one third of these complications occur antepartum; two thirds occur postpartum.

Aaro and Juergens[98] found that as many as 33% of pregnant or postpartum patients with deep vein thrombosis had a history of thromboembolism. If a patient has had a deep vein thrombosis, whether associated with contraceptive use, pregnancy, a surgical procedure, or an unknown factor, there is a 4% to 12% risk of recurrence.[99-101] Patients at risk may require prophylactic measures during the preconceptional, pregnancy, and postpartum periods.

BACKGROUND

Factors that place a patient at risk for deep venous thrombosis include obesity, sickle cell disease, a history of deep venous thrombosis, pregnancy, cesarean delivery, high parity, and advanced age. The incidence in pregnant women is greater than that in the general population. A recent cohort study of pregnant patients having their first venous thrombosis indicates that occurrence is equally distributed among the three trimesters of pregnancy.[102] More than 50% of postpartum cases appear within 3 days of delivery, but the condition may appear as late as 4 to 6 weeks after delivery. The risk associated with cesarean delivery is 10 times that associated with vaginal delivery. When deep venous thrombosis occurs during pregnancy and is adequately treated, less than 5% of patients develop pulmonary embolisms; 25% of untreated patients develop this complication, and the mortality rate in these patients is 5%.

A number of physiologic and functional changes that occur during pregnancy and in the postpartum period increase the risk of thrombosis: (1) elevated levels of many of the coagulation factors; (2) alteration in the venous wall, leading to increased venous distention; (3) reduced velocity of blood flow; and (4) rearrangement of elastic fibers in the veins, disrupting the underlying intima. Platelets may adhere to the damaged intima and release factors that activate the intrinsic coagulation pathway.[103] The increased venous pressure in the lower extremities and the interference of the pregnant uterus with venous return may lead to stasis of blood and thrombus formation. A postoperative cesarean course complicated by sepsis, prolonged bedrest, and dehydration increases the risk of deep venous thrombosis and pulmonary embolism.[104] Furthermore, the hypercoagulation state that exists during pregnancy continues for at least 6 weeks postpartum.[105]

Several prophylactic measures have been proposed to reduce the high incidence of recurrent deep venous thrombosis in pregnant patients. Anticoagulation therapy is indicated for those patients with a history of deep venous thrombosis or pulmonary embolism within 6 months before conception. For those who had a deep venous thrombosis during a past pregnancy, prophylactic anticoagulation therapy should begin 4 to 6 weeks earlier than the point at which the previous episode occurred. Heparin is the drug of choice because it does not cross into the fetal circulation. Taken during the first trimester, sodium warfarin (Coumadin) has been shown to have adverse fetal effects (i.e., saddle nose, nasal hypoplasia, frontal bossing, and short stature).[106,107] The use of warfarin drugs during late pregnancy has been associated with such fetal effects as skeletal dysplasia, optic atrophy, and hemorrhage.[108]

Anticoagulation prophylaxis for a pregnant woman with a history of a single deep venous thrombosis 6 months or more before conception is controversial. If the thrombosis occurred in a hyperestrogen milieu, such as during pregnancy or while oral contraceptives were being used, low-dose heparin prophylaxis, usually 5,000 units administered subcutaneously twice daily, is recommended. If a patient had a deep venous thrombosis 6 or more months before planned pregnancy, prophylactic treatment with heparin can be deferred until 4 to 6 weeks before her estimated delivery and continued for 4 to 6 weeks postpartum. The period may be extended in the presence of obesity, ante- or postpartum bedrest, febrile morbidity secondary to pelvic sepsis, cardiovascular disease, or an age greater than 35.[109]

The site of the thrombosis before pregnancy is important. In the case of a distal deep venous thrombosis, prophylaxis may be accomplished through low-dose heparin therapy; in the case of a proximal deep venous thrombosis (e.g., in the femoral vein) or a history of pulmonary embolism within 12 months of conception, therapeutic heparinization, usually requiring 20,000 to 24,000 units of heparin daily, is indicated.

Prolonged heparin therapy may lead to thrombocytopenia and osteoporosis. Thrombocytopenia occurs in 1% to 25% of patients. Because thrombocytopenia is thought to be an allergic reaction, a change in the drug lot or type of heparin may reverse the condition.[110-113] A recent study demonstrated roentgenographic evidence of osteopenia and spinal fractures immediately postpartum in women who received heparin during pregnancy.[114] Most findings were reversed by 6 to 12 months postpartum. It is unknown whether supplementation with calcium or initiation of other preventive therapies offers protection or whether there are postmenopausal consequences for women who had osteopenia at an early age. The length of heparin exposure can be reduced by substituting warfarin during the postpartum period. Evidence indicates that this action may also be appropriate for women who breast-feed: the drug has not been detected in breast milk and has not been found to induce an anticoagulant effect in infants.[115,116]

PRECONCEPTIONAL COUNSELING

The goal of preconceptional counseling for patients with a history of deep venous thrombosis is to introduce strategies that will decrease the risk of recurrence without jeopardizing normal fetal development in a subsequent pregnancy.

The patient who has had a recent deep venous thrombosis can reduce the risk of recurrence during pregnancy by waiting 6 to 12 months before conception. If the patient is on anticoagulation therapy and plans a pregnancy, the risk of a recurrence must be balanced against the potential complications of the anticoagulation therapy. Warfarin should not be used during the preconceptional period or during pregnancy because of its teratogenic effects on the fetus. Heparin is the safest anticoagulant for the prospective mother; unlike warfarin, heparin does not cross the placenta, and its effects can be easily reversed. However, the patient should be observed for abnormal bleeding, thrombocytopenia, and osteoporosis. If the patient has had a deep venous thrombosis during the past year and is not on anticoagulation therapy, she should be advised that anticoagulation therapy will be started during pregnancy and continued through the postpartum period.

The patient should be informed that close laboratory surveillance of her coagulation status will be necessary during pregnancy and that the parenteral dosage of heparin may need to be increased as pregnancy progresses. The use of warfarin may be considered in the postpartum period if the patient is not breast-feeding. Birth control pills and estrogen-containing medication for suppression of lactation should not be given in the postpartum period.

Patients and their partners should be advised of other prophylactic measures that can be taken to lessen the risk of deep venous thrombosis. In general, it is advisable for the patient to avoid prolonged standing, sitting, or dependency of the legs. The woman should rest on her side during pregnancy, rather than on her back, because resting on the back decreases venous return and promotes venous stasis of the legs. Flexing and extending the feet and legs intermittently during the day and elevating the foot of the bed 6 to 8 inches at night increase the venous return from the lower limbs. Long automobile rides should be interrupted by periods of walking every 2 hours to decrease edema and maintain collateral venous channels. The patient should be measured and fitted with elastic stockings, which she should wear throughout pregnancy and for at least 2 weeks postpartum. Locally constrictive garments, such as knee stockings or panty girdles, should be avoided. Dehydration should be prevented by keeping stays in the sun short and maintaining hydration during exercise.

Good general principles of health, such as proper diet, smoking cessation, weight control, and avoidance of alcohol, should be emphasized. Rubella immunization should be offered when appropriate, and the importance of early prenatal care should be stressed.

Kidney Disease

Pregnancy complicated by chronic renal disease places both the mother and the fetus at risk. The nature of the kidney disease, the functional status of the kidney, and the presence or absence of hypertension determine the pregnancy outcome. Prepregnancy renal evaluation and prospective plans for management may decrease the risks of pregnancy for the woman with kidney disease and for her fetus.

BACKGROUND

The kidney is actively involved in many of the homeostatic changes that occur during pregnancy. These physiologic changes may adversely affect patients with chronic renal disease, even those who are asymptomatic at conception.[117,118] The calices of the kidney pelves, as well as the ureters, dilate in response to the hormonal changes of pregnancy, resulting in an increased incidence of asymptomatic bacteriuria and pyelonephritis. Also contributing to the pregnant patient's susceptibility to urinary tract infection are bladder reflux and increased excretion of glucose.

By the second trimester of pregnancy, both the glomerular filtration rate and the renal plasma flow increase 30% to 50% above prepregnancy values.[117,118] The serum creatinine concentration decreases from an average prepregnancy value of 0.7 mg/dl to 0.5 mg/dl, and the blood urea nitrogen value decreases from 13 mg/dl to 9 mg/dl. Urinary protein excretion increases as much as 300 mg/day.

Pregnancy may not change the natural course of renal disease if renal function is well preserved and the serum creatinine concentration is equal to or less than 1.6 mg/dl at conception.[119] A 3- to 23-month follow-up in a study by Katz and colleagues[120] of 121 pregnancies in 89 women with kidney disease revealed that, if the initial serum creatinine concentration had been equal to or less than 1.4 mg/dl, a permanent decline in renal function occurred in only 10 of the 89 women. In 5 of the 10, however, the condition reached end-stage renal disease.

A woman with renal disease and normal blood pressure has an 85% chance of a successful pregnancy outcome. The conjunction of hypertension with moderate-to-severe renal insufficiency increases the risk of fetal loss, intrauterine growth retardation, and premature labor and delivery. Surian and colleagues[121] report that the rate of fetal loss, including stillbirth, second-trimester spontaneous abortion, and neonatal death, was 13.8% in patients with chronic renal disease without hypertension. If the patient was hypertensive, her blood urea nitrogen level at conception was equal to or greater than 30 mg/dl, and her serum creatinine concentration was equal to or greater than 3 mg/dl, the incidence of maternal complications, fetal death, and intrauterine growth retardation was markedly increased.[121]

Many patients with chronic renal disease as a result of such conditions as chronic pyelonephritis, nephrolithiasis, polycystic renal disease, or nephrotic syndrome can anticipate a normal pregnancy. In association with uncontrolled hypertension, however, any of these diseases places the mother and fetus at high risk. Even if the patient with chronic renal disease and hypertension is asymptomatic and normotensive (with or without medication) at the time of conception, pregnancy often exacerbates the hypertension. Regardless of its cause, chronic renal disease increases the risk of preeclampsia to 30%, and the presence of hypertension during early pregnancy further increases the risk.

Experience with patients who have become pregnant after renal transplantation secondary to kidney failure is limited. Penn, Makowski, and Harris[122] reported on 52 pregnancies in 37 women who had undergone renal transplantation. There were 44 live births and 8 abortions, 7 of which were therapeutic. Before pregnancy, renal function was normal or only slightly impaired. Renal function deteriorated during pregnancy in 2 patients and during the postpartum period in 2 more. Preeclampsia occurred in 27% of the patients, and 9 had cesarean deliveries.

Sciarra and colleagues[123] reported on 18 pregnancies in 12 patients who had renal transplants. In 6 of these patients, there were 5 therapeutic first-trimester pregnancy terminations and 1 spontaneous abortion. Of the 12 liveborn infants, 3 were small for gestational age, 7 were appropriate in size, and 2 were large. There were no serious congenital malformations in the infants. Preeclampsia and bacterial and viral infections were the only common medical problems. Renal function decreased in 3 of the women.

As of March 1985, researchers had reported on 1,200 pregnancies in women with renal transplants.[124] Analysis of these pregnancies indicates that pregnancy should be avoided 2 to 5 years after transplantation so that renal function can stabilize and immunosuppressive medication can be reduced to the lowest possible dosage before pregnancy. Immunosuppressive therapy typically consists of prednisone and azathioprine, which should be maintained during pregnancy to prevent kidney rejection. Both drugs cross the placenta poorly. Prednisone has not been associated with congenital malformation but has been associated in rare cases with hypoadrenalism in the offspring.[125] Chromosomal abnormalities have been reported in the offspring of patients receiving azathioprine,[126,127] but these aberrations reportedly clear within 20 to 32 months.[128] Azathioprine has also been associated with intrauterine growth retardation, but determining whether the underlying disease or the treatment is causative has been difficult.[129(p53)]

Bacterial and viral infections are common in the transplant recipient receiving immunosuppressive therapy. It has also been noted that transplant patients have an increase in the incidence of cytomegalovirus and hepatitis. Because these illnesses pose risks to the infant, patients should be monitored for their development, even when the patients are asymptomatic. Decompensation of renal function at any time during pregnancy may be deleterious to the continued survival of the transplant, and if this occurs termination of the pregnancy or premature delivery should be considered. Pregnancy after renal transplantation complicated by a poorly functioning graft or severe hypertension should be avoided.

PRECONCEPTIONAL COUNSELING
General Guidelines

The goal of preconceptional counseling for the patient with renal disease is to determine as accurately as possible the degree of renal impairment so that individualized assessments of potential risks to the mother and fetus can be offered and prospective plans for antenatal care developed. The preconceptional counselor should assess the short- and long-term effects that pregnancy may have on the disease process, the likelihood of pregnancy complications, and the chances of delivering a liveborn infant. If the patient chooses to attempt pregnancy, the counselor should offer guidance to optimize her chances for a good outcome.

Pregnancy can be considered a reasonably safe option in women who have a preconceptional serum creatinine level equal to or less than 1.6 mg/dl and diastolic blood pressure equal to or less than 100 torr. Because renal function in patients with chronic renal disease generally decreases with age, women with currently good renal function and normal blood pressure who are contemplating pregnancy should be encouraged to proceed with conception without unnecessary delay. A patient with severe renal insufficiency and hypertension must be advised not only that pregnancy could seriously jeopardize her health but also that the prognosis for a successful reproductive outcome is guarded.

To determine the patient's renal status, it is necessary to undertake a complete urinalysis and a thorough evaluation of kidney function, blood pressure, and all medications received. Consultation with the patient's nephrologist and other health care providers is appropriate.

The patient and her partner should be educated regarding the demands that pregnancy places on the renal system and advised that asymptomatic problems may become clinically evident as the pregnancy progresses. Careful monitoring for urinary tract infections and changing renal function will be necessary throughout pregnancy.

The patient with renal disease accompanied by hypertension should be informed of the possibly serious consequences of pregnancy and the importance of complying with the therapeutic regimen. The potential risks to the fetus of specific drugs must be balanced against the potential complications for the fetus of poorly controlled maternal hypertension. The patient should understand that termination of pregnancy may be recommended if there is a rapid deterioration of renal function or uncontrollable hypertension.

Good general principles of health, such as proper diet, smoking cessation, weight control, and avoidance of alcohol, should be emphasized. Rubella immunization should be offered when appropriate. Importance of early prenatal care should be carefully explained.

Specific Guidelines

There are many different forms of renal disease. Each carries a different level of risk and requires a different preconceptional intervention and education. The following information, in combination with the more general guidelines discussed earlier, may prove helpful in counseling patients about the risks of specific renal diseases.

Chronic Pyelonephritis

In general, the course of pregnancy is normal in the patient with chronic pyelonephritis, provided that adequate renal function is preserved and hypertension is not present. The patient with chronic pyelonephritis should be made aware, however, that she will require serial monitoring for kidney function and infection and that continuous antibiotic suppression therapy may be needed throughout her pregnancy.

Nephrolithiasis

Renal stone disease does not harm the pregnant patient, except that it increases the risk of urinary tract infection and attacks of renal colic. The preconceptional counselor should explain to the patient that pregnancy does not predispose her to further calculi formation but that she will be closely monitored for urinary tract infections during gestation.

Polycystic Renal Disease

Pregnancy in patients with polycystic renal disease is usually successful, even though the incidence of preeclampsia and pyelonephritis is slightly higher in these patients than in others. Pregnancy does not appear to affect the natural course of the disease adversely, although any signs of hematuria, hypertension, and recurrent urinary tract infection require close observation and monitoring of kidney function. It is important to inform patients that the adult form of the disease may have an autosomal dominant mode of inheritance and to offer consultation with a genetics counseling program.

Nephrotic Syndrome

In the absence of hypertension and significant renal function impairment, patients with nephrotic syndrome can be reassured about the prospect of a healthy pregnancy outcome. A decrease in serum albumin levels of less than 1 g/dl enhances the tendency toward fluid retention.

Permanent Urinary Diversion

Patients with permanent urinary diversion usually do well during pregnancy, although they should be informed preconceptionally of the associated increased incidence of acute pyelonephritis. The patient may develop an outflow obstruction secondary to compression of the ileal conduit by the enlarging uterus as pregnancy advances.

Solitary Kidney

Patients who have a solitary kidney as a result of nephrectomy for an infectious or renal structural problem usually tolerate pregnancy well. However serial surveillance for evidence of changing renal function is required during the antenatal period.

Pelvic Kidney

If kidney function is normal, a pelvic kidney is not associated with an increased rate of fetal loss. Patients should understand, however, that other urogenital tract malformations frequently coexist with pelvic kidneys. Such malformations sometimes make it impossible for the fetus to descend in labor and necessitate cesarean delivery.

Chronic Glomerulonephritis

Patients with a history of glomerulonephritis, normal or moderately depressed renal function, and normal blood pressure have an increased incidence of preeclampsia. Overall, however, the prognosis for the mother and fetus is favorable. Although most investigators do not believe that pregnancy accelerates the natural course of the disease,[130] some patients with preexisting renal disease have a significant worsening in renal function during gestation that does not improve after delivery. This occurrence is reportedly more frequent in women with diffuse glomerulonephritis, but it is not possible to predict which women will have the problem.[131] The patient should understand that severe hypertension or substantially decreased renal function before pregnancy may have adverse effects on both the mother and the fetus during pregnancy. The patient should also be aware that any deterioration of renal function during pregnancy may reflect the natural course of the disease or superimposed preeclampsia. Both conditions may require termination of pregnancy to prevent worsening maternal morbidity.

Renal Insufficiency

A serum creatinine concentration equal to or greater than 3 mg/dl and a blood urea nitrogen level equal to or greater than 30 mg/dl are usually associated with impaired fertility. In those pregnancies that do occur, the fetal survival rate is reduced if uncontrollable hypertension accompanies the renal insufficiency. However, chronic renal insufficiency may have little effect on the fetus when the patient is normotensive.[120] If her blood pressure is higher than 150/100 torr, the patient should be treated aggressively with antihypertensives, since blood pressure control is the cornerstone of the successful management of chronic renal disease during pregnancy.[131] If renal transplantation is an option, this decision should be made and, if considered appropriate, the procedure performed before pregnancy is attempted.

Renal Transplantation

The patient who has a renal transplant and is contemplating pregnancy should be advised that conception should be delayed for 2 to 5 years following transplantation and, even then, attempted only after a thorough evaluation of the risks involved. Ideally, the patient's blood pressure should be under control, and she should be free of significant proteinuria before attempting to conceive.[132] She should understand that she will continue her immunosuppressive therapy throughout pregnancy. She should also be aware that her renal status will be monitored closely and that any evidence of decompensation during the pregnancy may result in a recommendation to terminate the pregnancy. Screening for hepatitis, cytomegalovirus, and bacterial infections, with therapy as needed, should be provided during the preconceptional period and throughout pregnancy.

Systemic Lupus Erythematosus

N early one-half million individuals in the United States have systemic lupus erythematosus (SLE); most are women.[133] The disease may follow a subclinical course for years, manifested only in repeated early and late pregnancy wastage and reduced fecundity.[134,135] Maternal morbidity, mortality, and pregnancy outcomes typically relate to the activity of the disease at the time of conception. It has been reported that the changes in sex hormone levels and the physiologic changes of pregnancy aggravate SLE,[136] but more recent studies indicate that most patients with SLE do well during pregnancy, particularly if the patients are on immunosuppressive therapy.[137]

BACKGROUND

Like its response to pregnancy, the natural course of SLE is variable. It has been reported that 20% to 40% of patients with SLE experience an exacerbation of the disease during pregnancy or in the postpartum period,[138] but the data are conflicting. Hayslett and Lynn[136] reported on 56 pregnant women with SLE. The disease had been in remission for 6 months before pregnancy in 31 of these women; remission continued throughout pregnancy in 21 of them. In the 25 women with active disease at the time of conception, the disease worsened in 12 (48%), remained unchanged in 10 (40%), and improved in 3 (12%). Fourteen of these 25 pregnancies resulted in liveborn infants.

In a 1984 study, Lockshin and associates[139] compared 28 pregnant women with SLE (and a total of 33 pregnancies) with matched nonpregnant women with SLE. They found that the disease did not become more active during pregnancy or the postpartum period. In a prospective study of 75 SLE patients who had a total of 102 pregnancies from 1974 to 1983, Mintz and colleagues[135] found a 59.7% exacerbation rate during pregnancy. Most of the pregnancy-related episodes were mild. Of note, however, is that the authors treated all pregnant patients with at least 10 mg of prednisone as soon as pregnancy was confirmed. A recent review concludes that pregnancy, in the absence of active multisystem disease, does not worsen SLE.[140]

If the disease is inactive at the time of conception, fetal survival is approximately 85%, unless there are severe complications of the disease.[136] When pregnancy occurs in women with active SLE, however, fetal survival decreases to a rate of 50% to 75%.[136,141]

The incidence of preterm deliveries, fetal wastage, and small-for-gestational-age infants increases to 30% to 50% in patients who have evidence of chronic renal disease, such as hypertension or a serum creatinine concentration greater than 1.6 mg/dl.[134-136,142] Intensive antenatal and intrapartum surveillance of the mother and fetus has the potential to improve these statistics.

A recent prospective study followed 25 pregnancies of 21 women; 20 of the women had SLE and 1 had subacute cutaneous lupus erythematosus (SCLE).[143] The antenatal treatment schedule included low-dose aspirin, steroids at low to medium doses, and, if needed, azathioprine after 20 weeks of gestation. Steroid dosage was raised to 40 to 60 mg/day on the day of delivery and for the 2 subsequent days; steroids were then administered at the predelivery dose for the next month. Outcomes included 4 first-trimester spontaneous abortions and 21 liveborn infants. Nearly one third of the infants were premature (gestational age 33 to 35 weeks), and one third were small for gestational age. The authors note that exacerbation of the disease occurred no more frequently among the members of the study population than among nonpregnant patients and that, although obstetric complications were relatively frequent, careful monitoring prevented late fetal wastage.

Corticosteroids (prednisone) and azathioprine have not been associated with an increased rate of congenital malformation in humans.[135,144] Chromosomal abnormalities have occasionally been reported in the offspring of infants born to women receiving azathioprine,[144,145] but the abnormalities reportedly disappear by 20 to 32 months of age.[146] Use of the drug also has been associated with fetal growth retardation, but it is unclear whether the drug or another factor relating to the underlying disease is the major contributor.

Patients with SLE have been noted to have a variety of autoantibodies. For instance, 95% have antinuclear antibodies; 30% have anti-Ro(SS-A); and 70% have antiphospholipid antibodies, including 34% with lupus anticoagulant and 44% to 50% with anticardiolipin antibodies.[133] Evidence is accumulating that the presence of these antiphospholipid antibodies increases the risk of pregnancy wastage. A report on pregnancy outcomes from the Parkland Hospital Lupus Clinic found that 55% of the pregnancies of women with anticardiolipin antibodies ended in miscarriage, compared with 20% for women without these antibodies.[147] Low-dose aspirin in combination with prednisone has been demonstrated to markedly decrease fetal loss for this population.[148-150] Refer to Chapter 7 for further information.

In SLE, the placental transfer of maternal autoantibodies to the fetus may have transient or permanent fetal effects.[135,151] Usually, these maternal antibodies disappear from the infant's circulation within 4 months of birth; during this time, however, the newborn may display a transient discoid lupus rash and a hemolytic anemia. A more serious type of possible fetal injury is impairment of the fetal cardiac conduction system. A complete heart block has been observed in the offspring of women with established or subclinical SLE. These women develop an antibody to the tissue ribonucleoprotein antigen Ro(SS-A), which crosses the placenta and induces a reaction in fetal cardiac tissue. The reaction, however, is not universal.

PRECONCEPTIONAL COUNSELING

For the patient with SLE, the goal of preconceptional counseling is to assess the activity and complications of the disease in order to advise the patient and her partner of associated maternal and fetal risks.

Pregnancy does not usually increase the incidence of major systemic manifestations of SLE, but a woman with SLE is at a higher risk for complications during pregnancy and has a markedly reduced chance for a successful pregnancy outcome than do women in the general population. The risks are heightened if the disease is complicated by hypertension or renal dysfunction. Regardless of the previous manifestations of the disease, the patient has an improved prognosis for a successful outcome if the disease is in remission at the time of conception. Patients should be aware of the risks of pregnancy and the benefits of attempting to conceive during periods of remission. They should also be aware that extensive maternal and fetal monitoring is likely should pregnancy occur.

Prepregnancy assessment should include consultation with specialists in nephrology, rheumatology, and related disciplines. All women with SLE should undergo kidney function tests, such as determination of the creatinine clearance rate, and should be screened for Ro(SS-A) antibodies. The latter's potential significance in the development of fetal cardiac conduction defects should be discussed with women whose test results are positive, and the use of ultrasound electrocardiac monitoring during pregnancy should be explained to these women.

If the patient who seeks preconceptional counseling is receiving azathioprine or glucocorticoids for suppression of active disease, she should be reassured that no adverse fetal effects have been consistently associated with these drugs; she should be encouraged to continue them during the pre- and postconceptional periods. If she is receiving other types of chemotherapy, the fetal effects of these drugs should be evaluated and the results shared with the patient so that she can make an informed decision regarding continuation of the drug.

All patients with a medical history that includes recurrent spontaneous abortion or fetal death, thrombotic episodes, diagnosis of SLE, false-positive VDRL, Coombs-positive hemolytic anemia, or presence of Ro(SS-A) antibodies should be screened for lupus anticoagulant and anticardiolipin antibodies. If the results are positive, prepregnancy treatment with aspirin and glucocorticoids theoretically may increase the patient's chance of a good reproductive outcome.

Good general principles of health, such as proper diet, smoking cessation, weight control, and avoidance of alcohol, should be emphasized. Rubella immunization should be offered when appropriate, and education regarding the importance of early prenatal care provided.

Epilepsy

The most common neurologic problem seen during pregnancy is epilepsy; this condition has a prevalence of approximately 0.4% to 0.6%. Most patients with epilepsy must take anticonvulsants to remain seizure-free. During pregnancy, however, the possible teratogenic effects of these drugs must be addressed. For this reason, the prepregnancy period is an optimal time to review the diagnosis and classification of the patient's epilepsy. The effectiveness of therapeutic regimens in controlling seizures must be evaluated and then balanced against their potentially adverse effects on the fetus.

BACKGROUND

The effects of epilepsy on pregnancy have been extensively studied. Although early reports indicated that the risk of bleeding, preeclampsia, premature delivery, and perinatal death in pregnant women with epilepsy was double that in other pregnant women, more recent reports do not confirm this impression.[152-154]

Seizure Frequency during Pregnancy

There is general agreement that approximately 50% of women will have no change in their seizure frequency during pregnancy; approximately 10% will have fewer seizures; and approximately 40% will have an increase in seizure activity.[155,156] In a prospective study of 136 pregnancies in 122 epileptic women, Schmidt and colleagues[156] found that the number of seizures increased in 37% of the women, primarily because of medication noncompliance.

The likelihood of increased seizure frequency during pregnancy correlates with the history of seizure control during the year before conception. In the study by Schmidt and colleagues,[156] seizure frequency increased in only 25% of the women who had experienced no more than one seizure during the 9 months preceding conception. When the preconceptional seizure frequency is one or more seizures per month, however, seizure frequency can be expected to increase during pregnancy. The effect of pregnancy on the frequency of seizures during different pregnancies in the same patient is quite variable. Generally, seizure activity returns to the prepregnancy rate during the postpartum period.[157]

Increases in seizure frequency most often occur during the first trimester. It may be that the vomiting often associated with early pregnancy interferes with the ingestion and absorption of anticonvulsant medications, or it may be that the patient eliminates or reduces medication because of the fear that the drug(s) will adversely affect the fetus.

The physiologic changes of pregnancy may also affect seizure frequency. Increased plasma volume, increased glomerular filtration rate, and fetal or placental drug metabolism may all contribute to a decline in the blood level of anticonvulsants, leading to an increase in seizure activity. A nonpregnant epileptic patient who takes 300 to 400 mg of diphenylhydantoin daily, for example, usually has a therapeutic blood level of 10 to 20 μg/ml. As a result of the changes that occur during pregnancy, the same dosage may result in a blood level judged to be subtherapeutic by non-pregnancy standards. It has been suggested that the decreased concentration of medications is an indication for frequent blood measurements and adjustments in medication dosages. Because more nonprotein-bound diphenylhydantoin is available during pregnancy, however, the therapeutic effectiveness of the drug increases. Therefore, as many as 50% of patients who take diphenylhydantoin as instructed remain seizure-free, even when blood levels of the drug are theoretically subtherapeutic. The therapeutic effectiveness in seizure control and the safety of the drug are the criteria that should be used to determine which medication dosage is most efficacious during pregnancy—not the actual blood level of the drug.

Some patients on long-term therapy with diphenylhydantoin may have subnormal folate levels. Pregnancy may decrease the serum folate level further, potentially decreasing the effectiveness of the therapy and increasing the risk of seizures.[158] Hiilesmaa and colleagues[159] indicate, however, that there is no association between blood folate concentrations and seizure frequency.

The Effect of Epilepsy on Congenital Malformation

In animals, an induced deficiency of folic acid has been associated with congenital malformation.[160] Large human epidemiologic studies have linked an increased rate of congenital malformation of the central nervous system to folate deficiency and have shown that patients on anti–folic acid medication (e.g., aminopterin or methotrexate) during early pregnancy have an increased rate of severe fetal anomalies.[161-163] Women who increase their folic acid intake during the periconceptional period are known to have a decreased recurrence rate of neural tube defects in their offspring.[164,165] The association between folic acid deficiency and congenital malformation may partially explain the pathogenesis of congenital malformation in the offspring of patients receiving diphenylhydantoin therapy, as the drug is a folic acid antagonist; however, the etiology of congenital malformation in the infants of epileptic parents appears to be more complex.

Although the literature is not without exception, the risk of congenital malformation appears to be greater for infants whose mother or father or both have epilepsy, irrespective of fetal exposure to anticonvulsant therapy.[155,166-170] The incidence of congenital heart disease is increased twofold in these infants; the incidence of cleft lip and palate, eightfold.[171] In addition, skeletal, central nervous system, gastrointestinal, and urogenital abnormalities, in descending order of frequency, have been reported.[172-174] An increased incidence of facial clefts occurs in the offspring of epileptic fathers, indicating that there is a genetic predisposition to this condition.[175,176] The incidence of anomalies, the severity and duration of epilepsy, and the activity of disease during the index pregnancy also appear to be related.[152]

Various drugs are used to control seizures. Valproic acid (Depakene), approved in 1978, is presently used for tonic, clonic, myoclonic, and other types of epilepsy. It has been shown to be teratogenic in humans and animals, however; the offspring of patients on valproic acid have an 11% chance of neural tube defects and other craniofacial abnormalities.[177,178] Therefore, its use is contraindicated during pregnancy.

Diphenylhydantoin may produce fetal malformation when administered to some breeds of mice and rats at critical times in development.[174] In humans, maternal use of diphenylhydantoin may result in the fetal hydantoin syndrome,[169,170,171,179] most consistently manifested in prenatal growth retardation, craniofacial anomalies, hypoplastic nails, microcephaly, and, occasionally, borderline-to-mild mental deficiency. As many as 10% of fetuses exposed to hydantoin have enough clinical features of the syndrome to warrant its diagnosis at birth. Hydantoin effects, such as café au lait spots, inguinal hernias, and metatarsus varus, may be present in an additional 30% of exposed infants.[179,180]

A high incidence of a similar group of well-defined congenital anomalies is present in infants born to epileptic women treated with trimethadione (Tridione).[181] Thus the use of trimethadione is contraindicated during pregnancy. Phenobarbital is generally taken with other antiseizure medications, making its teratogenicity difficult to evaluate. Animal and human epidemiologic studies indicate that, if phenobarbital is a teratogen, it is very weak. Carbamazepine (Tegretol) has been suggested as the drug of choice in women who are likely to become pregnant and require anticonvulsant therapy, but current evidence indicates that this drug may also affect pregnancy outcomes adversely. A 1989 report that involved both retrospective and prospective data collection concluded that carbamazepine is associated with a pattern of congenital defects, including minor craniofacial anomalies, fingernail hypoplasia, and development delays.[182]

When the etiology of the mother's epilepsy is unknown, there is probably an increased risk that the child will become epileptic. This susceptibility is further increased when both parents have epilepsy or when the mother is epileptic and has a family history of epilepsy.[166] There is some controversy about whether the incidence of the disease in the offspring is higher than that in the general population if only the father has epilepsy.[166]

PRECONCEPTIONAL COUNSELING

The goals of preconceptional counseling for the woman with epilepsy are to keep her seizure-free and to decrease the incidence of congenital abnormalities in her offspring through appropriate drug therapy.

During the preconceptional visit of a patient with seizure disorders, the counselor should evaluate the patient's past and present history, as well as her treatment regimen and its effectiveness in controlling the seizure disorder. In collaboration with a neurologist, the prepregnancy workup may include skull roentgenograms, an electroencephalogram, and a computed tomography (CT) scan. A careful dietary and drug history that includes the use of alcohol and all medications—not only anticonvulsants—is essential.

The preconceptional counselor should inform the patient and her partner about the effects of epilepsy on pregnancy and offspring. The couple should understand that there is a 40% risk of more frequent seizures during pregnancy. It is important to inform them that the seizure activity during a pregnancy cannot be predicted from that during a previous pregnancy but that, if the patient is seizure-free on the lowest dosage of medication for at least 3 months before her pregnancy, she has a good chance of remaining seizure-free during pregnancy. The couple should also be aware that there appears to be a two- to threefold increase in the rate of congenital malformation compared with the rate in nonepileptics, irrespective of any treatment; however, the risk is probably decreased if there is no family history of other anomalies. Therefore, if a careful family history reveals no malformation, the patient should be advised that her chances of having a child without a major anomaly are probably greater than 90%.

The counselor should consider weaning the patient from anticonvulsant medication during the preconceptional period if she has not had a seizure for more than 2 years.[183] This requires consultation with the patient's neurologist and may take more than 6 months. Discontinuation of the medication should be recommended only after a discussion with the patient about the potential risks of recurrent seizures and the associated physical and emotional trauma. The effect of such an action on the patient's retention of her driver's license, which may vary from state to state, should also be considered. During the period without medication, the patient should remain on a contraceptive. If the patient remains seizure-free, she is likely to have no problems during pregnancy, and her chance of having a child with a serious malformation is reduced, although not eliminated.

The patient who has recurrent seizures whether or not she uses medication should be advised that treatment during pregnancy will be essential. The preconceptional counselor should explain that the adverse effects of seizures on the pregnancy are likely to be greater if anticonvulsants are not used. She should be made aware, however, of the risks associated with her medications. Consultation with the patient's neurologist is indicated to develop an individualized drug regimen that balances maternal seizure control with minimal fetal effects. Trimethadione and valproic acid should *not* be used during the preconceptional period or during pregnancy.

Folate supplementation as contained in normal prenatal vitamins is recommended, because there is some evidence that such supplementation may reduce the incidence or the severity of congenital malformation.[184] Prenatal vitamins should be given 2 to 3 months before conception is attempted.

Good general principles of health, such as proper diet, smoking cessation, weight control, avoidance of alcohol, and regular work and sleep habits, should be emphasized. Rubella immunization should be offered when appropriate, and education regarding the importance of early prenatal care should be provided.

Hemoglobinopathies

D isorders of hemoglobin structure and synthesis are the most common single gene defects worldwide. Populations from the eastern Mediterranean area, the Middle East, Southeast Asia, and Africa are most likely to be affected. The most common structural variant of hemoglobin is sickle hemoglobin, and the most common disorder in the synthesis of the globin chains is thalassemia.

In general, women who are heterozygous for either of these disorders do well during pregnancy and do not have appreciably poorer outcomes than does the general population. Their risk of bearing a child affected by the disease depends on their partner's genotype, because the disorders are autosomal recessive. Women who are homozygous for sickle cell disease or thalassemia are at increased risk for maternal morbidity and perinatal mortality if they become pregnant, and they should be aware of the problems they may encounter before they attempt pregnancy.

BACKGROUND

All normal human hemoglobin has a heme molecule that is attached to different pairs of globin chains: α, β, γ, and δ. These chains are under different genetic control. The α chain production takes place on chromosome 16 under the control of four genes, two inherited from each parent. The β, γ, and δ chains are determined by chromosome 11. The β chain production is under the control of only two genes, one inherited from each parent. Normal adults have a major hemoglobin A component (HbA) and a minor hemoglobin A component (HbA$_2$) attached to the β chains. In fetal life, the major hemoglobin is hemoglobin F (HbF), which is attached to the γ chains. The change from fetal to adult hemoglobin production begins at approximately 32 weeks of gestation but is not complete, since at term 60% to 80% of the cord blood is HbF.

Sickling Disorders

Hemoglobin S (HbS) is the most common and clinically important structural variant of normal hemoglobin. It differs from HbA by one amino acid substitution—glutamine in place of valine—on the β globin chain at the sixth position. The unique physical properties of HbS distort red blood cells so that they form the characteristic sickle shape. Sickling of the red blood cells may be exaggerated in the presence of lowered oxygen tension, infection, acidosis, or dehydration. This may precipitate a sickle cell crisis secondary to stasis in small blood vessels and thrombosis.

In black Americans, the sickling disorders and their prevalences include:
- homozygous state for sickle cell disease, 1 in 600 prevalence
- heterozygous state for sickle cell hemoglobin or sickle cell trait, 1 in 12 prevalence
- compound heterozygous state for HbS variants, such as sickle cell/hemoglobin C disease, 1 in 850 prevalence
- sickle cell thalassemia, 1 in 1,600 prevalence

Sickle cell disease is seen most commonly in black people of African origin. Pregnant and nonpregnant women with sickle cell disease have alternate periods of health and crises with severe anemia, cardiovascular symptoms, and joint pain. Women who have the sickle cell trait are usually asymptomatic, but they may have an increased incidence of urinary tract infections during pregnancy. Sickle cell/hemoglobin C disease is a variant of sickle cell disease; patients with this disorder have normal or near-normal levels of hemoglobin and may become symptomatic for the first time during pregnancy.

The combination of patient compliance and excellent medical care has decreased the incidence of complications of sickle cell disease and allowed women with this disorder to become pregnant. Despite advances in obstetrics, however, women with sickle cell disease still have increased rates of maternal morbidity and mortality secondary to complications of the disease itself. For example, these women have a higher incidence of vaso-occlusive disease, severe anemia, pneumonia, pyelonephritis, and congestive heart failure. In addition, they have an increased incidence of spontaneous abortion, preeclampsia, stillbirth, and intrauterine growth retardation.[185-187] The increased pregnancy loss is thought to be the result of uteroplacental insufficiency and decreased oxygen delivery to the fetus.[186]

In the early 1960s, it was suggested that prophylactic transfusion to maintain HbA at 60% to 70% in pregnant women with sickle cell disease might help to prevent sickle cell crises and improve oxygenation of the fetus.[188] After observing the results of a prophylactic transfusion regimen that began at 28 weeks of gestation, Morrison and colleagues[189] concluded that this technique improved maternal and fetal outcome more than previous series had shown. Cunningham and associates[190] retrospectively studied 24 pregnant women who had sickle cell disease and were given prophylactic transfusions from 1973 to 1982 and 24 historic controls who also had sickle cell disease and were not given transfusions during their pregnancies from 1955 to 1972. In the group that received transfusions, a significant reduction occurred in the incidence of intrauterine growth retardation, as well as in maternal and perinatal mortality. The investigators concluded that prophylactic transfusion was justified during early pregnancy for women with sickle cell disease. However, the use of prophylactic transfusions must be balanced against the risk of transmitting human immunodeficiency virus and the much greater risk of inducing the development of atypical red cell antibodies.

Tuck and colleagues[191] found no significant difference in pregnancy outcome for either mother or infant as a result of prophylactic transfusions. They also reported that the use of transfusion led to an immediate transfusion reaction in 14% of the patients and to the formation of red cell antibodies in 22%. Currently, prophylactic transfusion therapy does not appear to be routinely recommended. However, there are indications for therapeutic transfusion: (1) worsening anemia; (2) congestive heart failure; (3) major bacterial infection; and (4) complications of labor and delivery, such as bleeding, sepsis, or cesarean delivery.

Thalassemia

A group of hemoglobinopathies with variable clinical severity, thalassemia results from a quantitative decrease in the synthesis of the α or β chains of hemoglobin. Patients with α-thalassemia are generally from Southeast Asia. Patients with β-thalassemia are from Mediterranean countries, such as Italy and Greece; the Middle East; the Indian subcontinent; and Southeast Asia. The heterozygous state for α- and β-thalassemia in these areas ranges from 5% to 20%. The carrier state for α- and β-thalassemia is asymptomatic.

The offspring is not affected with β-thalassemia until early childhood, when hemoglobin synthesis switches from the γ to the β chain; at this point, the child may become symptomatic. Those with the heterozygous form, thalassemia minor, have only one β-thalassemia gene and are asymptomatic; those with the homozygous form of β-thalassemia, thalassemia major, have a marked deficiency of β chain production and severe, transfusion-dependent anemia. The latter develops during childhood, and early death from congestive heart failure is common. Even though patients with thalassemia major may live to their early twenties, pregnancy is rare in this group, and their reproductive outcome is poor. Patients with thalassemia minor may develop an anemia in the prenatal period, but in general they do well.

An inability to produce α globin chains characterizes α-thalassemia. During pregnancy, α-thalassemia patients may become very anemic, but their reproductive outcomes are good.

PRECONCEPTIONAL COUNSELING

The goals of preconceptional counseling for patients who are heterozygous or homozygous for a hemoglobinopathy are to offer prospective counseling regarding their offspring's risk of inheriting the disorder and to minimize the risk of pregnancy complications.

The hemoglobinopathies are single gene disorders inherited through mendelian principles. Prepregnancy counseling of patients who are carriers of α- or β-thalassemia or who are carriers of sickle cell hemoglobin should include a discussion of the newer techniques developed to diagnose hemoglobinopathies in utero. Fetal cord blood sampling, for example, can be performed as early as 14 to 16 weeks of gestation. In experienced hands, there is an approximately 2% rate of pregnancy loss from fetal exsanguination or premature labor.[192] Such procedures allow the obstetrician to give patients statistical probabilities of delivering an affected child.

Patients who are heterozygous for thalassemia and sickle cell disease do not have impaired reproductive outcomes attributable to their genotype. Aside from occasionally profound anemia and a high incidence of urinary tract infections in women who carry the sickle cell gene, these patients do not have higher-than-normal maternal morbidity.

Pregnancy is a significant risk for the woman with sickle cell disease. The anemia is likely to become more severe, and the episodes of crisis are likely to become more frequent. Patients who are homozygous for sickle cell disease are also at high risk for pregnancy complications and should be advised preconceptionally that intensive fetal surveillance is likely to be required. They should be aware that it may be necessary for them to curtail their usual work and leisure activities if signs of preterm labor or intrauterine growth retardation are observed. Complications of the pregnancy, such as pyelonephritis and placental abruption, may be erroneously attributed to a sickle cell crisis. Pregnant patients should be especially careful and persistent in reporting all symptoms of pain. Because infections are a frequent complication of pregnancy in women with sickle cell disease, every effort at primary prevention should be made. Appropriate steps include the preconceptional provision of the influenza and pneumococcal vaccines and the regular pre- and postconceptional analysis of urine cultures.

Patients with thalassemia major are unlikely to become pregnant. Should pregnancy occur, the risks to the mother and fetus are grave. For this reason, these patients should be advised not to attempt conception.

The effectiveness of prophylactic management of the patient with a homozygous hemoglobinopathy, such as sickle cell disease, by regular blood transfusions has not been scientifically proved.

Good general principles of health, such as proper diet, smoking cessation, weight control, and avoidance of alcohol, should be emphasized. Rubella immunization should be offered when appropriate, and the importance of early prenatal care should be stressed.

Cancer

C ancer is the second most common cause of death in women of childbearing age; malignancies complicate 1 in 1,000 pregnancies.[193] The malignancies most likely to affect women of childbearing age are thyroid, cervical, breast, ovarian, and colon cancers, as well as lymphoma, leukemia, and melanoma. Because the availability of accurate screening methods, effective radiation treatment techniques, and chemotherapy prolongs the lives of many women with these diseases, increasing numbers of women with a past or current history of cancer may seek preconceptional services.

BACKGROUND
Breast Cancer

Approximately 1 of every 10 women in the United States will develop breast cancer, with 15% of all breast cancer occurring in women under age 41[194]; Earley and colleagues[195] report the incidence of breast cancer to be 1.8% to 3% in women under 30. Approximately 3% of patients under the age of 40 with breast cancer are pregnant or lactating.

Breast cancer is often diagnosed late in pregnant women, and the disease has often spread to the lymph nodes. The vascular and lymphatic changes associated with pregnancy may increase the incidence of lymph node involvement. The elevated estrogen and progesterone levels and the immunologic changes that occur during pregnancy have also been implicated in the rapid growth and dissemination of breast cancer in gravid patients. Careful examination of the breast is an important preconceptional focus.

With early diagnosis and treatment, the prognosis for women with breast carcinoma during pregnancy or lactation is similar to that of comparable groups of women in the reproductive age group.[196] Among pregnant patients, in addition to early detection, the age of the patient at the time of the diagnosis is an important factor in the likelihood of long-term survival. When patients under 40 years old are compared with those over 40 years old, there is a decrease in the 5-year survival rate from 75% to 55%. Currently, the relationship of pregnancy and poor breast cancer outcome is believed to be related to age rather than to hormone levels.[197] Younger patients with breast cancer include those who are pregnant, and these patients have a greater proportion of estrogen and progesterone receptor-*negative*

147

tumors. This indicates that the tumors are hormonally insensitive and that termination of pregnancy would not alter tumor growth.[197,198]

Pregnancy does not appear to accelerate the course of breast cancer. In one series of 32 patients who became pregnant subsequent to treatment for breast cancer, 95% of those patients whose axillary nodes had been unaffected by the disease lived 5 years.[198] The 5-year survival rate dropped to 46% when the nodes were positive. In a study of 41 patients who had been treated for primary operable carcinoma of the breast before they became pregnant, Harvey and associates[199] concluded that pregnancy had no detrimental effect, even among patients whose axillary nodes had been affected by the disease or whose pregnancies occurred less than 2 years after their mastectomy. Peters and Meakin[200] report that 87% of 63 patients who conceived after treatment for breast cancer survived 3 years, 71% survived 5 years, 55% survived 10 years, and 43% survived 20 years. When the pregnancy occurred less than 1 year after treatment, 50% survived 5 years. When pregnancy occurred from 1 to 2 years after treatment, 83% survived 5 years; when pregnancy occurred more than 2 years after the diagnosis, 100% lived 5 years. Rissanen[201] states that pregnancy need not be avoided or terminated if it occurs more than 1 year after treatment and the patients are clinically free of recurrence following radiation treatment of breast cancer. Therefore, in the absence of recurrence or metastases, there is no indication for permanent avoidance of pregnancy. The excellent survival rates in some studies may be due to selection, however, in that women with poor prognoses do not live long enough to become pregnant. Although the studies indicate that pregnancy does not adversely affect survival, Landon[194] recommends that women without nodal involvement delay conception for 2 to 3 years after the original treatment, because one third of recurrences develop within this period. He extends the period of observation to 5 years in women who had positive nodes. In all women with a recent history of breast cancer, a full evaluation for metastatic disease should be undertaken before pregnancy.

Early Cervical Neoplasia

Carcinoma of the cervix is as common in pregnant women as is breast cancer, with approximately 3% of all cervical cancers occurring in the pregnant population.[202,203] In nonpregnant women, cervical cancer is treatable, with a 10-year survival rate of 45% to 50% for all stages. The cure rate in pregnant patients is similar to that reported in nonpregnant patients.[204]

The early diagnosis of cervical dysplasia and carcinoma in situ by use of widespread screening with the Papanicolaou smear and colposcopic biopsies has led to a decrease in the incidence of invasive cervical cancer. A relatively slow-growing malignancy, cervical carcinoma does not progress rapidly from dysplasia to invasive cancer.[205] On the basis of cytologic findings in 557 patients with dysplasia, Richart and Barron[206] report that the median transit time to carcinoma in situ ranged from 86 months in one patient with very mild dysplasia, to 58 months in patients with mild dysplasia, to 38 months in patients with moderate dysplasia, to 12 months in patients with severe dysplasia. The median transit time for all dysplasias to a diagnosis of carcinoma in situ was 44 months. Spontaneous regression and progression of all degrees of dysplasia can occur in nonpregnant and pregnant patients. It appears that the rate of progression of cervical dysplasia is comparable in the nonpregnant and the pregnant patient.[207-211]

The patient who was exposed in utero to diethylstilbestrol (DES) has the potential for vaginal or cervical squamous cell changes. Having examined 1,400 DES-exposed patients, Robboy and colleagues[212] report a prevalence of 2.1% of dysplasia, primarily mild dysplasia. Pregnancy does not affect the occurrence of dysplasia in patients who have had in utero DES exposure.

Today, many women who are contemplating pregnancy have a history of cervical intraepithelial neoplasia that has been treated conservatively. Available data concerning the outcome of pregnancy after conservative therapy with cautery, colposcopy, or conization are difficult to interpret. Cervical stenosis can develop after electrocoagulation, cryosurgery, or laser beam therapy to the cervix, but this has not been associated with adverse pregnancy outcomes. Some authors have reported a high rate of preterm labor and delivery after conization of the cervix.[213,214] A 1980 study by Jones and Buller[215] did not, however, show an increase in either abortion or premature delivery. The use of conization of the cervix has decreased dramatically as the use of colposcopy has become widespread.

Women should be reassured that pregnancy does not accelerate the natural course of cervical dysplasia and that the cervical changes that occur during pregnancy do not preclude adequate follow-up.[216] Vaginal delivery is not contraindicated in patients with a history of cervical cancer.[217]

Hodgkin's Disease

Characterized by the proliferation of lymphoid cells in lymph nodes and extranodal tissue involved with the immune system, Hodgkin's disease accounts for approximately 1% of cancer in humans and for approximately 40% of neoplastic lymphomas. Approximately one third of all cases occur in persons between the ages of 15 and 44, with an incidence during pregnancy of 1 in 5,000 births. Non-Hodgkin's lymphomas during pregnancy are usually associated with primary immunodeficiency states, such as acquired immunodeficiency syndrome (AIDS), or with chronic immunosuppressive therapy.

Nearly all patients with Hodgkin's disease have a long history of a persistent, painless enlargement of the lymph nodes that makes the nodes easily palpable. The cervical lymph nodes are involved 60% to 80% of the time.[218] The disease is indolent; the superficial nodes may be "actively" enlarged at times, but much smaller and barely noticeable at other times. In one study, researchers found that patients with Hodgkin's disease who became pregnant had a median survival of 90 months, compared with a median survival of 59 months for all reproductive-age patients and 52 months for a nonpregnant, age-corrected group.[219] It appears that pregnancy does not increase the disease activity; however, as in many diseases, there may be a postpartum exacerbation.[219,220]

The stage of Hodgkin's disease has a direct influence on the short-term and long-term prognosis:

- Stage I disease is confined to a single lymph node in an area above or below the diaphragm or to an extralymphatic site.
- Stage II disease is confined to two or more lymph node–bearing areas on the same side of the diaphragm or to one or more areas on the same side with contiguous spread to an extralymphatic organ.
- Stage III disease is manifested on both sides of the diaphragm.

The 5-year survival rate for patients with stage I disease is 90%. For patients with stage II disease, the 5-year survival rate is 82%; for patients with disseminated disease, the figure is 50%. Of stage I and stage II patients who relapse, 87% relapse within the first 3 years. Treatment of stage I and stage II Hodgkin's disease commonly consists of irradiation to a particular lymph node site at a rate of 1,000 rads/week for 4 weeks. Stage III Hodgkin's disease is treated with combination chemotherapy known as the MOPP regimen, which involves 2-week courses of mechlorethamine hydrochloride (Mustargen), vincristine (Oncovin), procarbazine hydrochloride, and prednisone.

Depending on the extent of the disease and the choice of therapy, Hodgkin's disease may adversely affect the patient's reproductive potential. Although the subsequent reproductive risk of a patient who receives mantle and abdominal radiation therapy is not definitely known, exposure of the ovaries to radiation may result in sterility and can theoretically lead to abnormal offspring because of either chromosomal abnormalities or gene mutations. Limited data on the effects of high-dose irradiation on human fertility have been obtained predominantly from studies of survivors of the atomic bombs at Nagasaki and Hiroshima. Blot and Sawada[221] investigated 2,345 women in these populations and found no subsequent reduction in the fertility rate, even when the estimated exposure was 100 rads. In their extensive research, Shaw and Damme[222] uncovered no evidence that irradiation of human gonads before conception increased the rate of congenital malformation. However, some human data based on case-control studies indicate that as little as 2 rads of preconceptional irradiation may increase the risk of aneuploid offspring.[223,224] In general, it appears that preconceptional irradiation to the ovaries is unlikely to result in abnormal offspring, but patients should be counseled that it is difficult to quantify the risks.

Horning and associates[225] reported amenorrhea in 52% and irregular menses in 28% of patients who received both pelvic irradiation and chemotherapy. Alone, chemotherapy resulted in amenorrhea in 15% and irregular menses in 29% of patients. The administration of chemotherapeutic agents appears to have age-related effects. Of patients under age 30 at the time of chemotherapy, 95% subsequently have normal ovarian function; of patients older than 30, however, only 39% return to normal ovarian function.[226] Therefore, chemotherapy may prevent future conception by causing ovarian failure.

In patients who did conceive after treatment with mantle irradiation and nitrogen mustard, vincristine, prednisone, and procarbazine hydrochloride, there was no demonstrated increase in fetal wastage or birth defects.[227] Patients who have received this chemotherapy during early pregnancy have usually had a favorable outcome, provided that concomitant radiation therapy was not administered. It is not recommended that patients conceive during the time of chemotherapy, however, but that they wait at least 2 years after the completion of the chemotherapeutic regimen before considering pregnancy.[228] After 2 years, the patient without evidence of any recurrence of Hodgkin's disease is considered cured.

Malignant Melanoma

In the United States, malignant melanoma accounts for 1% of all cancers diagnosed. Approximately 11,000 women develop the disease yearly.[229] The cancer may occur as a new lesion, or it may develop in a preexisting skin nevus. Thirty percent to fifty percent of malignant melanoma occurs in persons ages 20 to 40. Fair-skinned persons have the highest incidence, and blacks have the lowest. It most commonly occurs on the lower limbs of women, on the trunks of men, and on the upper limbs of both men and women.

Some controversy exists about the possibility that hormones may influence the occurrence and course of melanoma and specifically that pregnancy may accelerate a latent metastasis in a patient with a history of melanoma or cause a previously removed melanoma to recur and spread. Malignant melanoma is not generally regarded as a hormonally dependent neoplasm, but the presence of estrogen, progesterone, and other steroid receptors in the melanoma may influence its behavior.[230,231] Theoretically, the increased melanocyte-stimulating substances and areas of skin pigmentation during pregnancy may have an adverse effect on the tumor. There is no evidence, however, that the endocrine milieu of pregnancy or oral contraceptive use promotes malignant transformation of a benign nevus.[232]

The survival of patients with melanoma depends on the stage of their disease and the completeness of the surgical excision. In addition, the site of the lesion, the sex of the patient, and the depth of the primary tumor are important.[233] In stage I, the lesion is confined to the primary site. In stage II, there is evidence of regional lymph node metastasis.

When George and associates[234] studied 115 pregnant women with melanoma, they found that the prognosis for these patients did not differ significantly from the prognosis for a control group of 330 nonpregnant women. Shiu and colleagues[235] retrospectively reviewed 251 surgically treated cases of cutaneous melanoma during pregnancy; 165 patients had stage I melanoma, and 86 patients had stage II disease. There was no statistically significant difference in survival at 5 years associated with stage I melanoma in nulliparous patients, parous nonpregnant patients, and pregnant patients. For stage II melanoma, however, a significantly lower survival rate was observed after 5 years in pregnant patients (29%) and in parous patients whose lesion had become active during a previous pregnancy (22%) than was observed in nulliparous patients (55%) and other patients in the parous group (51%). Furthermore, pregnant women with stage II disease had a greater incidence of bleeding and ulceration, which strongly indicates an adverse influence of pregnancy.[235] In fact, activation of a lesion during a previous pregnancy, whether stage I or II, diminished the patient's chance of survival. It must be remembered that stage II disease is generally hazardous, and the risk for recurrence is high.

Sutherland and associates[236] studied two groups of patients with malignant melanoma who were treated from 1957 to 1983. Group I was made up of patients in whom melanoma was diagnosed during pregnancy, and group II was made up of patients in whom melanoma had been diagnosed before they became pregnant. The results of the study indicated that the majority of patients with a history of melanoma were not adversely affected by pregnancy but that patients who were pregnant at the time of diagnosis were more likely to have hormonally sensitive tumors. These findings indicate that the prognosis for patients with melanoma diagnosed during pregnancy is worse than that for patients with a history of melanoma.

Reintgen and colleagues[237] conducted a retrospective study of women of childbearing age who had been treated for stage I cutaneous melanoma at Duke University Comprehensive Cancer Center. They placed 58 women in whom melanoma had been diagnosed during pregnancy into group 1 and 43 patients who had become pregnant within 5 years of diagnosis of their melanoma into group 2. A control group of melanoma patients was matched for the clinical variables of age, primary site of involvement, stage of disease, and pathologic variables. Actuarial survival for patients in groups 1 and 2 did not differ from those of the controls. The results of the Reintgen study showed no difference in the survival rate for those patients whose melanoma had developed during a pregnancy or for those who became pregnant within 5 years of diagnosis when compared with the survival rate for the control group.

PRECONCEPTIONAL COUNSELING

The goal of preconceptional counseling for the patient with a history of cancer is to educate her and her partner about the effect that pregnancy may have on her prognosis and the fetal complications that may arise from current or past therapies.

Recommendations regarding pregnancy subsequent to successful treatment of breast cancer have changed in recent years. Apparently, pregnancy neither predisposes nor protects a woman from developing breast cancer, and there is no evidence that pregnancy accelerates the progression of breast cancer. The length of time since the initial cancer and the presence or absence of axillary metastases are the most important considerations in counseling. Most breast cancers that recur do so within the first 2 years after diagnosis. If the axillary nodes were unaffected by the disease, the patient should be advised not to become pregnant for 3 years after the initial diagnosis. If the axillary nodes were affected, this time should be extended to 5 years. Not only is there a higher incidence of recurrence in these patients, but also the risk of a second cancer in the remaining breast is higher. Before pregnancy, a mammogram of the remaining breast, a bone survey, and a careful physical examination should be performed.

Patients should be reassured that pregnancy does not accelerate the natural course of cervical dysplasia and that the cervical changes during pregnancy do not preclude adequate follow-up care for the dysplasia. When preinvasive and invasive cervical neoplasia have been ruled out, Papanicolaou smear surveillance and colposcopic examinations should be performed at 3-month intervals both before and during pregnancy. Aggressive treatment of vaginal/cervical infections is helpful in the prepregnancy and pregnancy cytologic evaluations. The patient should be advised that conservative therapy by means of cautery or conization of the cervix has been associated with an increased incidence of preterm labor and delivery but that the data remain controversial.

Patients who have been treated for Hodgkin's disease should be informed that pregnancy does not appear to affect the prognosis adversely. If radiation therapy was used in the treatment, the patient should be aware that her risk of bearing an abnormal offspring is difficult to quantify but that it does not appear to be significantly increased.

The patient undergoing chemotherapy should not be placed on hormonal contraceptive therapy, because the resumption of ovulation may be delayed by oral contraceptives and ovarian failure may be a gradual process after chemotherapy. In general, patients undergoing chemotherapy should be informed that there is a potential risk of infertility associated with chemotherapy, that pregnancy is contraindicated during treatment, and that it is advisable to wait at least 24 months after the completion of the chemotherapy before attempting to conceive. The patients should be counseled that genetic damage to the gametes in both men and women leads to abnormalities in approximately 4% of the offspring. This rate is slightly higher than that in the general population.[223-225,227] If further reassurance is necessary, the possibility of antenatal diagnosis by amniocentesis should be discussed.

In patients with a history of melanoma, the recommendations for or against pregnancy must be individualized according to the clinical stage and the anticipated course of the melanoma. It seems unnecessary to discourage pregnancy in patients with stage I melanoma, provided that they wait for a period of 3 to 5 years. In the patient who experienced an exacerbation of a melanoma during a previous pregnancy or who has stage II disease, pregnancy should be viewed as hazardous. The literature does not substantiate a causal association between oral contraceptives and the development or spread of melanoma, but barrier contraception is recommended for these patients.[238]

Good general principles of health, such as proper diet, smoking cessation, weight control, and avoidance of alcohol, should be emphasized. Rubella immunization should be offered when appropriate. Education regarding the importance of early prenatal care should be provided.

References

Diabetes Mellitus

1. Gabbe SG, Lowensohn RI, Wu PK, et al: Current patterns of neonatal morbidity and mortality in infants of diabetic mothers. *Diabetes Care* 1978;1:335-339.
2. Kucera J: Rate and type of congenital anomalies among offspring of diabetic women. *J Reprod Med* 1971;7:73-82.
3. Mills JL, Baker L, Goldman AS: Malformations in infants of diabetic mothers occur before the seventh gestational week: Implications for treatment. *Diabetes* 1979;28:292-293.
4. Pedersen J, Møolsted-Pedersen L: Congenital malformations: The possible role of diabetes care outside pregnancy, in *Pregnancy, Metabolism, Diabetes and the Fetus.* Ciba Foundation Symposium 63. New York, Excerpta Medica, 1979, pp 265-281.
5. Baker L, Egler JM, Klein SH, et al: Meticulous control of diabetes during organogenesis prevents congenital lumbosacral defects in rats. *Diabetes* 1981; 30:955-957.
6. Pedersen J: *The Pregnant Diabetic and Her Newborn: Problems and Management,* ed 2. Baltimore, Williams & Wilkins, 1977, pp 123-197.
7. Gonen B, Rubenstein AH, Rochman H, et al: Hemoglobin A_1: An indicator of the metabolic control of the diabetic patient. *Lancet* 1977;2:734-738.
8. Miller E, Hare JW, Cloherty JP, et al: Elevated maternal HbA_{1c} in early pregnancy and major congenital anomalies in infants of diabetic mothers. *N Engl J Med* 1981;304:1331-1335.
9. Ylinen K, Aula P, Stenman UH, et al: Risk of minor and major fetal malformations in diabetes with high haemoglobin A_{1c} values in early pregnancy. *Br Med J* 1984;289:345-346.
10. Fuhrmann K, Reiher H, Semmler K, et al: Prevention of congenital malformations in infants of insulin-dependent diabetic mothers. *Diabetes Care* 1983; 6:219-223.
11. Fuhrmann K, Reiher H, Semmler K, et al: The effect of intensified conventional insulin therapy before and during pregnancy on the malformation rate in offspring of diabetic mothers. *Exp Clin Endocrinol* 1984;83:173-177.
12. Steel JM, Johnstone FD, Smith AF: Five years' experience of a ''prepregnancy'' clinic for insulin-dependent diabetics. *Br Med J* 1982;285:353-356.
13. Kitzmiller JL, Gavin LA, Gin GD, et al: Preconception care of diabetes: Glycemic control prevents congenital anomalies. *JAMA* 1991;265:731-736.
14. Steel JM, Johnstone FD, Hepburn DA, et al: Can pregnancy care of diabetic women reduce the risk of abnormal babies? *BMJ* 1990;301:1070-1074.
15. Freinkel N: The Banting Lecture 1980: Of pregnancy and progeny. *Diabetes* 1980;29:1023-1035.
16. Coustan DR: Management of the pregnant diabetic, in Warshaw JB, Hobbins JL (eds): *Principles and Practice of Perinatal Medicine: Maternal, Fetal, and Newborn Care.* Menlo Park, Calif, Addison-Wesley, 1983, p 78-91.
17. Haysett JP, Reece EA: Effects of dia-

betic nephropathy on pregnancy. *Am J Kidney Dis* 1987;9:344.

18. Singerman LH, Aiello LM, Rodman HM: Diabetic retinopathy: Effects of pregnancy and laser therapy. *Diabetes* 1980;29:1.

19. Warren JH, Krolewski AS, Gottlieb MJ, et al: Difference in risk of insulin-dependent diabetes in offspring of diabetic mothers and diabetic fathers. *N Engl J Med* 1984;311:149-156.

20. Cahill GH, McDevitt HO: Insulin-dependent diabetes mellitus. The initial lesion. *N Engl J Med* 1981;304:1454-1458.

21. Milunsky A: Prenatal diagnosis of neural tube defects: The importance of serum alpha-fetoprotein screening in diabetic pregnant women. *Am J Obstet Gynecol* 1982;142:1030-1032.

22. *California Diabetes and Pregnancy Program: Guidelines for Care.* Maternal and Child Health, Department of Health Services, 1986.

Thyroid Disorders

23. Montoro M, Collea JV, Frasier SD, et al: Successful outcome of pregnancy in women with hypothyroidism. *Ann Intern Med* 1981;94:31-34.

24. Echt CR, Doss JF: Myxedema in pregnancy: Report of 3 cases. *Obstet Gynecol* 1963;22:615-620.

25. Raiti S, Holzman GB, Scott RL, et al: Evidence for the placental transfer of tri-iodothyronine in human beings. *N Engl J Med* 1967;277:456-459.

26. Mann EB: Maternal hypothyroxinemia: development of 4 and 7 year offspring, in Fisher DA, Burrows GN (eds): *Perinatal Thyroid Physiology and Disease.* New York: Raven Press, 1975, pp 117-132.

27. Cheron RG, Kaplan MM, Larsen PR, et al: Neonatal thyroid function after pro-

pylthiouracil therapy for maternal Graves' disease. *N Engl J Med* 1981; 304:525-528.

28. Burrow GN, Bartsocas C, Klatskin EH, et al: Children exposed in utero to propylthiouracil: Subsequent intellectual and physical development. *Am J Dis Child* 1968;116:161-165.

29. Halnan KE: Risks from radioiodine treatment of thyrotoxicosis. *Br Med J* 1983;287:1821-1822.

30. Sarkar SD, Beierwaltes WH, Gill SP, et al: Subsequent fertility and birth histories of children and adolescents treated with ^{131}I for thyroid cancer. *J Nucl Med* 1976;17:212-217.

31. Hill SC, Clark RL, Wolf M: The effect of subsequent pregnancy on patients with thyroid carcinoma. *Surg Gynecol Obstet* 1966;122:1219-1222.

32. Chopra IJ, Hershman JM, Pardridge VW, et al: Thyroid function in nonthyroidal illness. *Ann Intern Med* 1983;98:946-957.

33. Rossvoll RV, Winship T: Thyroid carcinoma and pregnancy. *Surg Gynecol Obstet* 1965;121:1039-1042.

34. Briggs GG, Freeman RK, Yaffe SJ: *Drugs in Pregnancy and Lactation,* ed 3. Baltimore, Williams & Wilkins, 1990, p 344.

Hyperphenylalaninemia

35. Friedman EG, Koch R: Report from the Maternal PKU Collaborative study. *Metab Curr* 1988;1:4-5.

36. Luke B, Keith LG. The challenge of natural phenylketonuria screening and treatment. *J Repro Med* 1990;35:667-673.

37. Lenke RL, Levy HL: Maternal phenylketonuria and hyperphenylalaninemia: An international survey of the outcome of untreated and treated pregnancies. *N Engl J Med* 1980;303:1202-1208.

38. Acosta PB, Wenz E: *Diet Management of PKU for Infants and Preschool Children.* US Dept Health, Education, and Welfare publication No. 77-5209. Washington, DC, US Government Printing Office, 1977.

39. Levy LH, Waisbren SE: Effects of untreated maternal phenylketonuria and hyperphenylalaninemia on the fetus. *N Engl J Med* 1983;309:1269-1274.

40. Platt LD, Koch R, Azen C, et al: Maternal phenylketonuria collaborative study, obstetric aspects and outcome: The first 6 years. *Am J Obstet Gynecol* 1992;166:1150-1162.

41. Kerr GR, Chamove AS, Harlow HF, et al: "Fetal PKU": The effect of maternal hyperphenylalaninemia during pregnancy in the Rhesus monkey *(Macaca mulatta). Pediatrics* 1968;42:27-36.

42. Levy HL: Maternal phenylketonuria, in Bickel H, Wachtel U (eds): *Inherited Disease of Amino Acid Metabolism.* New York, George Thieme, 1985, pp 175-185.

43. Lenke RR, Levy HL: Maternal phenylketonuria—Results of dietary therapy. *Am J Obstet Gynecol* 1982;142:548-553.

44. Koch R, Friedman EG, Wenz E, et al: Maternal phenylketonuria. *J Inher Metab Dis* 1986;9:159-168.

45. Farquhar DL, Simpson GK, Steven F, et al: Preconceptional dietary management for maternal phenylketonuria. *Acta Paediatr Scand* 1987;76:279-283.

46. Acosta PB, Blaskovics M, Cloud H, et al: Nutrition in pregnancy of women with hyperphenylalaninemia. *Research* 1982;80:443-450.

Asthma

47. Smith CV: Asthma and pregnancy: Should we be concerned?, in Cefalo RC (ed): *Clinical Decisions in Obstetrics*

and *Gynecology.* Rockville, Md, Aspen, 1990.

48. Mintz S: Pregnancy and asthma, in Weiss EB, Segal MS (eds): *Bronchial Asthma: Mechanisms and Therapeutics.* Boston, Little, Brown & Co, 1976, pp 971-982.

49. Cugell DW, Frank NR, Gaensler EA, et al: Pulmonary function in pregnancy: I. Serial observations in normal women. *Am Rev Tuberc* 1953;67:568-597.

50. Bahna SL, Bjerkedal T: The course and outcome of pregnancy in women with bronchial asthma. *Acta Allergol* 1972;27:397-406.

51. Rose CC, Murphy JG, Schwartz JS: Performance of an index predicting the response of patients with acute bronchial asthma to intensive emergency department treatment. *N Engl J Med* 1984;310:573-576.

52. Greenberger PA, Patterson R: Beclomethasone dipropionate for severe asthma during pregnancy. *Ann Intern Med* 1983;98:478-480.

53. Mabie WC, Barton JR, Wasserstrum N, et al: Clinical observations on asthma in pregnancy. *J Maternal-Fetal Med* 1992;1:45-50.

54. Fitzsimmons R, Greenberger PA, Patterson R: Outcomes of pregnancy in women requiring corticosteroids for severe asthma. *J Allergy Clin Immunol* 1986;78:349-353.

55. Shatz M, Zeiger RS, Harden KM, et al: The safety of inhaled beta-agonist bronchodilators during pregnancy. *J Allergy Clin Immunol* 1988;82:686-695.

56. Turner ES, Greenberger PA, Patterson R: Management of the pregnant asthmatic patient. *Ann Intern Med* 1980; 93(6):905-918.

57. Gluck JC, Gluck PA: The effects of pregnancy on asthma: A prospective study. *Ann Allergy* 1976;37:164-168.

58. Greenberger PA: Asthma in pregnancy. *Clin Perinatol* 1985;12:571-584.

59. Weinstein AM, Dubin BD, Podleski WK, et al: Asthma and pregnancy. *JAMA* 1979;241:1161-1165.

Heart Disease

60. Burwell CS, Metcalfe J: *Heart Disease and Pregnancy*. Boston, Little Brown, 1958.
61. McCenultz JH, Metcalfe J, Ueland K: Cardiovascular disease, in Burrow G and Ferris T (eds): *Medical Complications of Pregnancy*. Philadelphia, WB Saunders Co, 1982, pp 145-165.
62. Ueland K: What's the risk when the cardiac patient is pregnant? *Contemp Ob/Gyn* 1979;13:117-120.
63. Sullivan JM, Ramanathan KB: Management of medical problems in pregnancy—Severe cardiac disease. *N Engl J Med* 1985;313:304-308.
64. Szekely P, Snaith L: *Heart Disease and Pregnancy*. London, Churchill-Livingstone, 1974.
65. Arias F, Pineda J: Aortic stenosis and pregnancy. *J Reprod Med* 1978;20:229-232.
66. Hankins GD, Wendel GD, Leveno KJ, et al: Myocardial infarction during pregnancy: A review. *Obstet Gynecol* 1985;65:139-146.
67. Ueland K: Mitral valve prolapse: Alleviating your pregnant patients' anxiety. *Contemp Ob/Gyn,* December 1985, pp 47-51.
68. Neill C, Swanson S: Outcome of pregnancy in congenital heart disease. *Circulation* 1961;24:1003.
69. Batson GA: Cyanotic congenital heart disease and pregnancy. *J Obstet Gynaecol Br Commonw* 1974;81:549-553.
70. Spinnato JA, Kraynack BJ, Cooper MW: Eisenmenger's syndrome in pregnancy: Epidural anesthesia for elective cesarean section. *N Engl J Med* 1981;304:1215-1217.
71. Gleicher N, Midwall J, Hochberger D, et al: Eisenmenger's syndrome and pregnancy. *Obstet Gynecol Surv* 1979;34:721-741.
72. Dawkins KD, Burke CM, Billingham ME, et al: Primary pulmonary hypertension and pregnancy. *Chest* 1986;89:383-388.
73. Whittemore RH, Hobbins JC, Engle MA: Pregnancy and its outcome in women with and without surgical treatment of congenital disease. *Am J Cardiol* 1982;50:641-651.
74. Deal K, Wooley CF: Coarctation of the aorta and pregnancy. *Ann Intern Med* 1973;78:706-710.
75. Harrison EC, Roschke EJ, Ferenczi G, et al: Managing the pregnant patient with a heart valve prosthesis. *Contemp Ob/Gyn,* 1978;11:82-90.
76. Salazar E, Zajarias A, Gutierrez N, et al: The problem of cardiac valve prosthesis, anticoagulants and pregnancy. *Circulation* 1984;70:169-177.
77. Beadle EM, Luepker RV, Williams PP: Pregnancy in a patient with porcine valve xenografts. *Am Heart J* 1979;98:510-512.
78. Lockwood CJ: Preeclampsia and hypertensive disorders of pregnancy, in Cherry SH, Merkatz IR (eds): *Complications of Pregnancy: Medical, Surgical, Gynecologic, Psychosocial, and Perinatal,* 4th ed. Baltimore, Williams & Wilkins, 1991, pp 476-495.
79. Gladstone GH, Hordof A, Gersony WM: Propranolol administration during pregnancy: Effects on the fetus. *J Pediatr* 1975;86:962-964.
80. Opie LH: Drugs of the heart: IV. Antiarrythmic agents. *Lancet* 1980;1:861-867.
81. Hill LM, Malkasian GD: The use of quinidine sulfate throughout pregnancy. *Obstet Gynecol* 1979;54:366-368.
82. Ginsburg JS, Hirsh J. Use of antithrom-

botic agents during pregnancy. *Chest* 1992;102:385-390.

83. Dahlman T, Lindvall N, Hellgren M. Osteopenia in pregnancy during long-term heparin treatment: a radiological study postpartum. *Br J Obstet Gynecol* 1990;97:221-228.

84. Orme L'e, Lewis M, DeSwiet M, et al: May mothers given warfarin breast-feed their infants? *BMJ* 1977;1:1564-1665.

85. McKenna R, Cale ER, Vasan U: Is warfarin sodium contraindicated in the lactating mother? *J Pediatr* 1983;103:325-327.

Chronic Hypertension

86. Sibai BM, Anderson GD: Pregnancy outcome of intensive therapy in severe hypertension in first trimester. *Obstet Gynecol* 1986;67:517.

87. Sibai BM, Anderson GD: Hypertension, in Gabbe SG, Niebyl JR, Sempson JL (eds): *Obstetrics: Normal and problem pregnancies,* 2nd ed. New York, Churchill Livingstone, 1991.

88. Silverstone A, Trudinger BJ, Lewis PJ, et al: Maternal hypertension and intrauterine fetal death in mid-pregnancy. *Br J Obstet Gynaecol* 1980;87:457-461.

89. Lin CC, Lindheimer MD, River P, et al: Fetal outcome in hypertensive disorders of pregnancy. *Am J Obstet Gynecol* 1982;142:255-260.

90. Roberts JM: When the hypertensive patient becomes pregnant. *Contemp Ob/Gyn* 1979;13:47-55.

91. Barr M, Cohen M: ACE inhibitor fetopathy and hypocalvaria: the kidney skull connection. *Teratology* 1991;44:485-489.

92. Scott AA, Purohit DM: Neonatal renal failure. A complication of maternal antihypertensive therapy. *Am J Obstet Gynecol* 1989;160:1223-1224.

93. Watson WJ: chronic hypertension in

pregnancy, in Cefalo RC (ed): *Clinical Decisions in Obstetrics and Gynecology.* Rockville, Md, Aspen, 1990.

94. Sibai BM, Abdella TN, Anderson GD, et al: Plasma volume findings in pregnant women with mild hypertension. *Am J Obstet Gynecol* 1983;145:539.

95. Cockburn J, Ounsted M, Moar VA, et al: Final report of study on hypertension during pregnancy: the effects of specific treatment on the growth and development of the children. *Lancet* 1982;1:647.

96. Sibai BM, Abdella TN, Anderson GD: Pregnancy outcome in 211 patients with mild chronic hypertension. *Obstet Gynecol* 1983;61:571-576.

97. Surian M, Imbasciati E, Banfi G, et al: Glomerular disease and pregnancy. *Nephron* 1984;36:101-105.

Deep Venous Thrombosis

98. Aaro LA, Juergens JL: Thrombophlebitis and pulmonary embolism as complications of pregnancy. *Med Clin North Am* 1974;58:829-834.

99. Letsky EA, DeSwiet M: Thromboembolism in pregnancy and its management. *Br J Haematol* 1984;57:543-547.

100. Badaracco MA, Vessey MP: Recurrence of venous thromboembolic disease and use of oral contraceptives. *Br Med J* 1974;1:215-217.

101. Ginsberg JS, Hirsh J: Use of antithrombotic agents during pregnancy. *Chest* 1992;102:385-390.

102. Ginsberg JS, Brill-Edwards P, Burrows RF, et al: Venous thrombosis during pregnancy: Leg and trimester of presentation. *Thromb Haemost* 1992;67:519-520.

103. Lewis PJ, Boylan P, Friedman LA, et al: Prostacyclin in pregnancy. *Br Med J* 1980;280:1581-1582.

104. Fawer R, Dettling A, Weihs D, et al: Effect of the menstrual cycle, oral con-

traception and pregnancy on forearm blood flow, venous distensibility and clotting factors. *Eur J Clin Pharmacol* 1978;13:251-257.

105. Ratnoff OD, Holland TR: Coagulation components in normal and abnormal pregnancies. *NY Acad Sci* 1959;75:626-633.

106. Shaul WL, Emery H, Hall JG: Chondrodysplasia punctata and maternal warfarin use during pregnancy. *Am J Dis Child* 1975;129:360-362.

107. Fourie DT, Hay IT: Warfarin in pregnancy. *S Afr Med J* 1975;49:360-362.

108. Hall JG, Pauli RM, Wilson KM: Maternal and fetal sequelae of anticoagulation during pregnancy. *Am J Med* 1980; 68:122-140.

109. Baskett TF: *Essential Management of Obstetric Emergencies.* New York, John Wiley & Sons, 1985, pp 184-186.

110. Bonnar J: Venous thromboembolism and pregnancy. *Clin Obstet Gynecol* 1981;8:435-473.

111. Howel R, Fidler J, Letsky E, et al: The risks of antenatal subcutaneous heparin prophylaxis: A controlled trial. *Br J Obstet Gynaecol* 1983;90:1124-1128.

112. Kelton JG, Hirsch J: Venous thromboembolism disorders, in Burrow GN, Ferris TF (eds): *Medical Complications during pregnancy,* ed 2. Philadelphia, WB Saunders, 1982, pp 169-186.

113. Laros RK, Alger LS: Thromboembolism and pregnancy. *Clin Obstet Gynecol* 1979;22:871-887.

114. Dahlman T, Lindvall N, Hellgren M: Osteopenia in pregnancy during long-term heparin treatment: a radiological study postpartum. *Br J Obstet Gynecol* 1990;64:286-289.

115. Orme L'e, Lewis M, DeSwiet M, et al: May mothers given warfarin breast feed their infants? *BMJ* 1977;1:1564-1565.

116. McKenna R, Cale ER, Vasan U: Is warfarin sodium contraindicated in the lactating mother? *J Pediatr* 1983;103:325-337.

Kidney Disease

117. Lindheimer MD, Katz AI: Renal disease and pregnancy. *Perspect Nephrol Hypertens* 1976;3:237-254.

118. Davison JM, Lindheimer MD: Renal disease in pregnant women. *Clin Obstet Gynecol* 1978;21:411-419.

119. Bear RA: Pregnancy in patients with renal disease: A study of 44 cases. *Obstet Gynecol* 1976;48:13-18.

120. Katz AI, Davison JM, Hayslett JD, et al: Pregnancy in women with kidney disease. *Kidney Int* 1980;18:192-206.

121. Surian M, Imbasciati E, Banfi G, et al: Glomerular disease and pregnancy. *Nephron* 1984;36:101-105.

122. Penn I, Makowski EL, Harris P: Parenthood following renal transplantation. *Kidney Int* 1980;18:221-233.

123. Sciarra JJ, Toledo-Pereyra LH, Bendel RP, et al: Pregnancy following renal transplantation. *Am J Obstet Gynecol* 1975;123:411-425.

124. Hou S: Pregnancy in women with chronic renal disease. *N Engl J Med* 1985;312:836-839.

125. Penn I, Makowski E, Droegemueller W, et al: Parenthood in renal homograft recipients. *JAMA* 1971;216:1755-1761.

126. Leb DE, Weisskopf B, Kanovitz BS: Chromosome aberrations in the child of a transplant recipient. *Arch Intern Med* 1971;128:441-444.

127. The Registration Committee of the European Dialysis and Transplant Association. Successful pregnancies in women treated by dialysis and kidney transplantation. *Br J Obstet Gynecol* 1980;87:830-845.

128. Price H, Salaman J, Laurence K, et al: Immunosuppressive drugs and the fetus. *Transplantation* 1976;21:294.

129. Briggs GG, Freeman RK, Yaffe SJ: *Drugs in Pregnancy and Lactation,* ed 3. Baltimore, Williams & Wilkins, 1990.

130. Nageotte MP: How kidney impairments

affect obstetrical outcome. *Contemp Ob/Gyn,* January 1985, pp 179-194.

131. Samuels P: Renal disease, in Gabbe SG, Niebyl JR, Simpson JL (eds): *Obstetrics: Normal and Problem Pregnancies,* 2nd ed. New York, Churchill Livingstone, 1991.

132. Davison J, Lind T, Uldall P: Planned pregnancy in a renal transplant recipient. *Br J Obstet Gynaecol* 1976;83:518.

133. Cunningham FG: Connective-tissue disorders complicating pregnancy, in Cunningham FG, MacDonald PC, Gant NF (eds): *Williams Obstetrics,* 18th ed. Norwalk, Conn, Appleton & Lange, 1993.

Systemic Lupus Erythematosus

134. Fine LG, Barnett EV, Danovitch GM, et al: Systemic lupus erythematosus in pregnancy. *Ann Intern Med* 1981;94: 667-677.

135. Mintz G, Niz J, Gutierrez G: Prospective study of pregnancy in systemic lupus erythematosus: Results of a multidisciplinary approach. *J Rheumatol* 1986;13:732-739.

136. Hayslett JP, Lynn RI: Effect of pregnancy in patients with lupus nephropathy. *Kidney Int* 1980;18:207-220.

137. Meehan RT, Dorsey JK: Pregnancy among patients with systemic lupus erythematosus receiving immunosuppressive therapy. *J Rheumatol* 1987;14: 252-258.

138. Fraga A, Mintz G, Orozco J, et al: Sterility and fertility rates, fetal wastage and maternal morbidity in systemic lupus erythematosus. *J Rheumatol* 1974;1:293-298.

139. Lockshin MD, Reinitz E, Druzin ML, et al: Lupus pregnancy: Case-control prospective study demonstrating absence of lupus exacerbation during pregnancy. *Am J Med* 1984;77:893-898.

140. Out HJ, Derksen HWM, Christiaens GCML: Systemic lupus erythematosus and pregnancy. *Obstet Gynecol Surv* 1989;44:585-591.

141. Houser NT, Fish AJ, Tagatz GE, et al: Pregnancy and systemic lupus erythematosus. *Am J Obstet Gynecol* 1980; 138:409-413.

142. Tozman CS, Urowitz MB, Gladman DD: Systemic lupus erythematosus and pregnancy. *J Rheumatol* 1980;7:624-632.

143. Tincani A, Faden D, Tarantini M, et al: Systemic lupus erythematosus and pregnancy: a prospective study. *Clin Exp Rheumatol* 1992;10:439-446.

144. Briggs GG, Freeman RK, Yaffe SJ: *Drugs in Pregnancy and Lactation,* 3rd ed. Baltimore, Williams & Wilkins, 1990.

145. Leb DE, Weisskopf B, Kanovitz BS: Chromosome aberrations in the child of a transplant recipient. *Arch Intern Med* 1971;128:441-444.

146. Price H, Salaman J, Laurence K, et al: Immunosuppressive drugs and the fetus. *Transplantation* 1976;21:294.

147. Kutteh WH, Carr BR: Recurrent pregnancy loss, in Carr BR, Blackwell RC (eds): *Textbook of Reproductive Medicine.* Norwalk, Conn, Appleton & Lange, 1992.

148. Scott JR, Rote NS, Branch DW: Immunologic aspects of recurrent aboriton and fetal death. *Obstet Gynecol* 1987; 70:645.

149. Branch DW, Scott JR, Kochenour NK, et al: Obstetric complications associated with lupus anticoagulant. *N Engl J Med* 1985;313:1322.

150. Lubbe WF, Buttler WS, Palmer SJ, et al: Fetal survival after prednisone suppression of maternal lupus-anticoagulant. *Lancet* 1983;1:1361.

151. Hatakeyama M, Sumiya M, Gonda N, et al: Clinical study of systemic lupus

erythematosus and pregnancy. *Ryuma-chi* 1983;23:93-99.

Epilepsy

152. Buttino L Jr, Freeman RK: Seizure disorders of pregnancy. *Contemp Ob/Gyn*, June 1985, pp 62-68.
153. Hiilesmaa VK, Bardy A, Teramo K: Obstetric outcome in women with epilepsy. *Am J Obstet Gynecol* 1985;152: 499-504.
154. Teramo K, Hiilesmaa VK: Pregnancy and fetal complications in epileptic pregnancies: Review of the literature, in Janz D, Bossi I, Dam M (eds): *Epilepsy, Pregnancy and the Child.* New York, Raven Press, 1982, pp 53-60.
155. Dalessio DJ: Current concepts: Seizure disorders and pregnancy. *N Engl J Med* 1985;312:559-563.
156. Schmidt D, Canger R, Avanzini G, et al: Changes of seizure frequency in pregnant epileptic women. *J Neurol Neurosurg Psychiatry* 1983;46:751-755.
157. Remillard G, Dansky L, Andermann E, et al: Seizure frequency during pregnancy and the puerperium, in Janz D, Bossi I, Dam M (eds): *Epilepsy, Pregnancy and the Child.* New York, Raven Press, 1982, pp 15-26.
158. Speidel BD, Meadow SR: Maternal epilepsy and abnormalities in the fetus and newborn. *Lancet* 1972;2:839-843.
159. Hiilesmaa VK, Teramo K, Granstrom M-L, et al: Serum folate concentrations during pregnancy in women with epilepsy: Relation to antiepileptic drug concentrations, number of seizures, and fetal outcome. *Br Med J* 1983;287:577-579.
160. Armstrong RC, Monie IW: Congenital eye defects in rats following maternal folic acid deficiency during pregnancy. *J Embryol Exp Morphol* 1966;16:531.

161. Laurence KM, James N, Miller MH, et al: Increased risk of recurrence of pregnancies complicated by fetal neural tube defects in mothers receiving poor diets and possible benefits of dietary counseling. *Br Med J* 1980;281:1592-1594.
162. Kitay DZ: Folic acid and reproduction. *Clin Obstet Gynecol* 1979;22:809-817.
163. Scott DE, Whally PJ, Pritchard JA: Maternal folate deficiency and pregnancy wastage. *Obstet Gynecol* 1970; 36:26.
164. MRC Vitamin Study Research Group. Prevention of neural tube defects: Results of the Medical Research Council Vitamin Study. *Lancet* 1991;338: 131-137.
165. Centers for Disease Control. Use of folic acid for prevention of spina bifida and other neural tube defects 1983-1991. *MMWR* 1991;40:513-516.
166. Annegers JF, Houser WA, Elveback LR, et al: Seizure disorders in offspring of parents with a history of seizures— A maternal-paternal difference? *Epilepsia* 1976;17:1-9.
167. Janz D, Fuchs U: Are anti-epileptic drugs harmful when given during pregnancy? *Ger Med Mon* 1964;9:20-23.
168. Meadow SR: Anticonvulsant drugs and congenital abnormalities. *Lancet* 1968; 2:1296.
169. Fedrick J: Epilepsy and pregnancy: A report from the Oxford Record Linkage Study. *Br Med J* 1973;2:442-448.
170. Hill RM, Verniaud WM, Horning MG, et al: Infants exposed in utero to anti-epileptic drugs. *Am J Dis Child* 1974; 127:645-652.
171. Committee on Drugs, American Academy of Pediatrics: Anticonvulsants and pregnancy. *Pediatrics* 1979;63:331-333.
172. Friis ML, Hauge M: Congenital heart defects in liveborn children of epileptic parents. *Arch Neurol* 1985;42:374-376.

173. Eluma FO, Sucheston ME, Hayes TG, et al: Teratogenic effects of dosage levels and time of administration of carbamazepine, sodium valproate, and diphenylhydantoin on craniofacial development in the CD-1 mouse fetus. *J Craniofac Genet Dev Biol* 1984;4: 191-210.

174. Fabro S, Brown NA, Scialli AR: Valproic acid and birth defects. *Reprod Toxicol* 1983;2:9-12.

175. Shapiro S, Slone D, Hartz SC, et al: Anticonvulsants and parental epilepsy in the development of birth defects. *Lancet* 1976;1:272-275.

176. Dieterich E, Steueling A, Lukas A, et al: Congenital anomalies in children of epileptic mothers and fathers. *Neuropaediatric* 1980;11:274-283.

177. Gomez MR: Possible teratogenicity of valproic acid. *J Pediatr* 1981;98:508-509.

178. Bailey CJ, Pool RW, Poskitt EM, et al: Valproic acid and fetal abnormality. *Br Med J* 1983;286:190.

179. Hanson JW, Smith DW: The fetal hydantoin syndrome. *J Pediatr* 1975; 87:285-290.

180. Strickler SM, Miller MA, Andermann E, et al: Genetic predisposition to phenytoin-induced birth defects. *Lancet* 1985;2:746-749.

181. German J, Kowal A, Ehlers KH: Trimethadione and human teratogenesis. *Teratology* 1970;3:349-362.

182. Jones KL, Lacro RV, Johnson KA, et al: Pattern of malformation in the children of women treated with carbamazepine during pregnancy. *N Engl J Med* 1989;320:1661-1666.

183. Callaghan N, Garrett A, Goggin T: Withdrawal of anticonvulsant drugs in patients free of seizures for two years: A prospective study. *N Engl J Med* 1988;318:942-946.

184. Biale Y, Lewenthal H: Effect of folic acid supplementation on congenital malformation due to anticonvulsive drugs. *Eur J Obstet Gynecol Reprod Biol* 1984;18:211-213.

Hemoglobinopathies

185. Foster HW Jr: Sickle cell disease in pregnancy: An update. *Obstet Gynecol Annu* 1983;12:147-163.

186. Powars DR, Sandhu M, Niland-Weiss J, et al: Pregnancy in sickle cell disease. *Obstet Gynecol* 1986;67:217-228.

187. Fort AT, Morrison JC, Berreras L, et al: Counseling for patients with sickle cell disease about reproduction: Pregnancy outcome does not justify the maternal risk. *Am J Obstet Gynecol* 1971;111: 391-396.

188. Anderson R, Cassell M, Mullinax GL, et al: Effect of normal cells on viscosity of sickle cell blood. *Arch Intern Med* 1963;111:286-294.

189. Morrison JC, Propst MG, Blake PG: Sickle haemoglobin and the gravid patient: A management controversy. *Clin Perinatol* 1980;7:273-284.

190. Cunningham GF, Pritchard JA, Mason R: Pregnancy and sickle haemoglobinopathies: Results with and without prophylactic transfusions. *Obstet Gynecol* 1983;62:419-424.

191. Tuck SM, James CE, Brewster EM, et al: Prophylactic blood transfusion in maternal sickle cell syndromes. *Br J Obstet Gynaecol* 1987;94:121-125.

192. Hobbins JC, Mahoney MJ: In utero diagnosis of hemoglobinopathies: Techniques for obtaining fetal blood. *N Engl J Med* 1974;290:1065-1067.

Cancer

193. Koren G, Weiner L, Lishner M, et al: Cancer in pregnancy: Identification of unanswered questions on maternal and

fetal risks. *Obstet Gynecol Surv* 1990; 45:509.

194. Landon MB: Malignant diseases, in Gabbe SG, Niebyl JR, Simpson JL (eds): Obstetrics: Normal and Problem Pregnancies, ed 2. New York, Churchill Livingstone, 1991.

195. Earley TK, Gallagher JQ, Chapman KE: Carcinoma of the breast in women under thirty years of age. *Am J Surg* 1969;118:832-834.

196. Diekamp U, Bitran J, Ferguson DJ: Breast cancer in young women. *J Reprod Med* 1976;17:255-265.

197. Nugent P, O'Connell TX: Breast cancer and pregnancy. *Arch Surg* 1985;120:1221-1224.

198. Cooper DR, Butterfield J: Pregnancy subsequent to mastectomy for cancer of the breast. *Ann Surg* 1969;171:429-433.

199. Harvey JC, Rosen PP, Ashikari R, et al: The effect of pregnancy on the prognosis of carcinoma of the breast following radical mastectomy. *Surg Gynecol Obstet* 1981;153:725-732.

200. Peters MV, Meakin JW: The influence of pregnancy in carcinoma of the breast. *Prog Clin Cancer* 1965;1:471-506.

201. Rissanen PM: Pregnancy following treatment of mammary carcinoma. *Acta Radiol Ther* 1962;8:415-420.

202. Lutz MH, Underwood PB, Rozier JC, et al: Genital malignancy in pregnancy. *Am J Obstet Gynecol* 1977;129:536-542.

203. Sablinska R, Tarlowska L, Stelmachow J: Invasive carcinoma of the cervix associated with pregnancy: Correlation between patient age, advancement of cancer and gestation, and results of treatment. *Gynecol Oncol* 1977;5:363-373.

204. Hacker NF, Bereck JS, Lagasse LD, et al: Carcinoma of the cervix associated with pregnancy. *Obstet Gynecol* 1982; 59:735-746.

205. Gilotra PM, Lee FY, Krupp PJ, et al: Carcinoma in situ of the cervix uteri in pregnancy. *Surg Gynecol Obstet* 1976; 142:396-398.

206. Richart RM, Barron BA: A follow-up study of patients with cervical dysplasia. *Am J Obstet Gynecol* 1969;105:386-393.

207. Marsh M, Fitzgerald PJ: Carcinoma in situ of the human uterine cervix in pregnancy. *Cancer* 1956;9:1195-1207.

208. Rutledge CE, Christopherson WM, Parker JE: Cervical dysplasia and carcinoma in pregnancy. *Obstet Gynecol* 1962;19:351-354.

209. Kiguchi K, Bibbo M, Hasegawa T, et al: Dysplasia during pregnancy: A cytologic follow-up study. *J Reprod Med* 1981;26:66-72.

210. Creasman WT, Parker RT: Management of early cervical neoplasia. *Clin Obstet Gynecol* 1975;18:233-245.

211. Bertini-Oliveira AM, Keppler MM, Luisi A, et al: Comparative evaluation of abnormal cytology, colposcopy and histopathology in preclinical cervical malignancy during pregnancy. *Acta Cytol* 1982;26:636-644.

212. Robboy SJ, Keh PC, Nickerson RJ, et al: Squamous cell dysplasia and carcinoma in situ of the cervix and vagina after prenatal exposure to diethylstilbestrol. *Obstet Gynecol* 1978;51:528-535.

213. McLaren HC, Jordan JA, Glover M, et al: Pregnancy after cone biopsy of the cervix. *J Obstet Gynaecol Br Commonw* 1974;81:383-384.

214. Jones JM, Sweetnam P, Hibbard BM: The outcome of pregnancy after cone biopsy of the cervix: A case control study. *Br J Obstet Gynaecol* 1979;86:913.

215. Jones HW, Buller RE: The treatment of cervical intraepithelial neoplasia by

cone biopsy. *Am J Obstet Gynecol* 1980;137:882-886.

216. Sivanesaretnam B, Jayalaskshmi P, Loo C: Surgical management of early invasive cancer of the cervix associated with pregnancy. *Gynecol Oncol* 1993; 48:68.

217. DiSaia BJ, Creasman WT (eds): *Clinical Gynecologic Oncology*. St. Louis, Mo, Mosby-Year Book, 1993.

218. Richert TA, Moore JO: Hodgkin's disease, in Gleicher N (ed): *Principles of Medical Therapy*. New York, Plenum Medical Book Co, 1985, pp 1057-1063.

219. Barry RM, Diamond HD, Carver CF: Influence of pregnancy on the course of Hodgkin's disease. *Am J Obstet Gynecol* 1962;84:445-457.

220. Holmes GE, Holmes FF: Pregnancy outcome of patients treated for Hodgkin's disease: A controlled study. *Cancer* 1978;41:1317-1322.

221. Blot WJ, Sawada H: Fertility among female survivors of the atomic bombs of Hiroshima and Nagasaki. *Am J Hum Genet* 1972;24:613-622.

222. Shaw MW, Damme C: Legal status of the fetus, in Milunsky A, Annas GJ (eds): *Genetics and the Law*. New York, Plenum Press, 1976, pp 3-18.

223. Alberman E, Polani PE, Fraser-Roberts JA, et al: Parental exposure to x-irradiation and Down's syndrome. *Ann Hum Genet* 1972;36:195-208.

224. Uchida IA, Holunga R, Lawler C: Maternal radiation and chromosomal aberrations. *Lancet* 1968;2:1045-1049.

225. Horning SJ, Hoppe RT, Kaplan HS, et al: Female reproductive potential after treatment for Hodgkin's disease. *N Engl J Med* 1981;304:1377-1382.

226. Andrieu JM, Ochoa-Molina ME: Menstrual cycle, pregnancies and offspring before and after MOPP therapy for Hodgkin's disease. *Cancer* 1983;52: 435-438.

227. Blatt J, Mulvihill JJ, Ziegler JL, et al: Pregnancy outcome following cancer chemotherapy. *Am J Med* 1980;69:828-832.

228. McCann SR, Daly H, Hanratty TD, et al: Hodgkin's disease and pregnancy. *Acta Haematol* 1981;66:67-68.

229. Silverberg E, Lubera J: Cancer statistics, 1986. *Cancer* 1986;36:9-25.

230. McCarthy KS Jr, Wortman J, Stowers S, et al: Sex steroid receptor analysis in human melanoma. *Cancer* 1980;46: 1463-1470.

231. Sutherland CM, Wittliff JL, Fuchs A, et al: Hormonal studies in a pregnant patient with malignant melanoma. *J Surg Oncol* 1983;22:191-192.

232. Danforth DN Jr, Russell N, McBride CM: Hormonal status of patients with primary malignant melanoma: A review of 313 cases. *South Med J* 1982; 6:661-664.

233. Day CL Jr, Mihm MC Jr, Lew RA, et al: Cutaneous malignant melanoma: Prognostic guidelines for physicians and patients. *Cancer* 1982;32:113-122.

234. George PA, Fortner JG, Pack GT: Melanoma with pregnancy. *Cancer* 1960; 13:854-859.

235. Shiu MH, Schottenfeld D, MacLean B, et al: Adverse effect of pregnancy on melanoma: A reappraisal. *Cancer* 1976;37:181-187.

236. Sutherland CM, Loutfi A, Mather FJ, et al: Effect of pregnancy upon malignant melanoma. *Surg Obstet Gynecol* 1983; 157:443-446.

237. Reintgen DS, McCarty KS, Vollmer R, et al: Malignant melanoma and pregnancy. *Cancer* 1985;55:1340-1344.

238. Ellis DL: Pregnancy and sex steroid hormone effects on nevi of patients with dysplastic nevus syndrome. *J Am Acad Dermatol* 1991;25:467-482.

5

Infectious Disease

M aternal infections may have both short- and long-term effects on the mother and the fetus, by reason of either the disease itself or its therapy. Pregnancy alters a woman's immune response, which may lead to serious maternal infections that can be transmitted to the fetus. In approximately 2.5% of births, there is evidence of fetal infection.

Before 16 weeks of gestation, the fetus is not competent to mount an adequate immunologic response; therefore, a bacterium or virus can freely disseminate, frequently causing serious effects. Fetal infection after 16 weeks of gestation may not be evident at birth; it may remain latent, only to manifest its effects years later. The following infections may cause serious fetal problems: rubella; group B streptococcal disease; toxoplasmosis; herpesvirus; cytomegalovirus; *Chlamydia trachomatis;* human papillomavirus; gonorrhea; syphilis; viral hepatitis; and acquired immunodeficiency syndrome (AIDS).

For all infections, the goals of preconceptional counseling are the same: to identify potentially dangerous infections; to provide treatment, if possible, before conception; to educate the potential mother about preventive measures; and to discuss realistically the risks that current or future infection may pose to the patient and to her child, if she becomes pregnant.

To assess their risk of infection, the preconceptional counselor should ask all patients the following questions:

- Does the patient or her partner have a history of sexually transmitted disease, such as gonorrhea, hepatitis B, or infection with *Chlamydia,* herpes simplex virus, human papillomavirus, or human immunodeficiency virus?
- Do the patient and her partner now or have they in the past engaged in behavior that places them at high risk for hepatitis B or infection with the human immunodeficiency virus? For example, have they
  —used intravenous street drugs
  —had multiple sexual partners
  —had a sexual partner who is suspected or known to have hepatitis B or to be infected with the human immunodeficiency virus
  —had a sexual partner who is known or suspected to be bisexual, homosexual, or a user of intravenous street drugs

165

- Has the patient or her partner received a blood transfusion?
- Is the patient or her partner occupationally exposed to the blood or body secretions of others?
- Has the patient documented immunity to rubella?
- Is the patient exposed to cats?

Rubella

Although rubella is observed most often in children younger than 5 years, it occasionally occurs in adults. If acquired during the first 8 weeks of pregnancy, maternal rubella infection has a fetal infection rate of 50%. The risk of congenital rubella syndrome, which includes abnormalities of the heart, eye, or ear, is 20% if maternal infection occurs during early pregnancy.

BACKGROUND

Since the development of the rubella vaccine, there has been a concerted effort in the United States to vaccinate all children. This widespread vaccination of children, together with the vaccination of women of childbearing age, has decreased but not eliminated the wild virus. Between 1988 and 1991, a resurgence of rubella infection occurred in the United States.[1] Compared with the all-time low incidence of 225 cases reported to the Centers for Disease Control (CDC) in 1988, an average exceeding 1,000 cases was recorded in subsequent years. The greatest increase occurred among persons over 15 years of age. As might be anticipated, this upsurge in rubella increased the incidence of fetal infection. In 1989, only 2 cases of congenital rubella syndrome (CRS) were reported to the CDC[1]; in 1990, 17 confirmed or compatible cases of CRS and 5 provisional cases were reported to the CDC.[2] These figures may reflect significant under reporting. A recent report on the largest cluster of CRS in the United States during the last decade indicates that 23 infants with CRS and 2 infants with congenital rubella infection were born in four southern California counties in 1990.[3]

Data from a variety of population-based screening programs show that 6% to 25% of postpubertal women are seronegative for rubella antibody.[4] The major cause of rubella susceptibility is failure to immunize children.[1,2,5]

Many opportunities to immunize susceptible women after childhood are missed. An analysis of the outbreak of CRS in southern California revealed that more than one half of the cases could have been prevented if screening and immunization opportunities had been acted upon.[3] For instance, eight of the women (38%) had negative or equivocal rubella test results recorded during nine previous pregnancies delivered in the United States but did not receive postpartum immunization; an additional four women known to be seronegative did not receive immunization after having induced abortions. The authors conclude that rubella screening and vaccination should become routine activities in all health care programs that serve women.

Rubella vaccine RA 27/3 is a live, attenuated virus vaccine. A single dose of the vaccine at 15 months of age or older induces antibody formation in more than 95% of inoculated persons. Furthermore, this particular vaccine appears to confer immunity for a longer period of time than did previously used vaccines.

Because rubella vaccine is a live, attenuated virus, vaccination is contraindicated during pregnancy and for 3 months before conception. An analysis of data collected on German and American women who had been vaccinated within 3 months of pregnancy, during early pregnancy, or after the first trimester revealed no rubella-related defects in the offspring,[6] although the presence of immunoglobulin M antibody in several children suggested in utero infection. Follow-up studies of the children with immunoglobulin M rubella antibody over 2 years demonstrated normal growth and development. Between 1971 and 1988, the CDC collected data on 212 infants born to women who were immunized with the RA 27/3 vaccine during the 3 months preceding pregnancy or during the first trimester.[7] Three of the infants had laboratory evidence of in utero infection, but no illness or defects were identified. The observed risk is therefore zero, although the theoretical risk may be as high as 1.7%.[2]

PRECONCEPTIONAL COUNSELING

The primary purpose of the rubella immunization program is to prevent the severe fetal effects of wild rubella virus. Further decreases in the incidence of rubella and its devastating consequences for a fetus cannot be expected unless there is a continued effort to vaccinate adults, particularly women of childbearing age, as well as children.

Rubella vaccine is contraindicated during pregnancy because of the theoretical, albeit small, risk of congenital rubella syndrome. Therefore, reasonable precautions should be taken to preclude vaccination of pregnant women. Rubella vaccine is recommended for all children and for nonpregnant, nonimmune teenagers and adults. All preconceptional patients should have documented evidence of rubella immunity. If a patient is rubella-susceptible and does not plan to become pregnant for at least 3 months, a rubella vaccination should be recommended. If rubella vaccination does occur within 3 months of conception or even during early pregnancy, the teratogenic risk is negligible; thus, rubella vaccination is not in itself a reason to interrupt the pregnancy.

Group B Streptococcal Disease

G roup B streptococcus (GBS) can be cultured from the rectum and vagina of 15% to 40% of all pregnant women. Clinical infection in pregnant women is uncommon, although it may be associated with postpartum fever, endometritis, cystitis, pyelonephritis, and preterm labor. Neonatal complications include neurologic sequelae and death. Current estimates indicate that as many as 50,000 pregnant women and 12,000 infants suffer morbidity or mortality related to GBS annually.[8,9]

BACKGROUND

Group B streptococcal disease has been recognized in recent years as an important perinatal pathogen with prevention potential. It is currently identified as the leading cause of perinatal bacterial infection in the United States.[8] GBS is a common bacterium found in the genitourinary and lower gastrointestinal tracts of adults. Colonization rates vary with subpopulations; some reports have indicated higher rates in women who are younger than 20 years old, primigravid, medically indigent, black, or from Hispanic populations of Caribbean origin.[9] GBS has been identified, however, in women of all socioeconomic and cultural backgrounds. Evidence of colonization through culture of the rectum and vagina may be transient or chronic and is not affected by progressing gestation.

GBS is characterized by efficient vertical transmission, with 40% to 73% of neonates born to women who carry the bacteria being colonized.[10] Colonization may result in no consequences, early-onset disease (before or at 7 days after birth), or late-onset disease (7 days to 3 months of age). Each year approximately 1,600 infants die from GBS infection, and an equal number suffer long-term neurologic complications from GBS-associated meningitis.[9] Overall mortality is 15% for early-onset disease and 10% for late-onset disease. A number of maternal characteristics increase the risk of GBS sepsis in neonates:

- preterm delivery
- multiple gestation
- prolonged rupture of membranes
- GBS bacteriuria
- "heavy" GBS colonization
- low maternal levels of circulating antibodies to group B streptococci

Pregnant women with group B streptococcus in the urine may be at increased risk for premature rupture of the fetal membranes and premature delivery.[11] In a study that included 68 women with group B streptococci in their urine, 35% of these women had primary rupture of the membranes, and 20% had premature delivery. Of the 2,677 pregnant women in the series who did not have urinary evidence of group B streptococci, 15% had premature rupture of the membranes, and 8.5% had premature delivery. Five infants, all of whose mothers had streptococci in their urine, developed clinical infections; four of the infants died.[11]

Treatment of colonized women has failed to eradicate group B streptococci permanently because the reservoir of organisms in the rectum is resistant to chemotherapy. Antibiotics, administered orally or intravenously, eliminate group B streptococci from the vagina, but the organisms often return after treatment is discontinued.

PRECONCEPTIONAL COUNSELING

Patients who have had a previous child with group B streptococcal sepsis or who have experienced previous preterm labor should have cultures taken of the urine, the outer one third of the vagina, and the rectum. If group B streptococcus is found, the patient may be given prophylactic penicillin orally for the remainder of the pregnancy. If she has had a positive culture during pregnancy or a history of neonatal morbidity or mortality from group B streptococcal sepsis, she should receive penicillin intravenously at the time of labor. Erythromycin may be used for patients who are allergic to penicillin.

Toxoplasmosis

oxoplasmosis in humans is generally a mild disease that poses little threat to immunocompetent persons, except during gestation; acute toxoplasmosis complicates approximately 0.1% to 0.5% of all pregnancies,[12] with potentially devastating consequences for the infected fetus.

BACKGROUND

The etiologic agent of toxoplasmosis is the protozoan *Toxoplasma gondii*, which is an intracellular parasite found in a variety of warm-blooded animals. In animals, the usual route of transmission is oral; after entering the body, the parasite crosses the intestinal epithelium and multiplies in a variety of tissues.[13] Gradually, within a few weeks or months, parasite-containing cysts form in the brain, retina, and muscles.

Toxoplasmosis in humans is most commonly transmitted by contact with domestic cats; knowledge of this risk often causes exaggerated alarm in pregnant women and in women considering pregnancy. Cats who scavenge for food are at greatest risk for infection, because their prey, especially rodents and birds, are likely to harbor the trophozoite cysts in their muscle tissue. Once the cyst has been eaten, its wall is digested, releasing organisms that invade the epithelium of the cat's small intestine. Here the *Toxoplasma gondii* multiply and produce gametes that unite to form oocysts, which are discharged in the fecal stream. Garden soil and litter boxes contaminated by cat feces then become a source of human infection. Even though 30% to 80% of domestic cats are seropositive for toxoplasmosis, most are asymptomatic.[14,15] Another source of human infection is ingestion of meat that contains the infective tissue cysts.

In the United States, approximately 30% of the adult population have serum antibody to *Toxoplasma*.[12] The most common manifestations in adults are anterior cervical lymphadenopathy, rash, fever, malaise, and muscle pain that resolves in approximately 2 weeks. In this country, primary toxoplasmosis occurs in 1 to 5 per 1,000 pregnancies.

The greatest risk for the fetus follows first-trimester infection: although only 9% of the fetuses will be born with congenital toxoplasmosis, two thirds of those infected will have severe disease, and an additional 5% will die in the fetal or neonatal period.[16] Chorioretinitis, hydrocephaly, microcephaly, hepatosplenomegaly, thrombocytopenia, and intracranial calcifications are among the severe sequelae.[16,17] In comparison, 59% of infants who are exposed during the third trimester have evidence of perinatal infection, but the manifestations are subclinical or mild.[16]

Indirect fluorescent antibody tests for immunoglobulins G and M that are specific for toxoplasmosis are available to assist in the diagnosis. If primary toxoplasmosis is acquired during pregnancy, the patient may be treated with sulfonamides, pyrimethamine, and folic acid.

PRECONCEPTIONAL COUNSELING

Women who have owned cats that hunt are likely to be seropositive for toxoplasmosis, and infection poses no risk to their offspring. Similarly, women who own cats that never go outside are at low risk. However, all patients should be advised to avoid possible exposure to the infectious oocysts carried in cat feces. Cat litter boxes should be emptied daily and disinfected by washing with 50% ammonia hydroxide. To avoid contamination of soil, where oocysts survive for several months, it is best to dispose of cat feces by flushing them down the toilet. The patient should not allow her cat to jump on the kitchen counter or table. In addition, the patient should be advised to avoid eating raw or undercooked meats and to wash her hands after handling such meat. Pork, beef, and mutton heated to 105°F should pose no risk. Routine serologic testing for *Toxoplasma gondii* during the prepregnancy period is not recommended.

Herpesvirus Infections

The herpesvirus group consists of four subsets of viruses: (1) herpes simplex virus, types 1 and 2; (2) varicella-zoster virus; (3) Epstein-Barr virus; and (4) cytomegalovirus. These viruses become latent after a primary infection, persisting in various tissues even when levels of circulating antibody are high. On reactivation of these viruses, the host may become symptomatic and infectious. A pregnant woman can infect her fetus or neonate in the course of either a primary or a recurrent infection.

GENITAL HERPES SIMPLEX INFECTION
Background

It has been estimated that nearly 25 million people in the United States now suffer from herpes simplex genital infections, and the incidence is increasing dramatically among those of reproductive age. From 1981 to 1988, the annual number of initial visits to physicians' offices for diagnosis and treatment of genital herpes simplex virus type 2 (HSV-2) infections increased from approximately 58,000 to 169,000.[4] Antibodies to herpes simplex virus are present in 10% to 70% of women.[18] Symptomatic and asymptomatic carriers may transmit infection to susceptible individuals via inoculation on the skin or mucous membranes.

The major modes of transmission of herpes simplex virus type 1 differ from those of herpes simplex virus type 2. Type 1 is a common infection (cold sores) that may be transmitted orally. The infection is asymptomatic in the vast majority of patients, and the reasons for its reactivation are unknown. Type 1 is rarely a source of neonatal infection.

Herpes simplex virus type 2 may be the cause of an oral lesion, but lesions are more commonly located in the genital region. In most cases, HSV-2 is transmitted through sexual contact.[18] Depending on socioeconomic class, approximately 0.65% to 1% of pregnant women excrete the genital herpes virus.[19] According to retrospective estimates, approximately 1 in 7,500 liveborn infants will acquire HSV-2 through perinatal transmission.[20] More than 60% of women who give birth to infected infants are asymptomatic.[19,21]

Primary infection with genital herpes during pregnancy poses a significant risk to the fetus and to the newborn.[22] Spontaneous abortion and severe congenital anomalies have been associated with primary infection during the first trimester, and increased perinatal mortality and severe morbidity have been associated with primary infections during the second and, particularly, third trimesters. Lesser risk is posed to fetuses and neonates exposed to recurrent maternal HSV-2 infections. A recent report indicates a theoretic maximum infection rate of 8% in neonates exposed to recurrent HSV at the time of delivery.[23] Reliance on antenatal viral cultures to identify pregnant patients who are at risk has proved costly, has been associated with an increased cesarean birth rate, and has not reduced the incidence of neonatal herpes infection. This approach has, therefore, been abandoned as either an appropriate or an effective method of preventing neonatal infection.[22] Current techniques include careful inspection of the maternal genital tract at the onset of labor (with cesarean birth if suspicious lesions are identified); intrapartum HSV cultures of the external genitalia and cervix; and cultures of the newborn at birth, including the oropharynx, conjunctiva, and umbilicus.

Acyclovir has been administered orally and intravenously during all stages of pregnancy; no adverse fetal effects have been identified, but first-trimester data is extremely limited.[24]

Preconceptional Counseling

During the prepregnancy period, the patient who has recurrent genital herpes or whose partner has had documented herpes simplex virus infection should be informed about the risk that she and her partner will transmit the infection to each other and to their offspring. They should abstain from intercourse while genital lesions are present. The woman should learn to recognize her prodromal signs and symptoms. For example, she may experience tingling, burning, or itching a few hours to a day before lesions appear. The patient should consider herself infectious from the time she is first aware of symptoms until all lesions are completely healed.

Although it is unlikely that herpes simplex virus will survive on bath towels, bathtubs, or toilet seats, the use of separate towels during acute attacks is prudent, and chlorine-containing solutions (e.g., bleach) are excellent cleaning solutions for bathtubs and toilet seats. Hot tubs and swimming pools have not been found to be a source of genital herpes infection.

During the prepregnancy period, a patient with a history of recurrent herpes should be advised to inform her obstetric care provider of her or her partner's history of genital or oral herpes. The preconceptional counselor should explain to the patient the importance of definite diagnosis and preventive measures. The patient should be informed of the possibility of cesarean delivery if she has a recent positive culture (within 1 week) or active lesions at the time of labor. Her partner's use of a latex condom during sexual intercourse throughout her pregnancy may decrease the number of recurrent episodes of herpes.[25-27]

VARICELLA-ZOSTER VIRUS INFECTION
Background

Adults are generally seropositive for varicella-zoster virus, making varicella infection during pregnancy relatively rare, occurring in approximately 1 in 7,500 pregnant women.[12] Ten percent to thirty percent of women who contract varicella during pregnancy will develop varicella pneumonia; this complication is associated with a maternal mortality rate as high as 40%. Large studies in the United States and Britain have failed to document a significant risk of embryopathy secondary to varicella during the first 20 weeks of pregnancy,[28,29] although first-trimester infection has been associated with a congenital syndrome characterized by limb hypoplasia, cutaneous scars, chorioretinitis, cataracts, cortical atrophy, and microcephaly.[12] There is, however, a 30% chance that the fetus will be infected with varicella-zoster virus if the mother has chickenpox and delivers within 5 days of symptom development. Neonatal varicella is associated with a high mortality rate. The administration of zoster-immune globulin to the neonate upon delivery or within the first 24 hours significantly decreases this risk.

Preconceptional Counseling

In general, other than obtaining a thorough history that indicates whether the patient has had chickenpox, no preconceptional strategies are necessary regarding varicella-zoster virus. Serologic testing for varicella-zoster virus is not routine. However, an antibody test for varicella may be indicated for women with negative histories and small children who have not had varicella. Nurses and teachers who work with small children also are at risk.

EPSTEIN-BARR VIRUS INFECTION

The occurrence of infectious mononucleosis during pregnancy is rare. When it has occurred, it has not been associated with any increase in congenital anomalies or maternal complications. No specific preconceptional counseling is necessary.

CYTOMEGALOVIRUS INFECTION
Background

Approximately 0.2% to 2.2% of all liveborn infants are infected with cytomegalovirus. Most neonates are infected perinatally through exposure to contaminated maternal blood; urine; or cervical, vaginal, or breast secretions.[30] Even though 35% to 90% of women in their childbearing years are seropositive for cytomegalovirus, the virus can be cultured from the cervical tissue of 3% to 28% of pregnant women.[31] The excretion rates are highest in young, socioeconomically deprived, sexually promiscuous persons.[32]

Intrauterine transmission of cytomegalovirus after a primary maternal infection occurs in 40% to 50% of fetuses; 30% to 50% of these infections are clinically recognized at birth. Cytomegalovirus can be transmitted in utero through reactivation of a latent maternal infection, even in a seropositive woman, but a fetal infection acquired in this way is rarely evident at birth. Of congenitally infected infants without clinically apparent infection at birth, 5% to 15% develop late-appearing progressive deafness, learning disabilities, cerebral palsy, hydrocephalus, or eye problems.

Preconceptional Counseling

Asymptomatic infection with cytomegalovirus appears to be common in adults and children, although it does not appear to be highly contagious. Infection seems to require close contact with a person who is excreting the virus in the semen, saliva, urine, or blood. The person who has multiple sexual partners has an increased risk of exposure to cytomegalovirus. At particular risk for transmission and infection of the virus are children and susceptible workers in day-care centers. Data indicate that the cumulative infection rate of children who attend day-care centers may be as high as 80% by age 2.[33] The actual risk of exposure and spread of cytomegalovirus to day-care center personnel is not known. Day-care personnel who are considering pregnancy or who are pregnant should be informed of the potential risk of infection. Good personal hygiene measures, such as washing the hands after each contact with body secretions and careful handling and disposal of diapers contaminated with urine, are essential.

According to Balfour and Balfour,[34] primary acquisition of cytomegalovirus is not an occupational risk for renal transplant and neonatal staff nurses. Of the 943 nurses studied, 33% were seropositive for cytomegalovirus. The yearly conversion rate for these nurses was 1.84%, which did not differ significantly from that of control groups. It appears that the acquisition of cytomegalovirus by susceptible nurses in these environments requires prolonged intimate contact. Precautions such as the use of gowns and gloves and thorough hand-washing after each patient contact are good preventive measures.

During the prepregnancy period, routine culture or antibody identification for cytomegalovirus is not indicated. There is no known specific treatment for cytomegalovirus.

Chlamydial Infection

C *hlamydia trachomatis* is classified as a bacterium, but it has characteristics of both bacteria and viruses. Infection with this microorganism is a common disease that is sexually transmitted and affects approximately three to five million Americans each year.[35]

BACKGROUND

Chlamydia trachomatis infection is now recognized as the leading bacterial source of sexually transmitted disease in the United States.[36] Women risk serious reproductive consequences from infection, most notably pelvic inflammatory disease (PID) and its long-term sequelae, including infertility and ectopic pregnancy. More than one million cases of PID are reported annually.[1] Patients at highest risk for cervical infection with *C. trachomatis* are young (less than 25 years old), have multiple sexual partners, and usually do not use barrier contraception.

Approximately 50% to 70% of women with chlamydial infection are asymptomatic.[37] When symptoms do occur, women complain of burning and itching of the vagina; a persistent, purulent, yellow vaginal discharge; dysuria; or chronic pelvic pain. Perhaps 15% of women with pelvic inflammatory disease become infertile after a single infection with *Chlamydia,* even though the symptoms are clinically mild. In men, who are more often symptomatic, chlamydial infection may result in dysuria and penile discharge; infection in men is often diagnosed as nongonococcal urethritis.[38]

In the United States, the average prevalence of maternal chlamydial infection during pregnancy has been reported to be 5%,[39] although a range from 2% to 37% has been reported for subpopulations.[35]

Maternal infection with *C. trachomatis* during pregnancy is associated with postpartum endometritis, and some studies have shown an increased perinatal mortality rate secondary to premature rupture of the membranes.[40-43] This remains controversial, however, as do suggested associations of maternal infection with spontaneous abortion, preterm labor, and low birthweight. A patient with *Chlamydia* infection can transmit the disease to her infant during vaginal delivery. Estimates indicate that as many as 155,000 neonates are exposed to *Chlamydia* during the birth process, and 100,000 are infected.[4,44] *Chlamydia* is the most common cause of inclusion conjunctivitis, afebrile interstitial pneumonia, and broncheolitis in the neonate, as well as of repeated otitis media under 6 months of age.[35,45]

177

PRECONCEPTIONAL COUNSELING

Screening for infection with *Chlamydia* should be considered during the prepregnancy period for all women with a history of pelvic inflammatory disease, multiple sexual partners, or sexually transmitted disease. Cultures of the endocervix, if taken properly, are the gold standard and can detect 90% of the infections in nonpregnant and pregnant women. Positive cultures of the cervix or urogenital tract in nonpregnant women should be treated with doxycycline, 100 mg administered orally twice a day for 14 days. Sexual partners should be examined for other sexually transmitted diseases and treated for *Chlamydia* infection. It is recommended that the patient and her partner avoid sexual intercourse until both have completed treatment.

The patient should be informed that cultures may be repeated during pregnancy; if an antenatal culture is positive for *Chlamydia,* the treatment of choice is erythromycin, 500 mg administered orally 4 times a day for 14 days. It may also be advisable to administer prophylactic systemic erythromycin and erythromycin eye drops to the newborn. Barrier methods of birth control (e.g., latex condoms or a diaphragm with spermicidal agents) may provide some protection against chlamydial infection; the partner's use of latex condoms during sexual relations may be appropriate for a pregnant patient with a history of recurrent chlamydial infection.

Human Papillomavirus Infection

L ike chlamydial infection, human papillomavirus (HPV) infection is sexually transmitted, and, like the herpes simplex virus, subclinical infections are more common than symptomatic presentations.[4] It has reached epidemic proportions, with an estimated 40 million people now infected. During the last decade there was a 400% increase in the number of visits to physicians' offices for this condition. Estimates of the prevalence of HPV infection range from 5% to 27%, depending on the population tested.[4] Today, as many as 2% of all women tested by Papanicolaou smear have cytologic evidence of human papillomavirus infection. The human papillomavirus–DNA hybridization analysis has identified 46 different viral types.

BACKGROUND

Changes in the cervix as a result of human papillomavirus infection are associated with 90% of cervical dysplasia.[46,47] Infection with human papillomavirus proliferates during pregnancy, possibly secondary to an impairment in cell-mediated immunity. Lesions appear on the anogenital skin and mucous membranes. The infection may involve the cervix, vagina, and vulva so extensively that cesarean delivery is necessary to prevent severe maternal trauma during delivery. Furthermore, these lesions may result in viral transmission to the fetus, resulting in childhood laryngeal papillomas that are associated with recurrent respiratory infections.[48]

PRECONCEPTIONAL COUNSELING

As with all sexually transmitted diseases, the only absolute approach to prevention is a lifetime history of sex with only one partner who has also had no other partner. The use of latex condoms may afford some protection. During the prepregnancy period, lesions can be treated by a variety of techniques and medications: cryotherapy; electrocautery; carbon dioxide laser; and local applications of 10% or 25% podophyllin, trichloroacetic acid, or 5-fluorouracil.

During preconceptional counseling, the patient should be informed that treatment with topical trichloroacetic acid, cryotherapy, or vaginal antiseptic creams may be necessary during pregnancy. The chances of recurrence or continued growth are high, however. Unless the infection is extensive, cesarean delivery is not indicated. Transplacental passage of certain types of human papillomavirus continues to be a matter of controversy.

179

Gonorrhea

The most commonly reported sexually transmitted disease in the United States is gonorrhea, an infection caused by *Neisseria gonorrhoeae*. In 1989, approximately 740,000 cases were reported by the CDC, representing a decline from nearly 900,000 cases reported annually in the early 1980s.[49] Gonorrheal infections are often asymptomatic, thereby delaying diagnosis and treatment. Pelvic inflammatory disease, with the concomitant complications of infertility and ectopic pregnancy, are common consequences of infection. Depending on the population studied, the prevalence of gonorrhea in an obstetric clinic can be as high as 6%. Ophthalmia neonatorum as a consequence of maternal gonococcal infection has always been a serious concern. More recently, an association has been recognized between maternal gonococcal infection and disseminated gonococcal infection, amniotic fluid or membrane infection, preterm labor, and premature rupture of the membranes.[50] In pregnant women, gonococcal infection is most commonly asymptomatic. In any patient with a vaginal discharge, dysuria, and inflammation of the cervix accompanied by a mucopurulent discharge, however, gonorrhea should be considered.

PRECONCEPTIONAL COUNSELING

Because *Chlamydia* infection is common in those who have or have had gonorrhea, the patient with a history of gonorrhea should have during the prepregnancy period a *Chlamydia* culture of the cervix in addition to gonorrheal cultures of the anal canal, the urethra, and the endocervix. If the gonorrheal culture is positive, the CDC recommends that the patient and her partner be treated with ceftriaxone, a new antibiotic that kills penicillin-resistant strains of *Neisseria gonorrhoeae*. If the *Chlamydia* culture is also positive, tetracycline in the dosages outlined earlier should be prescribed.

Should pregnancy occur, gonorrheal cultures should be taken in the beginning of pregnancy as well as in the third trimester; ceftriaxone treatment should be prescribed if cultures are positive. The infant should be treated with eye drops that contain silver nitrate and tetracycline or erythromycin for protection not only against gonococcal infection but also against the frequently concomitant chlamydial infection.

Syphilis

The incidence of primary and secondary syphilis in the United States is increasing. The estimated annual rate of primary and secondary syphilis per 100,000 population rose from 10.9 to 13.3 cases between 1986 and 1987.[51] Comparing the first 3 months of 1986 with the first 3 months of 1987, the number of reported syphilis cases increased by 50% in New York City, by 86% in Florida, and by 97% in Los Angeles County.[51]

During the first 3 months of 1987, the CDC reported 8,274 cases of primary and secondary syphilis, compared with 6,725 cases reported during the same period in 1986.[51] Overall, this is the largest increase in the incidence of syphilis in 10 years.

Of women with primary or secondary syphilis, 80% are between the ages of 15 and 34, in the reproductive years. After an 8-year decline, the CDC reported that the number of cases of congenital syphilis rose from 166 in 1983 to 268 in 1985[51]; 1,751 cases were reported in 1989.[49] The latter figure reflects the upward trend noted throughout the 1980s but also reflects a 1989 change in case definition. The increasing occurrence of congenital syphilis indicates a lack of prenatal care or a failure of serologic testing, treatment, or follow-up during prenatal care.

BACKGROUND

Syphilis is a systemic infection with the spirochete *Treponema pallidum*. It may occur as a painless ulcer on the genitalia, pharynx, or rectum. Syphilitic ulcers can facilitate the spread of the human immunodeficiency virus because they may serve as portals of entry and reservoirs for the virus. If untreated, syphilis may progress to clinical syndromes, including secondary syphilis (associated with rash and lymphadenopathy) and tertiary syphilis (associated with cardiovascular and neurologic complications).

A pregnant woman with untreated syphilis at any stage can pass the disease to her fetus. Congenitally infected neonates may have rhinitis, vesicular cutaneous lesions, hepatosplenomegaly, lymphadenopathy, and anemia at birth, or they may show no sign of the infection until the third or fourth week of life. Patients with syphilis have an increased incidence of premature delivery.

Most states require prenatal screening for syphilis in the first trimester, but not in the third trimester. Thus, infections acquired later during pregnancy may not be detected and may cause fetal infections. To decrease the incidence of congenital syphilis, it is necessary to perform serologic screening tests in the first trimester, to repeat the tests in high-risk groups during the third trimester, and to provide prompt treatment and adequate follow-up of maternal cases.

PRECONCEPTIONAL COUNSELING

Women who are undergoing treatment for syphilis require close follow-up; their sexual partners may also need treatment. Follow-up care should include monthly determinations of serologic titers and physical examinations for evidence of clinical infection. Patients should be treated for a fourfold increase in their VDRL titer or for clinical recurrences. The patient should not consider pregnancy until treatment has been completed.

Should the patient become pregnant while under treatment, serial serologic testing is required. At the time of delivery, serologic tests of umbilical cord blood and examination of the neonate for evidence of congenital syphilis are advisable.[52]

Viral Hepatitis

O f the major causes of viral hepatitis, only hepatitis B virus (HBV) has been documented as transmissible to a fetus. The presence of hepatitis B surface antigen (HBsAg) in the serum of the patient establishes the diagnosis and identifies the patient as a potential source of infection for her family, her infant, and the medical personnel who care for her.[53]

Chronic HBV infection is a major cause of acute and chronic hepatitis, cirrhosis, and primary hepatocellular carcinoma. It affects as many as 200 million persons, or 5% of the world's population. The prevalence of this infection is as high as 20% in populations from Africa, Asia, and the Pacific Basin[53] but is generally low (0.5% to 1%) in the United States. Hepatitis B is the most common type of hepatitis in the United States, however, with 300,000 cases per year.[54] Hepatitis B occurs predominantly in homosexual men, parenteral drug users, and persons who have acquired the disease through heterosexual contacts. Five percent to ten percent of homosexuals and illegal drug users have HBsAg in their serum.

BACKGROUND

Data from the CDC indicate that each year nearly 19,000 women with HBV infection give birth in the United States. Approximately 46% of these women are Asian and foreign-born, 21% are white, 20% are black, and 11% are Hispanic.[4(p33)]

The incidence of in utero HBV infection has been variously estimated. Both pregnant women who have active disease and those who are chronic asymptomatic carriers can transmit the infection to their fetuses. Approximately 10% of patients with HBV infection become chronic carriers. Even though 90% of these chronic carriers are asymptomatic, they pose the greatest threat to the fetus. It is believed that the primary route for perinatal infection is through exposure to maternal blood and excreta.

The risk of infection in infants is directly related to the HBsAg titer or to the hepatitis B e antigen (HBeAg) titer in maternal blood. Approximately 90% of infants whose mothers have both antigens become infected, and most of these will be permanent carriers.[55] A newborn who becomes a carrier for HBV has a 25% risk of dying from a liver-related disease.[56] Infected infants born to women who are asymptomatic carriers, as well as those born to mothers who have acute HBV infection, remain HBsAg-positive for months to years. These children often have chronic hepatitis and high incidences of hepatoma and childhood liver carcinoma. The incidence of liver carcinoma and cirrhosis can be reduced by 75% in infants born to women who are HBsAg-positive, however, if hepatitis B immune globulin and hepatitis vaccine are administered within 48 hours of birth.[57]

In general, pregnancy does not alter the course of disease in a patient with HBV infection.

PRECONCEPTIONAL COUNSELING

Although all body fluids may contain HBV, the infection is predominantly a blood-borne and sexually transmitted disease. If patients or their sexual partners have a history of chronic hepatitis, multiple sexual partners, venereal disease, parenteral drug use, or household contact with dialysis patients or hemophiliacs, or if they work as nonimmunized health care providers, they should be considered to be at risk. Patients from Asia, Alaska, and the Pacific Islands are at a particularly high risk. All patients at risk should be tested for the presence of HBsAg and HBeAg; if the antigens are present, liver function should be assessed. If liver function is abnormal, additional rest and a high-calorie, high-protein diet should be prescribed during the preconceptional period. The patient should be informed that serial liver function tests will be needed during pregnancy and that the neonate will receive a hepatitis immune globulin and vaccine series that will begin within 48 hours of birth.

There is no increased incidence of congenital malformation in the offspring of mothers who are HBsAg-positive or HBeAg-positive. Fifteen percent to twenty percent of all health care workers have one or more serologic markers for hepatitis B, and 1% to 2% are HBsAg-positive. Active vaccination for all hospital personnel is critical as a preventive measure.

Human Immunodeficiency Virus Infection

S ince 1981, when the acquired immunodeficiency syndrome (AIDS) was first described in the United States, 133,233 persons have died from the infection; 13,863 of them were women.[58] AIDS is now a leading cause of death in women of reproductive age in the United States. According to the CDC, by the end of 1991, 202,921 cases of AIDS had been reported; 21,225 of these cases were in women.[58] The largest number of cases in females occurred in those who were 30 to 34 years of age (25%), with a slightly lower percentage occurring in those who were 25 to 29 (18%) and 35 to 39 (19%) years of age. Fifty percent of recognized infections in women are traced to exposure through injecting illicit drugs; of those who became infected through heterosexual contact (34%), more than 60% reported that their sexual partners injected illicit drugs. Eight percent of the total number of cases in women were linked to receipt of blood transfusions, blood components, or tissue, and 7% contracted the disease through undetermined routes. The number of AIDS cases associated with heterosexual transmission steadily increased during the 1980s.

Estimating the prevalence of the human immunodeficiency virus (HIV), which causes AIDS, is difficult. Most studies have been of special populations and cannot be generalized.[59,60] The CDC and others have attempted to establish prevalence estimates by testing populations undifferentiated by socioeconomic variables. Several of these studies have used neonatal blood samples that are screened anonymously to determine HIV exposure and, thus, maternal rates of infection. Gwinn and associates[61] estimate that 0.15% of women who gave birth in 1989 were infected; extrapolating this rate to all women of reproductive age, they estimate that as many as 80,000 women may already be infected.

BACKGROUND

The causative agent in AIDS is the retrovirus HIV.[62] This virus, which affects predominantly the T_4-helper lymphocytes, is capable of infecting body fluids, such as blood, breast milk, semen, urine, vaginal secretions, and saliva. The proportion of the virus in these fluids is related to the number of lymphocytes present; the proportion is high in semen, for instance, and low in saliva and tears. HIV possesses an enzyme called reverse transcriptase, which enables it to make a DNA copy in the

185

host germ cell. This leads to latency and permanency.[62] Eventually, HIV depletes the T_4-helper lymphocytes, resulting in defects in cell-mediated immunity and in the onset of opportunistic infections. These infections indicate progression to AIDS. The mean interval between HIV infection and the onset of AIDS is 7 years.

A large increase in the number of AIDS cases reported to the CDC through its surveillance program occurred in 1993 after its case definition was revised. Effective January 1, 1993, HIV-infected persons with severe immunosuppression and no evidence of opportunistic infection, as well as those with pulmonary tuberculosis, recurrent pneumonia, or invasive cervical cancer, were added to the number of AIDS cases. Of the 35,799 AIDS cases reported to the CDC during the first 3 months of 1993, 60% were reported as a result of the expanded definition. Most (89%) were added because of severe HIV-related immunosuppression.[63]

Transmission of HIV

The three major ways in which HIV can be transmitted are
1. through heterosexual or homosexual contact
2. through injection of blood or infectious body fluids, such as semen
3. through perinatal infection

A small but increasingly important factor is perinatal transmission from mostly asymptomatic HIV-positive mothers to their offspring. There is some evidence to indicate that in utero transmission may occur. Virus-infected cells were found in the tissue of children born by cesarean delivery to mothers who died of AIDS within a few hours of delivery.[64,65] Casual contact with HIV from food or environmental surfaces does not transmit the virus, and patient contact by health care personnel who use reasonable precautions has not been documented as a cause for seroconversion.[66] Accidental injury with needles contaminated with blood from HIV-infected people results in a less than 1% risk of transmission of the infection.[67]

The risk for HIV disease in women, like other sexually transmitted diseases, is dependent on the number of their sexual partners and the incidence of clinical or serologic evidence of HIV among them.[68] Women who are seropositive for HIV are nearly five times more likely than are seronegative women to have had more than 100 sexual contacts with an infected man. In addition, women who use or have used illicit drugs intravenously or who come from countries where the heterosexual transmission of HIV is common (e.g., countries of central and east Africa and Haiti) are at significant risk for HIV infection. The efficiency of HIV male-to-female sexual transmission varies by the source of male infection and has been reported to be 6% among the partners of hemophiliacs, 16% among the partners of men with transfusion-associated infection, 23% among the partners of bisexual men, and 35% among the partners of male intravenous drug users.[69]

Human immunodeficiency virus is much less likely to be transmitted through a single sexual contact than is *Neisseria gonorrhoeae* or hepatitis B virus. The incidence of gonorrhea is estimated at 22% to 25% after a single exposure of a man to an infected woman and 50% after a single exposure of a woman to an infected man. Hepatitis B virus is 30 to 100 times more infectious than is HIV. Approximately 6% of people infected with hepatitis B virus become chronic carriers, however, compared with 100% of those infected with HIV.

Manifestations of HIV Infection

Most patients who acquire HIV infection have a positive serologic test for the virus, but they may remain asymptomatic for years. For every one person with AIDS, there are approximately 50 to 100 asymptomatic seropositive persons. There is a 50% to 60% likelihood that a person will develop AIDS within 5 years of laboratory evidence of infection.[70]

During the asymptomatic period, the person is infectious through sexual contact, contact with blood (e.g., through needle sharing), and pregnancy. This asymptomatic period may be followed by a mononucleosis-type illness, with fever, weight loss, lymphadenopathy, lethargy, and a marked lymphopenia. AIDS-related complex (ARC) occurs in a patient who is seropositive for HIV antibody and has persistent, nonspecific symptoms and lymphadenopathy for longer than 6 months for no demonstrable reason, despite appropriate medical workup. Multiple defects in natural immunity against diseases are characteristic of AIDS. In the later stages, patients may develop major opportunistic infections, such as *Pneumocystis carinii* pneumonia (protozoa), persistent herpes simplex (virus), tuberculosis (bacteria), or neoplasms, such as Kaposi's sarcoma or lymphoma.

It is not yet known whether the immunologic changes of pregnancy affect the progression of HIV disease. Some reports have indicated a declining status with pregnancy,[71,72] but most studies have not included a nonpregnant control population. One study that compares pregnant and nonpregnant patients indicates little or no difference in the rate of immunologic or clinical deterioration between the two groups.[73]

Many of the factors associated with the perinatal transmission of HIV are unknown. Apparently, the mother who has had subclinical disease for many years may or may not transmit the disease to her offspring. There is one documented instance of postpartum transmission, possibly via breast-feeding.[74] Nearly all mothers are asymptomatic when they deliver their first infected children.[62]

In a study of 16 mothers who had 22 infants with AIDS or ARC, Scott and colleagues[71] found that all except one of the mothers were clinically free of AIDS at the time of delivery. Five of these mothers developed clinically apparent AIDS 12 to 30 months after giving birth to a child infected with HIV. Clinical manifestations in the infants were hepatitis, toxoplasmosis, and other infections. An average of 4 months elapsed after delivery before the clinical signs of AIDS-related complex became manifest in the infant. Some mothers remained clinically well, despite evidence that they were carriers of the disease. Six of the sixteen mothers whose serologic tests strongly suggested immunodeficiency syndrome have subsequently given birth to children who did not have the syndrome.

PRECONCEPTIONAL COUNSELING

Prepregnancy counseling for HIV-infected patients must include strategies for reducing or eliminating their risk of acquiring *all* sexually transmitted diseases. In general, those men and women known to have sexually transmitted disease should not plan a pregnancy until they have undergone treatment and examination indicates that the infection is no longer present. Unfortunately, many patients with sexually transmitted disease remain infectious, even after they have become asymptomatic.

Patients can reduce or eliminate their risk of acquiring sexually transmitted disease by avoiding sexual partners who are likely to have such disease and by limiting the number of their sexual partners. A study of men with recurrent gonorrhea indicated that those who were free of infection during a 9-month period had reduced the number of their sexual partners, whereas those who became reinfected had multiple contacts.[75]

The correct and consistent use of latex condoms effectively prevents the transmission of most sexually transmitted diseases.[75-78] In a prospective study, researchers found that men who always used condoms were less likely to be infected with *Neisseria gonorrhoeae* and herpes simplex virus than were those who had never used condoms.[79] Women whose sexual partners use condoms have a significantly lower risk of hospitalization for pelvic inflammatory disease than do women who use no method of contraception.[80,81] In addition, in vitro studies have shown the latex condom to be impermeable to the herpes simplex virus, cytomegalovirus, *Chlamydia trachomatis,* and HIV.[26,82,83]

The use of a spermicide in conjunction with a latex condom or diaphragm further protects men and women against sexually transmitted disease.[84] Spermicides have been shown in vitro to inhibit *N. gonorrhoeae* and *Trichomonas vaginalis,* to inactivate culture of herpes simplex virus type 2 and HIV, and to decrease the infectivity of *Treponema pallidum.*[85,86] Used alone, vaginal spermicides that contain nonoxynol-9 appear to decrease the risk of gonorrhea, but not as effectively as they do when combined with the use of a condom. In a large, randomized clinical trial, the reinfection rate for women recently treated for gonorrhea who used nonoxynol-9 foam for 6 months was one-tenth that of a control group.[87] Comparisons with women who use an oral contraceptive or those who have undergone surgical sterilization have shown that women who use a spermicide are at one-tenth the risk of contracting gonorrhea.[88]

The preconceptional counselor should provide pertinent information to men and women whose behavior has placed them at risk for an HIV infection. They need extensive information not only on their own current health status but also on measures to prevent infection in themselves and their offspring.[89-91] Historical screening, monitoring, and counseling for patients at risk for HIV should be part of sexually transmitted disease clinics, drug abuse programs, family planning clinics, women's health and preconceptional clinics, and prenatal care programs. Although not all-inclusive, the following are indications for HIV screening:

- persistent candidiasis of the mouth and pharynx
- presence of *Mycobacterium tuberculosis*
- herpes simplex virus infections that persist for more than 1 month
- present or former intravenous drug use
- nonmonogamous relationships
- emigration from a country that has high heterosexual transmission rates, such as Haiti and countries in east and central Africa
- sexual partners who are intravenous drug users, bisexuals, hemophiliacs, or those who have evidence of HIV infection

Screening for HIV antibodies, which indicates whether the patient has a current infection, is usually performed with a highly sensitive and specific enzyme-linked immunosorbent assay (ELISA). Test results are generally validated by Western Blot immunofluorescence assays.[92] It should be made clear to patients that the antibody to HIV may not be detectable for 4 to 6 months after exposure and infection. Therefore, it may be necessary to repeat the test periodically for those who have been exposed. Those at risk who remain serologically negative should be advised to modify their behavior and to take appropriate precautions against becoming infected.

The strategies recommended for preventing transmission of HIV are based on the knowledge that the virus is present in many body fluids, including blood, semen, vaginal and cervical secretions, saliva, tears, and urine. The following principles are relevant to preventive counseling:

- A monogamous sexual relationship in which both partners know whether they are infected with HIV and take precautions, if necessary, decreases sexual transmission rates.
- Women infected with HIV should inform their sexual partners of the infection and the availability of HIV testing.
- Women infected with HIV should be informed that they are unlikely to transmit the infection to household members with whom their contact is nonsexual. It is recommended, however, that HIV-infected patients keep separate items that can become contaminated with blood (e.g., toothbrushes and razors). Household areas that may become contaminated with blood should be cleaned with a freshly prepared 1:10 bleach:water solution.
- It is unknown whether pregnancy in an HIV-infected patient will exacerbate the disease. If she chooses to continue the pregnancy, the woman should understand that the infection is passed to 25% to 35% of exposed fetuses and that rapid progression to AIDS and death for the infected infant is likely. She

should also understand that diagnosis of the neonate is hampered by the presence of passively acquired maternal antibodies, which may persist up to 15 months of age.[73]

- Those at risk for HIV infection should not donate blood and should avoid pregnancy until serologic tests have been negative for at least 6 months after the last potential exposure.
- Men should use latex condoms during sexual intercourse. Condoms should be well lubricated with a non-oil-based lubricant. Oil-based lubricants (petroleum jellies) may weaken latex and cause the condom to tear. Some spermicides with nonoxynol-9 have been found to kill the virus in laboratory experiments; thus, the use of spermicides with latex condoms or a diaphragm or both may provide a greater margin of safety. Those in long-standing, mutually monogamous relationships in which neither partner uses intravenous drugs and neither partner is HIV-positive need not use condoms or spermicides.
- Health care workers should use gloves when touching mucous membranes or nonintact skin of all patients and use other appropriate barrier methods (e.g., masks, eye coverings, gowns, and aprons) when assisting in invasive procedures and when handling instruments contaminated with blood or body secretions.[93]

References

Rubella

1. Centers for Disease Control, Immunization Practices Advisory Committee: Increase in rubella and congenital rubella syndrome—United States, 1988-1990. *MMWR* 1991;40:93-99.
2. American College of Obstetricians and Gynecologists: *Rubella and Pregnancy.* Technical Bulletin 171. Washington, DC, ACOG, 1992.
3. Lee SH, Ewert DP, Frederick PD, et al: Resurgence of congenital rubella syndrome in the 1990s: Report on missed opportunites and failed prevention policies among women of childbearing age. *JAMA* 1992;267:2616-2620.
4. Horton JA (ed): *The Women's Health Data Book.* Washington, DC, The Jacobs Institute of Women's Health, 1992.
5. The National Vaccine Advisory Committee: The measles epidemic. The prob-

lems, barriers, and recommendations. *JAMA* 1991;266:1547-1552.
6. Enders G: Rubella antibody titers in vaccinated and nonvaccinated women and result of vaccination during pregnancy. *Rev Infect Dis* 1985;7:103-107.
7. Centers for Disease Control: Rubella vaccination during pregnancy—United States, 1971-1988. *MMWR* 1989;38:289-292.
8. American College of Obstetricians and Gynecologists: *Group B Streptococcal Infections in Pregnancy.* Technical Bulletin 170. Washington, DC, ACOG, 1992.
9. Committee on Infectious Diseases and Committee on Fetus and Newborn: Guidelines for prevention of Group B streptococcal (GBS) infection by chemoprophylaxis. *Pediatrics* 1992;90:775-778.
10. Baker CJ, Edwards MS: Group B strep-

tococcal infections: perinatal impact and prevention methods. *Ann NY Acad Sci* 1988;549:193-202.

11. Møller M, Thomsen AC, Borch K, et al: Rupture of fetal membranes and premature delivery associated with group B streptococci in urine of pregnant women. *Lancet* 1984;2:69-70.

Toxoplasmosis

12. American College of Obstetricians and Gynecologists: *Perinatal Viral and Perinatal Infections.* Technical Bulletin 177. Washington, DC, ACOG, 1993.
13. Frenkel JK, Dubey JP, Miller NL: *Toxoplasma gondii* in cats: Fecal stages identified as coccidian oocysts. *Science* 1970; 167:893-896.
14. Ladiges WC, DiGiacomo RF, Yamaguchi RA: Prevalence of *Toxoplasma gondii* antibodies and oocysts in pound-source cats. *J Am Vet Med Assoc* 1982; 180:1334-1335.
15. Frenkel J: Toxoplasmosis in cats and man. *Feline Practice* 1975;5:28-41.
16. Remington JS, Desmonts G: Toxoplasmosis, in Remington JS, Klein JO (eds): *Infectious Diseases of the Fetus and Newborn Infant,* 2nd ed. Philadelphia, WB Saunders Co, 1983.
17. Desmonts G, Couvreur J: Congenital toxoplasmosis: A prospective study of 378 pregnancies. *N Engl J Med* 1974; 290:1110-1116.

Herpesvirus Infections

18. Nahmais AJ, Roizman B: Infection with herpes simplex viruses 1 and 2. *N Engl J Med* 1973;289:667-670.
19. Stagno S, Whitley RJ: Herpes virus infections of pregnancy: II: Herpes simplex virus and varicella-zoster virus infections. *N Engl J Med* 1985;313: 1327-1330.

20. Isada NB, Grossman III JH: Perinatal infections, in Gabbe SG, Niebyl JR, Simpson JL (eds): *Obstetrics—Normal and Problem Pregnancies,* 2nd ed., New York, Churchill Livingstone, 1991, p. 1249.
21. Guinan ME, Wolinsky SM, Reichman RC: Epidemiology of genital herpes simplex virus infection. *Epidemiol Rev* 1985;7:127-146.
22. Baker DA: Herpes and pregnancy: New management. *Clinical Obstet Gynecol* 1990;33:253-257.
23. Prober CJ, Sullender W, Gasakawa LL, et al: Low risk herpes simplex virus in neonates exposed to the virus at the time of vaginal delivery to mothers with recurrent genital herpes simplex virus infections. *N Engl J Med* 1987;316:240.
24. Briggs G, Freeman RK, Yaffe SJ: *Drugs in Pregnancy and Lactation,* 3rd ed. Baltimore, Williams & Wilkins, 1990.
25. Kish LS, McMahon JT, Bergfeld WF, et al: An ancient method and a modern scourge: The condom as a barrier against herpes. *J Am Acad Dermatol* 1983;9: 769-770.
26. Conant MA, Spicer DW, Smith CD: Herpes simplex virus transmission: Condom studies. *Sex Transm Dis* 1984;11:94-95.
27. Postic B, Singh B, Squeglia NL, et al: Inactivation of clinical isolates of herpes virus hominus, types 1 and 2, by chemical contraceptives. *Sex Transm Dis* 1978;5:22-24.
28. Siegel M: Congenital malformations following chicken pox, measles, mumps, and hepatitis. *JAMA* 1973;226:1521-1524.
29. Paryani SG, Arvin AM: Intrauterine infection with varicella-zoster virus after maternal varicella. *N Engl J Med* 1986; 314:1542-1546.
30. Alford CA, Stagno S, Pass RF: Natural history of perinatal cytomegaloviral infection. *Ciba Found Symp* 1979;77: 125-147.

31. Stagno S, Pass RF, Dworsky ME, et al: Maternal cytomegalovirus infection and perinatal transmission. *Clin Obstet Gynecol* 1982;25:563-576.

32. Stagno S, Pass RF, Cloud G, et al: Primary cytomegalovirus infection in pregnancy. *JAMA* 1986;256:1904-1908.

33. Pass RF, Hutto SC, Reynolds DW, et al: Increased frequency of cytomegalovirus infection in children in group day care. *Pediatrics* 1984;74:121-126.

34. Balfour CL, Balfour HH: Cytomegalovirus is not an occupational risk for nurses in renal transplant and neonatal units: Results of a prospective surveillance study. *JAMA* 1986;256:1909-1914.

Chlamydial Infection

35. Schachter J, Hanna L, Hill EC, et al: Are chlamydial infections the most prevalent venereal disease? *JAMA* 1975;231:1252-1258.

36. Cates W, Jr, Wasserheit JN: Genital chlamydia infections: epidemiology and reproductive sequelae. *Am J Obstet Gynecol* 1991;164:1771-1781.

37. Holmes KK: Lower genital tract infections in women: Cystitis/urethritis, vulvovaginitis, and cervicitis, in Holmes KK, Mardh P-A, Sparling PF, et al (eds): *Sexually Transmitted Diseases.* New York, McGraw-Hill, 1984, pp 557-589.

38. Holmes KK, Handsfield HH, Wang SP, et al: Etiology of nongonococcal urethritis. *N Engl J Med* 1975;292:1199-1205.

39. Schachter J, Grossman M, Sweet R, et al: Prospective study of perinatal transmission of *Chlamydia trachomatis.* *JAMA* 1986;255:3374-3378.

40. Martin DH, Koutsky L, Exchenbach DA, et al: Prematurity and perinatal mortality in pregnancies complicated by maternal *Chlamydia trachomatis* infections. *JAMA* 1982;247:1585-1588.

41. Sweet RL, Landers DW, Walker C, et al: *Chlamydia trachomatis* infection and pregnancy outcome. *Am J Obstet Gynecol* 1987;156:824-833.

42. Harrison HR, Alexander ER, Weinstein L, et al: Cervical *Chlamydia trachomatis* and mycoplasmal infections in pregnancy: Epidemiology and outcomes. *JAMA* 1983;250:1721-1727.

43. Gravett MG, Nelson P, De Rouen T, et al: Independent associations of bacterial vaginosis and *Chlamydia trachomatis* infection with adverse pregnancy outcome. *JAMA* 1986;256:1899-1903.

44. McGregor JA, French JI: *Chlamydia trachomatis* infection during pregnancy. *Am J Obstet Gynecol* 1991;164:1782-1789.

45. Centers for Disease Control: *Chlamydia trachomatis* infections: Policy guidelines for prevention and control. *MMWR* 1985;34:53S.

Human Papillomavirus Infection

46. Meisels A, Morin C: Human papillomavirus and cancer of the uterine cervix. *Gynecol Oncol* 1981;12:111-123.

47. Kaufman RH, Adam E: Herpes simplex virus and human papillomavirus in the development of cervical carcinoma. *Clin Obstet Gynecol* 1986;29(3):678-692.

48. Mounts P, Shah KV: Respiratory papillomatosis: Etiological relation to genital tract papillomavirus. *Prog Med Virol* 1984;29:90-114.

Gonorrhea

49. Centers for Disease Control: *Sexually transmitted disease surveillance, 1989.* DHHS Publ No. 91-736-854R. Washington, DC, US Government Printing Office, 1991.

50. Minkoff H, Grunebaum AN, Schwarz RH, et al: Risk factors for prematurity and premature rupture of membranes: A prospective study of the vaginal flora in

pregnancy. *Am J Obstet Gynecol* 1984; 150:965-972.

Syphilis

51. Centers for Disease Control: Increase in primary and secondary syphilis—United States. *MMWR* 1987;36:393-397.
52. Mascola L, Pelosi R, Blount JH, et al: Congenital syphilis: Why is it still occurring? *JAMA* 1984;252:1719-1722.

Viral Hepatitis

53. Heathcote J, Sherlock S: Spread of acute type-B hepatitis in London. *Lancet* 1973; 1:1468-1470.
54. Shapiro CN, Margolis HS: Hepatitis B epidemiology and prevention. *Epidemiol Rev* 1990;12:221-227.
55. Beasley RP, Trepo C, Stevens CE, et al: The e antigen and vertical transmission of hepatitis B surface antigen. *Am J Epidemiol* 1977;105:94-98.
56. Beasley RP, Hwang LY, Lee GC, et al: Prevention of perinatally transmitted hepatitis B virus infections with hepatitis B immune globulin and hepatitis B vaccine. *Lancet* 1983;2:1099-1102.
57. Centers for Disease Control: Recommendations for protection against viral hepatitis. *MMWR* 1985;34:313-318.

Human Immunodeficiency Virus Infection

58. Centers for Disease Control: *HIV/AIDS surveillance: year-end edition.* Atlanta, CDC, 1992.
59. Burke DS, Brundage JF, Goldenbaum M, et al: Human immunodeficiency virus infections in teenagers. Seroprevalence among applicants for U.S. military service. *JAMA* 1990;263:2074-2077.
60. St. Louis ME, Conway GA, Hayman CR, et al: Human immunodeficiency virus infection in disadvantaged adolescents. *JAMA* 1991;266:2387-2391.
61. Gwinn M, Pappaioanou M, George JR, et al: Prevalence of HIV infection in childbearing women in the United States. *JAMA* 1991;265:1704-1708.
62. Ho DD, Pomerantz RJ, Kaplan JC: Pathogenesis of infection with human immunodeficiency virus. *N Engl J Med* 1987;317:278-286.
63. Centers for Disease Control: Impact of the expanded AIDS surveillance case definition on AIDS case reporting—United States, First Quarter, 1993. *MMWR* 1993;42:308-310.
64. Cowan MJ, Hellman D, Chudwin D, et al: Maternal transmission of acquired immune deficiency syndrome. *Pediatrics* 1984;73:382-386.
65. Lapointe N, Michaud J, Pekovic D, et al: Transplacental transmission of HTLV-III virus. *N Engl J Med* 1985;312:1325-1326.
66. McCray E: Occupational risk of the acquired immunodeficiency syndrome among health care workers. *N Engl J Med* 1986;314:1127-1132.
67. Centers for Disease Control: Acquired immunodeficiency syndrome: Precautions for health-care workers and allied professionals. *MMWR* 1983;32:450-451.
68. Curran JW, Morgan WM, Hardy AM, et al: The epidemiology of AIDS: Current and future prospects. *Science* 1985;229:1352-1357.
69. Padian N, Marquis L, Francis DP, et al: Male-to-female transmission of human immunodeficiency virus. *JAMA* 1987;258:788-790.
70. Weber DJ, Redfield RD, Lemon SM: Acquired immunodeficiency syndromes; Epidemiology and significance for obstetrician and gynecologist. *Am J Obstet Gynecol* 1986;155:235-239.
71. Scott GB, Fischl MA, Klimas N, et al: Mothers of infants with the acquired immunodeficiency syndrome: Evidence

for both symptomatic and asymptomatic carriers. *JAMA* 1985;253:363-366.

72. Pinching AJ, Jeffries DJ: AIDS and HTLV-III/LAV infection: Consequences for obstetrics and perinatal medicine. *Br J Obstet Gynaecol* 1985;92:1211-1217.

73. American College of Obstetricians and Gynecologists: Human immunodeficiency virus infections. Technical Bulletin 169. Washington, DC ACOG, 1992.

74. Zeigler JB, Cooper DA, Johnson RO, et al: Postnatal transmission of AIDS-associated retrovirus from mother to infant. *Lancet* 1985;1:896-898.

75. Tucker CW: Gonorrhea recidivism in Richard's County, South Carolina. Contract No: 200-76-0672. Atlanta, Centers for Disease Control, 1977.

76. Barlow D: The condom and gonorrhoea. *Lancet* 1977;2:811-813.

77. Pemberton J, McCann JS, Mahoney JD, et al: Sociomedical characteristics of patients attending a VD clinic and the circumstances of infection. *Br J Vener Dis* 1972;48:391-396.

78. Hart G: Factors influencing venereal infection in a war environment. *Br J Vener Dis* 1974;50:68-72.

79. Smith OL, Oleske J, Cooper R, et al: Efficacy of condoms as barriers to HSV-II in gonorrhea, in *Program and Abstracts for Sexually Transmitted Disease.* San Juan, Puerto Rico, World's Congress, Latin American Union Against Venereal Disease, 1981.

80. Kelaghan J, Rubin GL, Ory HW, et al: Barrier-method contraceptives and pelvic inflammatory disease. *JAMA* 1982; 248:184-187.

81. Austin H, Louv WC, Alexander WJ: A case-control study of spermicides and gonorrhea. *JAMA* 1984;251:2822-2824.

82. Katznelson S, Drew WL, Mintz L: Efficacy of the condom as a barrier to the transmission of cytomegalovirus. *J Infect Dis* 1984;150:155-157.

83. Connant M, Hardy D, Sernatinger J, et al: Condoms prevent transmission of AIDS-associated retrovirus. *JAMA* 1986; 255:1706.

84. Quinn RW, O'Reilly KR: Contraceptive practices of women attending the Sexually Transmitted Disease Clinic in Nashville, Tennessee. *Sex Transm Dis* 1985; 12:99-102.

85. Singh B, Cutler JC, Utidjian HM: Studies on the development of vaginal preparation providing both prophylaxis against venereal disease and other genital infections and contraception. *Br J Vener Dis* 1972;48:57-64.

86. Hicks DR, Martin LS, Getchell JP, et al: Inactivation of HTLV-III/LAV-infected cultures of normal human lymphocytes by nonoxynol-9 in vitro. *Lancet* 1985;2: 1422-1423.

87. Culter JC, Singh B, Carpenter U, et al: Vaginal contraceptives as prophylaxis against gonorrhea and other sexually transmissible diseases. *Adv Planned Parenthood* 1977;12:45-56.

88. Jick H, Harran MT, Stergachis A, et al: Vaginal spermicides and gonorrhea. *JAMA* 1982;248:1619-1621.

89. Peterman TA, Curran JW: Sexual transmission of human immunodeficiency virus. *JAMA* 1986;256:2222-2226.

90. Bayer R, Levine C, Wolf SM: HIV antibody screening: An ethical framework for evaluating proposed programs. *JAMA* 1986;256:1768-1774.

91. Francis D, Chin J: The prevention of acquired immunodeficiency syndrome in the United States. *JAMA* 1987;257:1357-1366.

92. Fleming DW, Cochi SL, Steece RS, et al: Acquired immunodeficiency syndrome in low-incidence areas: How safe is unsafe sex? *JAMA* 1987;258:785-787.

93. Centers for Disease Control: Human immunodeficiency virus in health care worker exposed to blood of infected patients. *MMWR* 1987;36:285-288.

6

Medication History

R esearchers have estimated that 2% of all congenital anomalies are attributable to drugs and chemicals. The preconceptional patient should be educated regarding the indications, benefits, safety, and risks of any medications that she takes. Every effort should be made to obtain the most current information available for this educational process and to place the benefit to risk ratio of all medications into the proper perspective. Sound medical practice dictates that only essential drugs should be prescribed in the preconceptional period and during pregnancy and that during the postpartum period those drugs should be taken in the minimum effective dosage.

In taking the preconceptional history, the counselor should include the following two questions:

1. Does the patient routinely or occasionally take any prescribed medications?
2. Does the patient routinely or occasionally take any over-the-counter medications?

BACKGROUND

A teratogen may adversely affect the preembryo, embryo, or fetus. In the past, all birth defects were thought to have a genetic pathogenesis, but the thalidomide tragedy made it clear that drugs can produce congenital malformation. Teratogens are usually associated with major and minor defects that form patterns of malformation. A drug such as thalidomide, which is strongly teratogenic, reveals itself rather quickly; a weak teratogen, however, may not be detectable for an extended period of time because a larger exposed population is needed to demonstrate an increased incidence of the abnormal effect. For example, if the background incidence of a malformation is 1 in 10,000 in unexposed pregnancies and 2 in 10,000 in exposed pregnancies, more than 200,000 pregnancies are required to confirm a difference in the rate of malformation.

The physiologic changes associated with pregnancy may affect the distribution, metabolism, and excretion of drugs. For example, the increased plasma volume and body fat in pregnant women may dilute fat-soluble drugs. Decreased plasma albumin concentrations may affect the ratio between the inactive and the active fractions of a drug in the maternal circulation. Increased hepatic blood flow and changes in liver function may alter drug metabolism. Increased renal plasma flow and glomerular filtration rate may hasten the excretion of drugs.

Drugs easily pass through the placental membrane if they are (1) lipid soluble, (2) nonionized, and (3) of low molecular weight (less than 700). The placenta may metabolize and detoxify drugs by the mechanisms of oxidation, hydroxylation, acetylation, deamination, and reduction.

Gestational age is an important factor in the effect that a drug or its metabolites have on the developing conceptus. The critical stage of organogenesis occurs between day 17 and day 56 postfertilization. During this stage, the fetus is extremely sensitive to teratogens, and the potential for major structural malformation is great. After day 56, the danger of structural malformation is considerably reduced, but functional abnormalities may develop in normally formed organs.

Identification of Teratogens

Very few drugs have been proved teratogenic. To be classified as a teratogen, a drug must meet the following criteria as outlined by Brent[1]:

> 1) The drug produces a unique group of identifiable malformations (syndrome) which are demonstrated to occur in a much higher incidence in the exposed population; and/ or 2) the drug has been demonstrated to be associated with an increase in a malformation in the exposed population; 3) there is an animal model that mimics the human malformation with the effects being dose-related and as the dose increases, the effects increase; and 4) there is a reasonable biological explanation and understanding of the pathophysiology and the mechanism of the teratogenesis.

Animals are generally more susceptible to the teratogenic effects of drugs, the environment, starvation, and other factors than are humans.[2] On occasion, however, a drug has fewer teratogenic effects in animals than it does in humans. Such was the case with thalidomide, which was tested on mice and rats before it was used in humans and appeared to produce no ill effects. After thalidomide was identified as a human teratogen, animal studies were again undertaken. The new investigations involved monkeys and rabbits. These animals exhibited some malformations after in utero exposure to thalidomide, but not the full syndrome observed in humans. Extrapolation from animal data to human risk is, therefore, difficult. Because of species variation, applicable and precise knowledge about the effects of drugs on the human fetus is often lacking, making proper assignment of risk difficult.

Since the thalidomide tragedy, the Food and Drug Administration (FDA) has established many safeguards that will theoretically prevent the widespread use of teratogens by women of reproductive age. The FDA now requires both primate and nonprimate toxicologic and teratologic studies before it gives approval for clinical trials of a drug in humans. Preliminary studies of the drug must have involved two or more species, the administration of the drug at several concentrations, and an evaluation of fertility and general reproductive performance for both sexes over three generations. Embryo toxicity and teratogenicity studies are required in three species, as are perinatal and postnatal evaluations to assess late effects.[3]

In 1980, the FDA recommended that all drugs be categorized as A, B, C, D, or X to indicate their possible adverse fetal effects.[4] Category A indicates that controlled studies of the drug in humans have demonstrated no fetal risks in the first trimester and that the risk of fetal harm appears to be remote. Category B includes drugs for which human and animal data have not demonstrated a significant risk. Many drugs taken during pregnancy are in category C, which includes drugs for which human or animal studies are inadequate or for which animal studies have shown adverse fetal effects, but no human data are available. Category D drugs are those for which data indicate a fetal risk, but whose benefits (i.e., the management of life-threatening situations in which safer drugs are unavailable) are thought to outweigh the risk. Drugs in category X are those with proved fetal risks in humans and animals, whose risks clearly outweigh possible benefits; these drugs are contraindicated during pregnancy.

Unfortunately, availability of evidence on risk does not guarantee elimination of unnecessary exposure. For example, since its introduction, isotretinoin (Accutane) has been classified as a category X drug. This classification was based on findings in laboratory animals that indicated a risk of developmental toxicity. Shortly after isotretinoin (Accutane) was licensed for use in the treatment of severe cystic acne, there were reports that mothers who had received this drug during pregnancy had delivered infants with anomalies of the cranium, ears, face, heart, limbs, or liver. Stern and colleagues[5] reported on 35 exposed pregnancies that resulted in 6 normal infants, 19 spontaneous abortions, and 10 malformed infants. The most common anomaly in these infants involved the ears. Eight of the ten children had hydrocephaly or microcephaly, and five had heart defects.

In 1985, Lammer and colleagues[6] reported on 154 pregnancies in which the fetuses had been exposed to isotretinoin. Of these, 95 were electively terminated. Twelve (20%) of the remaining 59 pregnancies ended in spontaneous abortion. Of the 47 continuing pregnancies, 3 resulted in stillbirths of anomalous infants, 18 in live births of anomalous infants, and 26 in live births of apparently normal infants. Central nervous system defects and craniofacial defects occurred in 80% of the abnormal infants, and cardiac defects occurred in more than 50%.

In 1988, Lammer and colleagues[7] calculated a 23% risk of malformation for exposed fetuses that reached 20 weeks' gestation. Preliminary results of a long-term follow-up study indicate that 52% of children who were exposed in utero during the first trimester of gestation have intellectual impairment at age 5; 37.5% of these have no serious malformation.[8]

Despite strong efforts to publicize the potent teratogenicity of isotretinoin, the FDA estimates that 65,000 women of reproductive age receive a prescription for this drug annually, but less than 4,000 women have an approved indication.[9] In 1991, the Teratology Society recommended that the manufacturers of isotretinoin develop a plan to distribute the drug only to patients with an FDA-approved indication and that female recipients of the drug be strongly encouraged to use injectable or implantable progesterone contraceptive agents to avoid unplanned pregnancies.[9]

Use of Medication during the Preconceptional Period

The health care provider who prescribes medication for a woman who is planning a pregnancy should keep several principles in mind. First, few drugs have been proved to be either teratogenic or totally safe for human development, because the variation in response is great and research is difficult to conduct and interpret. Second, the maternal condition being treated may itself have adverse effects on fetal development. Third, the assigned classification regarding fetal risk is not always the most conservative and is subject to change. Fourth, there are many instances in which the benefits of potentially harmful drugs outweigh the risks. Finally, when therapy is required, alternatives should be explored and a drug chosen that has the least likelihood of adverse fetal effects.

Anticoagulants

Heparin should be substituted for warfarin in preconceptional patients who require anticoagulation therapy. Warfarin has a low molecular weight and readily crosses the placenta, often causing significant adverse fetal effects. The use of warfarin during the first trimester may lead to the fetal warfarin embryopathy syndrome in 15% to 20% of exposed fetuses.[10] The syndrome may include facial defects, epiphyseal stippling, optic atrophy, microcephaly, mental retardation, and other central nervous system abnormalities.[10-12] Heparin is a large molecule that does not cross the placenta and has not been associated with congenital malformation. Therefore, despite the fact that heparin requires subcutaneous injection, it is the anticoagulant of choice for the woman who is considering pregnancy.

Anticonvulsants

Treatment of maternal epilepsy with diphenylhydantoin during pregnancy has been associated with a twofold to threefold increase in the occurrence of major birth defects or in the constellation of defects known as the fetal hydantoin syndrome. This syndrome may include mental retardation, prenatal and postnatal growth retardation, cleft palate, microcephaly, midface hypoplasia, hypoplastic fingernails, or café au lait spots. In their prospective study of 468 infants who were exposed in utero to diphenylhydantoin, Kelly and colleagues[13] found evidence of minor cranial, facial, and digital abnormalities in 30% of the infants, but they found no increased incidence of mental retardation or major malformation. The full fetal hydantoin syndrome is reported to occur in less than 10% of exposed infants. In fact, whether diphenylhydantoin causes the syndrome remains controversial.[14,15] It is possible that a genetic predisposition to anomalies in the offspring of epileptics is the causal factor, because the hydantoin syndrome has been reported in the offspring of epileptic mothers who were either untreated or treated with a different drug.[16]

Trimethadione (Tridione), another drug used in the treatment of epilepsy, has been associated with growth retardation, microcephaly, short stature, cardiac and eye anomalies, and other findings similar to those of the fetal hydantoin syndrome.[17] Although trimethadione has been classified as a category D drug, both animal studies and human epidemiologic data have shown the drug to be highly embryotoxic and teratogenic; it should not be used during pregnancy.[17,18]

Valproic acid (Depakene) has been used to treat the seizures of petit mal epilepsy, as well as generalized tonic, clonic, and myoclonic seizures. The use of valproic acid during pregnancy has been associated with a 1% to 2% incidence of neural tube defects and an increased risk of microcephaly.[19-23] Jäger-Roman and colleagues[24] noted a pattern of malformation that included brachycephaly, craniofacial anomalies, long, thin fingers, and hyperconvexed nails in fetuses whose mothers had taken valproic acid. In addition, these infants were more likely than were other infants to have fetal distress during labor. Although the FDA has classified valproic acid as a category D drug, it should be recognized as a teratogen and is, therefore, contraindicated during pregnancy.

Because phenobarbital is usually prescribed in combination with other anticonvulsants, its teratogenic potential is difficult to evaluate. Animal studies and human epidemiologic studies indicate that in utero exposure to phenobarbital slightly increases the risk of cleft palate and congenital heart disease.[25,26] In addition to its teratogenic potential, phenobarbital is associated with barbiturate withdrawal and an increased incidence of hemorrhagic disease in neonates exposed in utero. The drug is classified as category D.

In animal studies, carbamazepine (Tegretol) was found to be less likely than was diphenylhydantoin to result in craniofacial defects.[27] Dr. K.L. Jones, Director of the California Teratogen Registry, has collected outcome data on human fetuses whose mothers received carbamazepine (Tegretol) (personal communication, 1987). In a retrospective study of 9 infants, Jones found 2 with intrauterine growth retardation, 3 with microcephaly, 2 with cardiac defects, and 4 with hypoplastic fifth fingernails; all of the 3 infants followed beyond the newborn period had developmental delays. Four of the 9 infants had been exposed to Tegretol alone. The remaining 5 had been exposed to additional epileptic medications, including phenobarbital (2 infants), clonazepam and phenobarbital (1 infant), valproic acid and phenobarbital (1 infant), and valproic acid and primidone (1 infant). Of 31 patients who were followed prospectively, 23 had been exposed prenatally to Tegretol alone and 8 had been exposed to carbamazepine (Tegretol) and phenobarbital. One pregnancy ended in a spontaneous abortion, 3 were voluntarily terminated, and 4 were lost to follow-up. In studying 15 of the remaining 23 infants, Jones found no intrauterine growth retardation or microcephaly, but 3 of the 23 children had fifth finger hypoplasia, 1 had a ventricular septal defect, and 1 had a cleft uvula.

A concurrent prospective control study compared 72 women treated with carbamazepine during early pregnancy with 73 pregnant nonepileptic women. The incidence of infants born with major anomalies and with two minor abnormalities was similar in the two groups; children born with three or more minor defects were more common in the exposed group. Based on their retrospective and prospective studies, the researchers concluded that carbamazepine is associated with a pattern of neonatal defects that includes craniofacial anomalies, fingernail hypoplasia, and developmental delay.[28]

This review of the fetal effects of drugs used in the treatment of maternal epilepsy makes it clear that choosing a totally safe preconceptional therapeutic regimen for the control of seizures is not possible; none of the drugs has been proved harmless, and the classification of some of the drugs appears too lenient. Yet to avoid all potentially dangerous anticonvulsants could place the woman's health in serious jeopardy. In addition, epilepsy itself may alter normal organogenesis. One option to decrease fetal teratogenic risks caused by using anticonvulsant drugs is to evaluate the need for continued use by the prospective mother. Callaghan and colleagues[29] suggest that as many as 65% of patients who have been free of seizures for at least 2 years will not have a relapse after gradual withdrawal of their medications.

Contraceptives

Briggs and colleagues[30] have identified oral contraceptives as category X drugs. They have also indicated, however, that there is no firm evidence to establish a causal relationship between the use of oral contraceptives and the occurrence of various congenital anomalies, except in the instance of modified development of the sexual organs. The teratogenic potential of oral contraceptives is not well established, as data are contradictory. Some retrospective and a few prospective studies appear to show an increased incidence of cardiovascular anomalies and limb reduction deformities,[31-34] but other studies reveal no such association.[35,36] In 1981, an extensive review of available laboratory and epidemiologic data revealed that inadvertent exposure to sex steroids during animal and human pregnancy caused developmental abnormalities in nongenital organs and tissues.[36] In 1986, Lammer and Cordero[37] reported the results of a case-control study of first-trimester sex hormone exposure among 1,091 infants with 12 defect categories. Estrogen/progestin exposure occurred in 3.5% of the mothers interviewed. These authors found no statistically significant relationship between any malformation category and oral contraceptive exposure.

Two studies indicated that vaginal spermicides were associated with an increased risk of spontaneous abortion and congenital malformation, including limb reduction defects, neoplasms, Down syndrome, and hypospadias.[38,39] The findings were considered tentative because of the small number of affected infants and the significant limitations in study design. Subsequent studies have shown that the risks of poor reproductive outcomes for mothers who used spermicides around the time of conception are not elevated.[40-43] Although these later studies were large enough to permit the detection of any association between spermicides and the overall risk of bearing a malformed child, they were too small to reveal any association between spermicides and specific malformations. The National Institutes of Health recently provided reassuring information regarding the safety of using vaginal spermicides during the periconceptional period (1 month before through 1 month after the last menstrual period), during the first trimester of pregnancy, and at any time during the reproductive years.[44]

PRECONCEPTIONAL COUNSELING

The goal of preconceptional counseling regarding the use of medications is to minimize any adverse effects on the embryo or fetus while maximizing maternal health. If the patient requires medication for her own well-being, the counselor must help her to assess realistically the conceptus' risk during pregnancy and, if she chooses to attempt pregnancy, to effect a balance between her own health status and embryonic/fetal exposure. The patient should be given up-to-date information on the indications, benefits, safety, and risks of any medications she is taking. Such educational efforts require a considerable amount of research by the counselor, especially if the drug is one not commonly used.

All preconceptional counselors should have ready access to a reference such as *Drugs in Pregnancy and Lactation,* by Briggs, Freeman, and Yaffe,[30] which includes reviews of the reproductive literature relevant to drugs and provides classifications of safety during pregnancy as outlined by the FDA. Counselors should also be familiar with and use other resources, such as teratology hotlines, to help assess risk to benefit ratios. Examples of such resources are listed in Appendix B.

The importance of continually reassessing the literature and spending time explaining the findings to patients cannot be overstressed. New studies can significantly alter the recommendations offered to patients and their perceptions of risk, should inadvertent periconceptional exposure occur. For example, informing patients of early reports that oral contraceptives were teratogenic without reviewing the subsequently discovered evidence with them could create unjustified anxiety and possibly unnecessary pregnancy termination, if exposure occurs.

The following general guidelines provide a framework for preconceptional counseling regarding medications:

- It is impossible to state categorically that any medication used before or during pregnancy, including topical preparations, is completely safe, but there are relatively few drugs that are definitely known to be teratogenic in humans.
- All medications, including over-the-counter remedies, should be reviewed and assessed for their risk to benefit ratio.
- Many variables, including the teratogenicity of the specific drug, the timing and dosage of exposure, the genetic characteristics of the mother and embryo, and environmental factors, interact to determine the effect of a drug on the development of a specific conceptus.

- Category X drugs should be avoided for all women likely to become pregnant. The list of proved human teratogens is surprisingly short; it includes alcohol, thalidomide, some folic acid agonists (e.g., aminopterin), isotretinoin, and some of the sex steroids (e.g., DES). Several other medications are listed in category X by some authorities or by their manufacturers: oral contraceptives, valproic acid, some live virus vaccines (e.g., rubella vaccine), radioactive iodine, trimethadione, some synthetic estrogens, quinine, and disulfiram.[30,45]
- When possible, category D drugs should be avoided during pregnancy. If this is impossible, the lowest possible dosage that is therapeutically effective should be used.
- Investigation of a drug's fetal effects should not be limited to its teratogenicity. The potential nonteratogenic adverse effects on the fetus should also be evaluated and discussed with the patient. Examples include the premature closure of the ductus arteriosus associated with antiprostaglandins and the intrauterine growth retardation associated with prolonged use of β-adrenergic blockers.
- When a choice of effective therapies is available, the drug that has been in use the longest without epidemiologic evidence of human fetal harm should be chosen.
- Recommendations for changed therapy should be discussed with the prescribing physician before being suggested to the patient.
- Women who require medication for their own health needs should be made aware that, while the general rule is to avoid medications, drug therapies are beneficial to pregnancy outcome in some circumstances. In such cases, the safest choice is to take prescribed drugs as recommended.
- Most congenital anomalies are the result of multifactorial influences. Excellent maternal and paternal health habits, including good nutrition and the avoidance of alcohol and tobacco exposure, may provide some protection for the fetus exposed to potentially harmful maternal medications.
- Drug metabolism and elimination may change during pregnancy. Therefore, differing dosages may be needed to maintain therapeutic levels after conception. Patients should be aware that it may be necessary to monitor blood levels of their medications and to change dosages during pregnancy.
- Even in the absence of any drug exposure, there is no guarantee of a perfect reproductive outcome. Women and their partners should be aware that spontaneous abortion, congenital malformation, and low birthweight can occur under optimal conditions.

References

1. Brent RL: Weak teratogens, letter. *Teratology* 1978;17:183.
2. Lenz W: Thalidomide and congenital abnormalities, letter. *Lancet* 1962;1:45.
3. Kurzel RB, Cetrulo CL: Chemical teratogenesis and reproductive failure. *Obstet Gynecol Surv* 1985;40:397-424.
4. Pregnancy categories for prescription

drugs. *Federal Register* 1980;44:37434-37467.

5. Stern RS, Rosa F, Baum C: Isotretinoin and pregnancy. *J Am Acad Dermatol* 1984;10:851-854.

6. Lammer EJ, Chen DT, Hoar RM, et al: Retinoic acid embryopathy. *N Engl J Med* 1985;313:837-841.

7. Lammer EL, Hayes AM, Schunior A, et al: Unusually high risk for adverse outcomes of pregnancy following fetal isotretinoin exposure. *Am J Hum Genet* 1988;43:A58.

8. Adams J: High incidence of intellectual deficits in 5 year old children exposed to isotretinoin "in utero." *Teratology* 1990;41:614.

9. The Teratology Society: Recommendations for isotretinoin use in women of childbearing potential. *Teratology* 1991; 44:1-6.

10. Hall JG, Pauli RM, Wilson KM: Maternal and fetal sequelae of anticoagulation during pregnancy. *Am J Med* 1980;68: 122-140.

11. Warkany J: Warfarin embryopathy. *Teratology* 1976;14:205-209.

12. Barr M Jr, Burdi AR: Warfarin-associated embryopathy in a 17-week-old abortus. *Teratology* 1976;14:129-134.

13. Kelly TE, Edwards P, Rein M, et al: Teratogenicity of anticonvulsant drugs: II. A prospective study. *Am J Med Genet* 1984;19:435-443.

14. Friis ML, Hauge M: Congenital heart defects in live-born children of epileptic parents. *Arch Neurol* 1984;42:374-376.

15. Shapiro S, Hartz SC, Siskind V, et al: Anticonvulsants and parental epilepsy in the development of birth defects. *Lancet* 1976;1:272-275.

16. Dalessio DJ: Seizure disorders and pregnancy. *N Engl J Med* 1985;312:559-563.

17. Zackai EH, Mellman WJ, Neiderer B, et al: The fetal trimethadione syndrome. *J Pediatr* 1975;87:280-284.

18. Brown NA, Shull G, Fabro S: Assessment of the teratogenic potential of tri-methadione in the CD-1 mouse. *Toxicol Appl Pharmacol* 1979;51:56-71.

19. Centers for Disease Control: Valproate: A new cause of birth defects. Report from Italy and follow-up from France. *MMWR* 1983;32:438-440.

20. Gomez MR: Possible teratogenicity of valproic acid. *J Pediatr* 1981;98:508-509.

21. Dalens B, Raynaud EJ, Gaulme J: Teratogenicity of valproic acid. *J Pediatr* 1980;97:332-333.

22. Robert E: Valproic acid in pregnancy: Association with spina bifida. A preliminary report. *Clin Pediatr* 1983;22:336.

23. Bailey CJ, Pool RW, Poskitt EM, et al: Valproic acid and fetal abnormality. *Br Med J* 1983;286:190.

24. Jagër-Roman E, Deichl A, Jakob S, et al: Fetal growth, major malformations, minor anomalies in infants born to women receiving valproic acid. *J Pediatr* 1986;108:997-1004.

25. Sullivan FM, McElhattan PR: A comparison of the teratogenic activity of the antiepileptic drugs carbamazepine, clonazepam, ethosuximide, phenobarbital, phenytoin, and primidone in mice. *Toxicol Appl Pharmacol* 1977;40:356-378.

26. Annegars JF, Elveback LR, Hauser WA, et al: Do anticonvulsants have a teratogenic effect? *Arch Neurol* 1974;31:364-373.

27. Eluma FO, Sucheston ME, Hayes TG, et al: Teratogenic effects of dosage levels and time of administration of carbamazepine, sodium valproate, and diphenylhydantoin on craniofacial development in the CD-1 mouse fetus. *J Craniofac Genet Dev Biol* 1984;4:191-210.

28. Jones KL, Lacro RV, Johnson KA, et al: Pattern of malformations in the children of women treated with carbamazepine during pregnancy. *N Engl J Med* 1989; 320:1661-1666.

29. Callaghan N, Garrett A, Goggin T: Withdrawal of anticonvulsant drugs in patients free of seizures for two years: A

prospective study. *N Engl J Med* 1988; 318:942-946.

30. Briggs GG, Freeman RK, Yaffe SJ: *Drugs in Pregnancy and Lactation,* ed 3. Baltimore, Williams & Wilkins, 1990.

31. Heinonen OP, Slone D, Monson RR, et al: Cardiovascular birth defects and antenatal exposure to female sex hormones. *N Engl J Med* 1977;296:67-70.

32. Janerich DT, Piper JM, Glebatis DM: Oral contraceptives and congenital limb-reduction defects. *N Engl J Med* 1974; 291:697-700.

33. Janerich DT, Dungan JM, Standfast SJ, et al: Congenital heart disease and prenatal exposure to exogenous sex hormones. *Br Med J* 1977;1:1058-1060.

34. Kasan PN, Andrews J: Oral contraception and congenital abnormalities. *Br J Obstet Gynaecol* 1980;87:545-551.

35. Royal College of General Practitioners Oral contraceptive study: The outcome of pregnancy in former oral contraceptive users. *Br J Obstet Gynaecol* 1976; 83:608-616.

36. Wilson JG, Brent RL: Are female sex hormones teratogenic? *Am J Obstet Gynecol* 1981;141:567-580.

37. Lammer EJ, Cordero JF: Exogenous sex hormone exposure and the risk of major malformations. *JAMA* 1986;255:3128-3132.

38. Jick H, Walker AM, Rothman KJ, et al: Vaginal spermicides and congenital disorders. *JAMA* 1981;245:1329-1332.

39. Huggins G, Vessey M, Flavel R, et al: Vaginal spermicides and outcome of pregnancy: Findings in a large cohort study. *Contraception* 1982;25:219-230.

40. Mills JL, Harley EE, Reed GF, et al: Are spermicides teratogenic? *JAMA* 1982; 248:2148-2151.

41. Cordero JF, Layde PM: Vaginal spermicides, chromosomal abnormalities and limb reduction defects. *Fam Plann Perspect* 1983;15:16-18.

42. Linn S, Schoenbaum SC, Monson RR, et al: Lack of association between contraceptive usage and congenital malformations in offspring. *Am J Obstet Gynecol* 1983;147:923-928.

43. Warburton D, Newgut RH, Lustenberger A, et al: Lack of association between spermicide use and trisomy. *N Engl J Med* 1987;317:478-482.

44. Louik C, Mitchell AA, Werler MM, et al: Maternal exposure to spermicides in relation to certain birth defects. *N Engl J Med* 1987;317:474-478.

45. Gilstrap LC, Cunningham FG: Drugs and medications in pregnancy. *Williams Obstetrics Supplement* No. 13, July/August 1987.

7

Reproductive History

O ne of the primary reasons that couples seek preconceptional counseling is a previous poor reproductive outcome. The preconceptional reproductive history is an important tool for identifying factors that contributed to the earlier poor outcome and that may be amenable to intervention. Factors such as uterine malformation, maternal autoimmune disease, endocrine abnormalities, and genital infection lend themselves to diagnosis and therapy that may lessen the risk of recurrent fetal and neonatal loss. In general, 70% to 80% of couples with a history of pregnancy loss will eventually have a successful pregnancy, even if the underlying cause of the earlier loss(es) has not been determined.

As part of the preconceptional screening process, the counselor should ask whether the patient has had

- a history of uterine or cervical abnormalities
- two or more pregnancies that ended in first-trimester miscarriage
- one or more fetal deaths
- one or more pregnancies that ended in second-trimester delivery
- one or more infants who weighed less than 2,500 g at birth
- one or more infants who required care in a neonatal intensive care unit
- one or more infants with a birth defect

BACKGROUND
First-Trimester Pregnancy Loss

Habitual abortion has traditionally been defined as the occurrence of three or more pregnancy losses before the twentieth week of gestation. Currently, however, it is believed that a woman with two consecutive losses should be considered for preconceptional counseling. Recurrent consecutive pregnancy loss is a clinical problem in approximately 0.5% to 1% of couples. Gant's[1] synthesis of information on spontaneous abortion indicates that more than 80% of these abortions occur during the first 12 weeks of pregnancy and that more than 50% of the early losses are associated with chromosomal abnormalities. The risk of spontaneous abortion increases with parity and with advancing maternal and paternal age.

In 1964, Warburton and Fraser[2] calculated recurrence risks for spontaneous abortion after zero, one, two, three, or four previous occurrences (Table 7-1). The risk for recurrence of spontaneous abortion may be influenced by (1) the presence or

Table 7-1 Estimate of abortion risk in pregnancies after a given number of abortions

No. of Previous Abortions	% of Abortions
0	12.3
1	23.7
2	26.2
3	32.2
4	25.9

From *American Journal of Human Genetics* (1964; 16:1–25), University of Chicago Press.

absence of liveborn offspring; and (2) the chromosomal status of previous abortuses. If the woman has had one normal pregnancy in addition to three consecutive spontaneous abortions, for example, she has a 70% chance of a subsequent successful pregnancy outcome. Moreover, the chance of successful pregnancy is 35% to 50% if three abortuses were chromosomally normal and the mother has no liveborn offspring.[3]

It appears that there is at least a 10% to 15% rate of pregnancy loss between fertilization and in utero implantation, which approximates the percentage of loss observed in clinically recognized pregnancies. Opitz and colleagues[4] report that 58% of fertilized ova do not survive long enough to result in a missed period, with 16% of the fertilized ova not cleaving and another 15% being lost during the first postovulatory week. Of the ova that survive the first missed period, approximately 15% will abort spontaneously. Using immunoradiometric assay to determine human chorionic gonadotropin (hCG) levels in daily urine specimens, Wilcox and associates[5] assessed early pregnancy loss. Over 707 menstrual cycles were followed for 221 women. Of the 198 pregnancies identified by the assay, 22% ended before the pregnancies were clinically detected; the overall rate of pregnancy loss was 31%.

Genetic Factors

Chromosomal abnormalities have traditionally been considered a major cause of early pregnancy loss. As a result of their chromosomal analysis of 23 human preovulatory oocytes, Wramsby and colleagues[6] suggest that as many as 50% of oocytes may have an abnormal karyotype. Yamomoto and colleagues[7] found chromosomal defects associated with 50% to 60% of first-trimester spontaneous abortions and with 7.3% of therapeutic abortions. Using chorionic villus sampling (CVS) to obtain tissue for cytogenetic analyses immediately after ultrasound diagnosis of first-trimester fetal demise, Guerneri and associates[8] found chromosomal abnormalities in 77% of the cases.

Gestational age at the time of miscarriage relates to the incidence of chromosomal abnormality. As noted earlier, more than 80% of spontaneous abortions occur during the first 12 weeks of pregnancy; chromosomal abnormalities cause approximately 53% of these losses, compared with 36% of second-trimester abortions and 5% of third-trimester stillbirths, and are present in 0.6% of liveborns.[1,9] The most common chromosomal abnormality associated with first-trimester loss is autosomal trisomy, which is detected in nearly 25% of early losses.[1,10] The trisomies may result from a maternal or paternal balanced translocation, a balanced chromosomal inversion, or an isolated nondisjunction.[11]

In 1975 and in 1981, Alberman and colleagues[12,13] reported that the risk of an abnormal karyotype (e.g., trisomy) in a pregnancy is increased if such a karyotype occurred in an earlier pregnancy. Abortuses in a particular family show nonrandom distribution of chromosomal abnormalities: if the complement of the first abortus is abnormal, the likelihood is as high as 80% that the complement of a second abortus will be abnormal.[10,14]

In 4.8% to 5.5% of phenotypically normal couples with two or more consecutive spontaneous abortions, one of the parents can be expected to have a chromosomal abnormality, such as reciprocal translocation, Robertsonian translocation, or inversion.[15] A balanced translocation chromosomal complement has been noted in 6.2% of women and 2.6% of men.[16] If either the mother or father has a balanced translocation, meiotic segregation may lead to unbalanced gametes, which are associated with spontaneous abortion, congenital anomalies, or healthy children.[17]

Immunologic Factors

Among the immunologic factors that have been suggested as causes of repetitive early abortion are systemic lupus erythematosus, presence of antiphospholipid antibodies in the mother, and abnormal maternal alloimmune responses to the pregnancy. The latter might be triggered by histocompatibility between the mother and her partner, such as an increased sharing of maternal and paternal human leukocyte antigens (HLAs)[1] or increased homozygosity for HLA loci.[18,19] According to Gant,[1(p5)] "There is strong evidence that *histoincompatibility* is essential to successful human pregnancy and that if mother and fetus are 'too compatible' then reproduction failure develops."

The proposed link between histocompatibility and spontaneous abortion resulted in a prevention initiative involving maternal immunization with paternal or third-party leukocytes; the intent was to induce maternal antipaternal antibodies that would block immune rejection of the embryo or fetus.[20-24] Some successful outcomes have been reported for this intervention, but many of the studies have lacked a sufficient number of subjects or appropriate comparison groups to allow adequate evaluation. Furthermore, the role and mechanisms of the human immune response in pregnancy are not fully understood. One recent study investigated numerous aspects of immunologic responses after conception in women with a history of repeated spontaneous abortion, compared with a control group. Using serum samples, the researchers were unable to identify consistent patterns of response in either group or significant differences between them.[20] Whether maternal serum accurately reflects uterine immune responses is unknown. Cauchi and colleagues[25] undertook a double-blind randomized controlled investigation of the efficacy of maternal leukocyte immunization and demonstrated that immunization did not affect continuing pregnancy rates. Too many questions remain to view leukocyte immunization as a reasoned alternative for habitual aborters. Until it is determined whether and how this technique affects pregnancy and whether it has long-term health consequences for exposed mothers and children, the technique should be viewed as experimental and limited to research centers involved in carefully designed studies.

Another interesting but unproved explanation for recurrent pregnancy loss is immunologic interaction between trophoblasts remaining from a previous conception and tissues of a new pregnancy, resulting in resorption of the latest embryo.[26]

The incidence of antiphospholipid antibodies, including the lupus anticoagulant and anticardiolipin antibodies, in the general obstetric population is 3% to 5%.[27] Some but not all of these women have more frequent occurrences of vascular thromboses, thrombocytopenia, false positive serologic tests for syphilis, repeated spontaneous abortion, and fetal wastage.[27] In one review, a 91% fetal loss rate was reported for 242 pregnancies in 65 patients with lupus anticoagulant.[26] Other studies have demonstrated antiphospholipid antibodies in 10% to 40% of "healthy" women with recurrent abortions.[28]

Recurrent pregnancy loss associated with the antiphospholipid antibodies may relate to thrombosis of placental vessels secondary to an imbalance of prostacyclin and thromboxane A_2. Low-dose aspirin in combination with prednisone has been demonstrated to markedly decrease fetal loss for women with antiphospholipid antibodies.[26,29,30] Effectiveness may relate to the ability of prednisone to reduce concentration of the autoantibodies and of aspirin, in small doses, to inhibit thromboxane synthesis. This combination discourages thrombosis formation, but benefits of the treatment are neither universal nor without risk. In one study, nearly one half of treated women developed complications, most notably gestational diabetes, following corticosteroid therapy.[31] A recent multicenter randomized trial demonstrated that a combination therapy of low-dose aspirin and heparin is more effective than an aspirin and prednisone combination in preventing fetal loss and maternal morbidity.[32] No data available to date indicate that the preconceptional use of low-dose aspirin, alone or combined with either prednisone or heparin, improves pregnancy outcome or decreases the incidence of maternal complications.

Endocrine Factors

Disorders of the thyroid, diabetes mellitus, and luteal phase defects have been suggested as endocrine causes of early pregnancy loss. Thyroid dysfunction as a cause of repeated spontaneous abortion is controversial. Glass and Golbus[33] suggest that thyroid dysfunction plays only a small role, if any. Similarly, well-controlled or moderately well-controlled diabetes is no longer believed to be associated with increased abortion rates. When Crane and Wahl[34] studied the incidence of spontaneous abortion among 154 diabetic pregnant patients and compared them with matched nondiabetic controls, they found that the incidence of both spontaneous abortion and repetitive abortion (two or more) was not different in the two groups. They concluded that diabetes mellitus, if well controlled, is not a frequent cause of repetitive early pregnancy loss. It is still generally believed, however, that patients with uncontrolled type I diabetes mellitus have a greater incidence of repetitive pregnancy loss.

A defect in corpus luteum function may account for 3% to 4% of recurrent abortions. Tho, Byrd, and McDonough[35] report that 21 of 23 patients with habitual abortion caused by a luteal phase defect had excellent reproductive outcomes when they were treated with a progesterone replacement regimen. When ovulation was detected, the patient received progesterone in oil, 12.5 mg administered intramuscularly each day, or progesterone vaginal suppositories, 25 mg administered twice a day. If pregnancy was confirmed, the patient received 17-hydroxyprogesterone caproate ester, 250 mg administered intramuscularly each week until placental steroidogenesis was established.

Current recommendations for diagnosis of corpus luteum defects include two endometrial biopsies performed late in the luteal phase that demonstrate at least a two-day lag from the expected histologic dating features.[36] Luteal phase deficiency can be treated with progesterone or with clomiphene citrate. Either regimen requires a repeat endometrial biopsy to determine whether the defect has been corrected.[34] Unfortunately, well-controlled prospective studies are unavailable to determine whether treatment of luteal defects results in a decreased rate of pregnancy loss.

Anatomic Factors

Congenital uterine anomalies and uterine leiomyomas have been observed in 10% to 15% of patients with recurrent early abortion; however, these are more likely to be associated with second-trimester loss.[35] Congenital uterine anomalies may vary from a double cervix or uterus to a septate or arcuate uterus. A defect in the vascular supply to the endometrium, decreased uterine cavity size, and abnormal cervix have all been implicated in the pathophysiology. Of the various anomalies, the septate uterus is most frequently associated with early pregnancy loss. Hysteroscopic lysis of uterine septa has replaced metroplasty as the preferred treatment.[36]

Uterine leiomyomas may prohibit normal pregnancy development because they grow rapidly secondary to the hormones of pregnancy or because they are associated with a defect in the endometrial vasculature that causes uterine contractions and subsequent abortion. A hysteroscopy may be both diagnostic and therapeutic in a patient with recurrent pregnancy loss if a hysterosalpingogram indicates the presence of a leiomyoma. A submucosal fibroid may be removable by resectoscope. Present reports are anecdotal, however, and long-term studies are needed before it is known whether hysteroscopic resection of a submucosal leiomyoma improves subsequent pregnancy outcomes.

The presence of uterine adhesions or synechiae may also cause early reproductive loss. This diagnosis should be suspected when the patient has a history of uterine trauma (e.g., induced abortion, septic abortion, repeated or postpartum curettage) followed by scanty menses and recurrent pregnancy loss. It is confirmed by hysterosalpingogram or hysteroscopy. Treatment consists of dilation and curettage or hysteroscopy to lyse the adhesions, followed by the administration of estrogens for approximately 3 months before pregnancy is attempted. Jewelewicz and colleagues[37] reported a 50% conception rate and a 16% uncomplicated full-term delivery rate in 36 patients with a history of recurrent abortion and findings consistent with uterine synechiae. A report by Valle and Sciarra[38] indicates that women with a history of pregnancy wastage have nearly a 90% likelihood of conceiving after hysterscopic lysis, with 90% of those women carrying their pregnancies to term.

Other Factors

Infections with *Listeria monocytogenes, Toxoplasma, Mycoplasma hominis,* herpes simplex virus, and *Ureaplasma urealyticum* have all been associated with early pregnancy loss. Carefully controlled studies that prospectively identify microorganisms and determine the effect of various treatments are needed before preconceptional antibiotic therapy can be recommended as a widespread preventive approach to pregnancy loss. However, some evidence is accumulating that antimicrobial therapy may be beneficial. Administration of antibiotics to women who had experienced at least one spontaneous abortion reduced the rate of recurrent loss to 10% in the treated group, compared with 38% in a control group.[39] Quinn and colleagues[40] significantly reduced the pregnancy loss rate in patients with asymptomatic genital tract *Mycoplasma* infection by treating them with doxycycline before conception. Stray-Pedersen and associates[41] treated women with *Ureaplasma urealyticum* and their sexual partners with doxycycline and demonstrated improved pregnancy outcomes; however, the study lacked a control group.

A tubal pregnancy is a significant cause of first-trimester loss. During the past 25 years, the incidence of ectopic pregnancy has been steadily increasing; the Centers for Disease Control report an increase from 4.5 to 16.8 per 1,000 pregnancies.[42] This increase in ectopic pregnancy is thought to be related to the increased incidence of pelvic inflammatory disease.[43] The recurrence rate for ectopic tubal pregnancy ranges from 8% to 25%,[44] and the incidence of involuntary infertility in patients who have had an ectopic pregnancy is approximately 50%.[45] After two ectopic pregnancies, the incidence of a third ectopic pregnancy and the incidence of involuntary infertility are both further increased.[46]

Second- and Third-Trimester Pregnancy Loss and Neonatal Death

In general, second-trimester abortuses have normal chromosomal complements. The possibility of genetic defects should be explored, however, particularly if the patient has a history of both first- and second-trimester loss. Usually, repeated second-trimester losses result from such factors as uterine anomalies, incompetent cervix, antiphospholipid antibodies, severe preeclampsia, and abruptio placentae. The most common causes of neonatal death are premature birth and congenital malformation.

Goldenberg and associates[47] confirmed that one of the best predictors of a poor outcome in a current pregnancy is a poor outcome in the preceding gestation. In their study, which examined pregnancy outcome after a previous second-trimester loss, 39% of women who had a loss at 13 to 24 weeks' gestation had a preterm delivery in the next pregnancy; 5% had a stillbirth, and 6% had a neonatal death. All of these findings were worse than for two comparison groups.

Abnormalities in the Reproductive Organs

A congenital uterine anomaly may first be suspected after a second-trimester loss. In patients with a septate uterus, Semmens[48] recorded a 30% spontaneous abortion rate, a 20% incidence of breech presentation, a 10% incidence of transverse lie, a 20% incidence of premature labor, and a 15% incidence of postpartum hemorrhage. Other series have indicated that the rate of fetal wastage associated with a septate uterus is 58% to 85%.[49]

Diagnosing a specific uterine anomaly requires thorough investigation. Careful laparoscopic and hysteroscopic examinations are helpful diagnostic tools. Hysteroscopy may also be used therapeutically for removal of the septum in women with a septate uterus. Rock and Jones[50] found a significant reduction in pregnancy wastage after surgical correction of the uterus.

The reproductive organ abnormalities induced by in utero exposure to diethylstilbestrol (DES) result from impaired development of the müllerian duct system. Likely anomalies include an irregular uterine contour, a T-shaped uterine cavity, deformity of the cervix and endocervical canal, and a hypoplastic uterus.[51] Compared with nonexposed daughters, exposed daughters have an increased rate of spontaneous abortion (26% vs. 16%), ectopic pregnancy (4% vs. 1%), premature labor (8% vs. 4%), and stillbirth (4% vs. 1%).[52] The poor outcomes tend to occur most often in women who were exposed to DES before the nineteenth week of their mother's pregnancy.[53] The uterine and cervical anomalies of DES-exposed daughters appear to increase the likelihood of adverse reproductive outcomes, especially in the first pregnancy, but do not adversely affect fertility.[52] Daughters exposed to DES who have either radiographically or grossly apparent uterine anomalies have a higher incidence of cervical incompetence.[52,54,55] For these women, a cervical cerclage during early pregnancy may be indicated.

An incompetent cervix has been reported to be associated with 0.1% to 1% of all deliveries and as many as 20% of midtrimester abortions.[56] Cervical incompetence may be secondary to cervical trauma or laceration in a previous labor, induced second-trimester abortion, cone biopsy of the cervix, or in utero DES exposure. Rarely, congenital connective tissue defects, such as those that occur in Ehlers-Danlos syndrome, result in cervical incompetence. The diagnosis is usually evident in the history. A classic presentation is silent cervical effacement, spontaneous rupture of the membranes, and rapid second-trimester delivery. In addition, easy passage of a #8 Hegar dilator through the cervix is considered diagnostic, as is the identification of a cervical defect on a hysterogram.

A classic history, alone or in combination with these diagnostic tests, is sufficient to warrant a therapeutic surgical procedure. Shirodkar[57] achieved an 81% fetal salvage rate after operative intervention for cervical incompetence. As described by McDonald,[58] cervical cerclage is usually performed at 14 to 16 weeks of pregnancy and has been reported to increase the salvage rate of viable fetuses from 30% to 88%. A multicenter randomized trial of cervical cerclage was undertaken to determine whether cerclage placement in women believed to be at risk of cervical incompetence resulted in prolonged pregnancy and improved fetal and neonatal outcome. Those having cerclage had fewer deliveries before 33 weeks, fewer infants with birthweights less than 1,500 g, and fewer miscarriages and fetal and neonatal deaths. The results were only marginally significant, however, leading the researchers to caution against enthusiatic interpretation of the data.[59]

Autoimmune Disorders

As noted under "First-Trimester Pregnancy Loss," placental thrombosis and infarction leading to uteroplacental insufficiency has been associated with reproductive loss in patients with antiphospholipid antibodies. The presence of these antibodies should be investigated in the woman who has a history of pregnancy loss in the late second trimester or third trimester,[60,61] particularly when associated with intrauterine growth retardation, idiopathic prematurity, severe preeclampsia, or recurrent stillbirth. In addition, the presence of lupus anticoagulant should be suspected in patients with SLE, recurrent first-trimester loss, false-positive VDRL, and repeated or unusual presentations of preeclampsia. Current therapies, discussed in the preceding section, have been demonstrated to favorably affect pregnancy outcomes for women with antiphospholipid antibodies.

Fetal and Neonatal Mortality

Intrauterine fetal death after 20 weeks of gestation occurs in approximately 1% of pregnancies. In 1963, the British Perinatal Mortality Study revealed a marked increase in reproductive loss in pregnancies that followed a perinatal death.[62] Analysis of computerized birth records in British Columbia revealed that, after one stillborn child, a couple's risk of stillbirth or severe perinatal morbidity in a subsequent pregnancy more than doubled, from 6.8% to 15.4%; after two previous perinatal deaths, the risk rose to 34.3%.[63] Freeman and colleagues[64] have shown that a history of previous stillbirth places a subsequent pregnancy at high risk for perinatal complications, including abnormal fetal heart tracings consistent with fetal distress.

For the woman with a history of previous fetal or neonatal death, a review of related prenatal, intrapartum, and neonatal records and the autopsy, if available, may provide valuable information. An autopsy indicates the cause of a fetal or neonatal death in 50% of cases. Postmortem examination may reveal evidence of erythroblastosis fetalis, congenital anomalies, fetal infection, cord or placental complications, medical complications, fetal hypoxemia, or abnormal chromosomal typing. Only 5% to 10% of stillbirths are associated with an abnormal karyotype. Findings in as many as 50% of cases indicate multiple maternal or fetal causes. Maternal exposures and disease, for example, are possible contributory factors (see Chapters 2 and 4).

A history of low-birthweight infants may be the result of induced or spontaneous labor, congenital anomalies, or a suboptimal uterine environment. In the United States, 7% to 8% of all liveborn infants have a low birthweight. The most common cause of low birthweight, which is well recognized for its association with infant mortality and morbidity, is preterm delivery.

Preterm delivery. Although the etiology of preterm birth is not completely understood, many factors are known to play roles. Previous pregnancy outcomes and current pregnancy complications, such as placenta previa, cervical incompetence, uterine distention, infections of the cervix and vagina, and socioeconomic and psychosocial stress factors, appear to contribute in varying degrees to the risk of preterm labor and delivery. A study of more than 6,000 women indicates that the likelihood of preterm delivery increases from 5% to 15% for women who have had one preterm delivery; after two spontaneous preterm deliveries, the risk is increased to 32%.[65] Other considerations in risk assignment include maternal age and a history of spontaneous abortion. Although late second-trimester spontaneous abortion is associated with an increased incidence of preterm delivery in subsequent pregnancies,[66] first-trimester abortion is not.[67] Women at the beginning or at the end of their reproductive years, particularly teenage mothers who are having second and third pregnancies, are at greater risk.[68]

Many studies have attempted to implicate amniotic, vaginal, and cervical infections in the pathogenesis of preterm labor and premature rupture of the membranes.[69-71] The importance of these studies lies in the possibility that the detection and treatment of vaginal or cervical infection may decrease the incidence of preterm labor. The evidence that infection is a cause of premature delivery includes the following: (1) the incidence of clinically manifested infection is increased in preterm neonates and their mothers; (2) various vaginal organisms are associated with premature delivery and premature rupture of the membranes; (3) the microbiology of the amniotic fluid has been related to preterm labor; and (4) small studies have indicated that antibiotic trials reduce the rate of preterm birth.[72] Prospective controlled randomized studies have not yet scientifically confirmed this impression, however.

McGregor's[73] recent review of the infectious microorganisms that have been associated with preterm birth highlights the variety of specific organisms that have been identified prenatally within the genital tract. Among the various organisms that have been reported to be related to preterm birth are *Neisseria gonorrhoeae,* group B streptococci, *Chlamydia trachomatis, Mycoplasma hominis, Ureaplasma urealyticum, Trichomonas vaginalis,* and other anaerobic and aerobic organisms. This indicates that, although vaginal, cervical, amniotic membrane, or amniotic fluid infection may be a cause of preterm labor and birth, the presence of specific pathogens may not be necessary to initiate the process of preterm labor. The normal flora of the cervix and vagina may produce substances that help to induce labor.

Both normal and abnormal inhabitants of the lower reproductive tract produce the phospholipases A_2 and C. In turn, these phospholipases produce arachidonic acid, which is essential for the production of prostaglandins, such as E_2 and $F_{2\alpha}$. These prostaglandins are important for both the initiation and the maintenance of uterine activity. In addition, neutrophils and macrophages in the genital tract produce a variety of proteases, including collagenase and elastase, that can diminish the local tactile strength of the chorionic membranes and lead to rupture. However, evidence for the existence of many of the bacterial relationships in preterm labor and rupture of the membranes is circumstantial at this time.

Because the pathophysiologic process that triggers preterm labor is not fully known, it is difficult to design preventive strategies. The risk of repetitive preterm labor may be lessened not only by aggressive local and systemic antibiotic treatment regimens but also by restrictions of work, travel, and exercise and by more frequent rest periods. Women with jobs that involve prolonged standing have a relatively higher risk for preterm delivery than do others; those with professional occupations have intermediate risk, while unemployed homemakers have lower risk.[74]

Psychosocial stress also plays an important but difficult to quantify role in preterm birth.[75] Large epidemiologic studies indicate that lifestyle factors, particularly alcohol consumption and smoking, have some causal relationship to preterm delivery.[68,76] The relationship between nutrition and preterm delivery has been extensively examined. For example, the Collaborative Perinatal Study has shown that increased maternal weight gain is inversely associated with the risk for low birthweight.[77] Other studies report that, although the risk of another preterm delivery is high in patients who have experienced a previous preterm delivery, a subsequent child has approximately a 90% chance of survival after either expectant treatment or judicious use of cervical cerclage.[78,79]

Labor induction. Preeclampsia is a common indication for labor induction, which often results in a low-birthweight infant. In 1958, MacGillivray[80] reported that the risk of recurrent preeclampsia in a second pregnancy is related to its severity and the associated reproductive outcome in the first pregnancy. Results of a recent study indicate that women who develop preeclampsia as nulliparas have a 33.7% risk of having the same complication in a subsequent pregnancy. This compares with 7.7% for women whose previous pregnancy was normotensive.[81] The same study found that women who had severe preeclampsia before 30 weeks' gestation had a 76% recurrence rate, compared with 38% for those who had onset of disease at or later than 37 weeks' gestation. Two reports by Sibai and colleagues[81,82] indicate that women who have experienced severe preeclampsia have an increased risk of later developing chronic hypertension; the highest risk (55%) is for women who have had recurrent severe preeclampsia during the second trimester.

A disease of many causes, preeclampsia appears to have a higher incidence in patients who are pregnant for the first time or are pregnant for the first time with a new partner[83] and a relatively high incidence in daughters of mothers who had preeclampsia, compared with their mothers-in-law and controls.[84]

Maternal vaginal bleeding during the late second and early third trimesters is another reason for effecting delivery of the low-birthweight infant. At times the bleeding is so profuse that a cesarean delivery must be performed. The major causes of vaginal bleeding during pregnancy are abruptio placentae and placenta previa.

Abruptio placentae, which can lead to fetal demise in utero, occurs in 0.3% to 3% of pregnancies. The wide range in reported incidence is secondary to variations in presentation and to inconsistencies in documentation of the signs and symptoms of the disease. Many times the patient with abruptio placentae also has severe preeclampsia; in fact, abruptio placentae may further complicate as many as 5% of preeclamptic pregnancies, with a fetal loss rate of 28%. If a patient has an abruption in one pregnancy, she has approximately a 6% risk of recurrence in each subsequent gestation.[85] Unfortunately, recurrent episodes of abruption appear to be more severe than the initial episode.[86]

The pathogenesis of abruptio placentae is not clear, although many relationships have been reported. Controversial relationships have been proposed between abruptio placentae and maternal age, parity, smoking, folate deficiency, and socioeconomic status. In addition, the presence of chronic hypertension, preeclampsia, uterine anomalies, previous premature labor, and unexplained second-trimester elevation in maternal serum α-fetoprotein have been reported.[87] The patients at greatest risk for abruptio placentae and its recurrence appear to be those who are older than age 35, have chronic hypertension, and smoke cigarettes. Mothers who stop smoking have a 23% lower rate of abruption and a marked decrease in fetal and neonatal death caused by abruptio placentae than do those who continue to smoke.[87]

Placenta previa occurs in 0.2% to 0.5% of pregnancies. If the mother or fetus cannot tolerate the bleeding that is associated with symptomatic placenta previa, premature termination of pregnancy may be indicated. Increased maternal age or parity, smoking, previous cesarean delivery, and multiple induced abortions appear to increase the incidence of both primary and recurrent placenta previa. Although the etiology may not be known in all cases, there is a 4% to 8% recurrence rate.[88]

Congenital malformation. Of the 4 million infants born in the United States each year, 250,000 (6.25%) will suffer from a birth defect.[89] Over time, birth defects have become an increasingly important cause of infant mortality while other causes, such as infectious disease, have been dramatically reduced. Birth defects are currently identified as the direct cause of 21% of infant deaths in this country and are recognized as the leading cause of infant mortality and the fifth leading cause of shortened life expectancy before the age of 65. The full effect of congenital anomalies on reproductive outcomes is not known, because many infants who are stillborn or who die shortly after birth do not undergo autopsy to uncover or confirm a diagnosis. Identifying anomalies; understanding the pathogenesis, when possible; and practicing good maternal health habits during the periconceptional period are reasonable but unproved preventive steps.

PRECONCEPTIONAL COUNSELING

The goals of preconceptional counseling for patients who have had a pregnancy loss are to investigate the factors that may have contributed to the previous outcome, to assuage guilt and resolve grief, to provide recommendations that may prevent the recurrence of such a loss in a subsequent pregnancy, and to inform patients realistically regarding their likelihood of successful childbearing.

Those who have experienced a pregnancy loss may express frustration and anger during the preconceptional period. It is crucial for the preconceptional counselor to provide empathy and emotional support and to allow the couple to express their feelings, fears, and fantasies. The counselor should, if possible, repeatedly reassure the couple that they are not to blame for their loss. Couples should be seen together in a nonhurried manner in order to increase comprehension and reduce anxiety.

The preconceptional counselor should be aware of the dynamics of the grieving process. Because unresolved grief may be manifested as depression, sexual dysfunction, or a physical symptom, the couple may not recognize it. Unresolved grief may also occur as an emotionally charged desire for another pregnancy. This is unlikely to be the most psychologically beneficial action, however; in fact, it could be detrimental to the resolution of the previous loss. To provide proper support and recommendations, the counselor must determine the couple's stage of mourning.

The preconceptional counselor's approach to a couple with a history of pregnancy loss or compromised neonatal outcomes should begin with a thorough medical history, including coexistent illnesses, infectious diseases, and environmental exposures of the couple. A complete and detailed reproductive summary of all pregnancy outcomes is necessary. Patients should be questioned concerning any history of pelvic infection, use of intrauterine contraceptive devices, or repeated dilation and curettage. The family history should include the health status of first-degree (i.e., siblings, parents, and offspring), second-degree (i.e., aunts, uncles, nieces, nephews, and grandparents), and third-degree (i.e., first cousins) relatives of both husband and wife. The occurrence of mental retardation, congenital anomalies, and early adult deaths among family members should be thoroughly investigated.

It is important to categorize the losses as early or late spontaneous abortion, second- or third-trimester fetal death, preterm birth, or neonatal death, because each category indicates different areas for preconceptional exploration:

- early pregnancy loss
  - chromosomal defect
  - immunologic disorder (e.g., leukocyte compatibility; lupus anticoagulant anticardiolipin antibodies)
  - corpus luteum defect
  - uterine anatomic abnormality (e.g., intrauterine adhesions, septate uterus)
  - infection (e.g., *Chlamydia, Mycoplasma,* herpes, *Ureaplasma urealyticum*)
  - ectopic pregnancy
- second- and third-trimester loss
  - immunologic disorder (e.g., lupus anticoagulant)
  - infection (e.g., group B streptococci, *Mycoplasma hominis, Listeria, Hemophilus influenzae*)
  - uterine or cervical anatomic abnormality (e.g., cervical incompetence, septate uterus, DES uterine anomaly)
  - placental abruption
  - placenta previa
  - maternal disease (see Chapter 4)
  - chromosomal defect
- neonatal loss
  - premature delivery or premature rupture of membranes
  - congenital malformation
  - in utero infection (e.g., group B streptococci, *Neisseria gonorrhoeae*)

A history of early pregnancy loss mandates a complete physical examination of the woman, including close inspection of the cervix for signs of infection or surgical or obstetric trauma consistent with an incompetent cervix or DES exposure. Further investigational studies may include routine blood work; urinalysis; aerobic, anaerobic, and viral cultures of tissue from the cervix; serologic studies; endometrial biopsy; determination of progesterone levels; and basal body temperature charts.

If a corpus luteum defect is diagnosed, consideration may be given to the periconceptional administration of progesterone. Thyroid function studies may be performed. Hysterosalpingogram or hysteroscopy may be necessary to identify a fixed anatomic defect; because hysteroscopy has both diagnostic and therapeutic capabilities, it is superior to a blind dilation and curettage. Hysteroscopy appears especially useful in efforts to exclude uterine anomalies and in the diagnosis and treatment of submucosal fibroids and septate uteri. This approach may obviate the need for major surgery.

Repeated early abortions suggest that the parents may have a balanced translocation; karyotyping should be done. In general, nearly 3% of couples who experience two consecutive pregnancy losses have a chromosomal defect; with three consecutive abortions, there is a 3% to 8% chance that one parent has an abnormal karyotype with high-resolution banding.

Because overt or subclinical maternal autoimmune disease may be responsible for recurrent miscarriage, an antinuclear antibody determination and screening for lupus anticoagulant and anticardiolipin antibodies should be included in the test battery for patients with recurrent pregnancy loss. If these antibodies are detected, a diagnosis of SLE should be considered and preconceptional treatment with aspirin (60 mg daily) and steroids (40 to 80 mg daily) may be advisable. Replacing prednisone with heparin in the treatment regimen may be advantageous.

Patients with lupus anticoagulant or autoimmune disease should be informed that they may develop hypertension and other signs of preeclampsia during the second trimester and that fetal growth may be delayed. Consequently, close monitoring of blood pressure and urine albumin levels, as well as monthly ultrasonographic evaluations of fetal growth, will be necessary. Patients should also understand that tests of fetal well-being, including fetal movement monitoring by the mother, biophysical profiles, and contraction stress testing, are likely to be initiated at the point in gestation when there is a reasonable chance of newborn survival.

A late pregnancy loss requires investigation for uterine abnormalities, incompetent cervix, infection, and immunologic abnormalities, as discussed earlier. The possibility of uteroplacental compromise and underlying maternal disease should also be investigated, particularly if previous pregnancies were associated with intrauterine growth retardation (see Chapter 4).

A chronically hypertensive patient who has had a previous abruption should be advised not to consider another pregnancy until her blood pressure is under control. A balanced diet, a decrease in stress, and an increase in bedrest during pregnancy may further decrease her risk of a recurrent episode of abruptio placentae. The patient must be aware, however, that another poor pregnancy outcome may not be totally preventable.

There do not appear to be any preventive measures that can be taken to decrease the incidence of placenta previa other than to recommend that the patient stop smoking and to limit the number of cesarean deliveries, either by allowing the patient to attempt a vaginal delivery or by performing a sterilization procedure after a repeat cesarean delivery.

Preterm delivery has a tendency to be a repetitive problem. Underlying causes, such as uterine anomalies, cervical incompetence, circulating lupus anticoagulant, and infection, should be investigated. If the cause of a previous preterm delivery was pregnancy-induced hypertension, the preconceptional counselor should undertake a thorough review of previous records to confirm the diagnosis and classification. Patients who had severe preeclampsia should be reassured that the risk for recurrence appears to be only 7.5% in a second pregnancy.

A history of silent cervical effacement and spontaneous rupture of the membranes with rapid midtrimester delivery indicates an incompetent cervix, and the possibility of cervical cerclage may be suggested. A patient who experienced spontaneous preterm labor and delivery in a previous pregnancy should be advised of the likely antenatal recommendations regarding rest, work, travel, exercise, tobacco

use, and coitus during a subsequent pregnancy so that she can weigh their accepta-
bility and prepare accordingly. However, except for tobacco use, which has been
clearly shown to be related to preterm labor, these factors have not been definitely
associated with shortened gestation. Infections of the vagina, cervix, and urinary
tract should be treated with appropriate antibiotics. Patients should be aware that it
will be important to have frequent examinations during pregnancy to assess silent
cervical changes. Instructing patients that preterm labor is frequently associated with
many subtle signs and symptoms that, if identified before significant cervical dilation
has occurred, make it possible to interrupt labor often proves reassuring.

When a woman seeks preconceptional counseling after a stillbirth, the counselor
should make every effort to obtain the prenatal records and a copy of the autopsy,
if one is available. If an autopsy was performed, a cause of death can be identified
50% of the time. The counselor can use such information as a guide in making
recommendations.

For all women with a less than optimal reproductive history, good general principles of health, such as proper diet, smoking cessation, weight control, and avoidance of alcohol, should be emphasized. Rubella immunization should be offered
when appropriate and education provided on the importance of early prenatal care.
The preconceptional counselor should help couples realize that 70% to 80% of couples with a history of recurrent reproductive loss eventually have successful pregnancy outcomes.

References

1. Gant NF: Recurrent spontaneous abortion. Suppl 21 to Pritchard JA, MacDonald PC, Gant NF (eds) *Williams Obstetrics*, ed 17. Norwalk, Conn.: Appleton &
   Lange, Dec/Jan, 1989.
2. Warburton D, Fraser FC: Spontaneous
   abortion risks in man: Data from reproductive histories collected in a medical
   genetics unit. *Am J Hum Genet* 1964;16:
   1-25.
3. Roman E: Fetal loss rates and their relation to pregnancy order. *J Epidemiol
   Community Health* 1984;38:29-35.
4. Opitz JM, Shapiro SS, Uehling DT:
   Genetic causes and workup of male and
   female infertility: I. Prenatal reproductive loss. *Postgrad Med* 1979;65:247-
   252.
5. Wilcox AJ, Weinberg CR, O'Conner JF,

et al: Incidence of early loss of pregnancy. *N Engl J Med* 1988;319:189-194.
6. Wramsby H, Fredga K, Liedholm P:
   Chromosome analysis of human oocytes
   recovered from preovulatory follicles in
   stimulated cycles. *N Engl J Med* 1987;
   316:121-124.
7. Yamomoto M, Fujimore R, Adachi K, et
   al: Surveillance system of chromosomal
   abnormalities in early embryonic stage
   of induced abortions. *Tohoku J Exp Med*
   1975;115:197-198.
8. Guerneri S, Bettio D, Simoni G, et al:
   Prevalence and distribution of chromosome abnormalities in a sample of first
   trimester internal abortions. *Hum Repro*
   1987;2:735.
9. Warburton D, Stein Z, Kline J, Susser M:
   Chromosome abnormalities in sponta-

neous abortion: Data from New York City study, in Porter IH, Hook EB (eds): Human Embryonic and Fetal Death. New York, Academic Press, 1980.

10. Simpson JL: Genetic causes of spontaneous abortion. *Cont OB/GYN* 1990; September:25-40.

11. Cunningham FG, MacDonald PC, Gant NF (eds): Williams Obstetrics, ed 18. Norwalk, Conn.: Appleton & Lange, 1989, pp 561-593.

12. Alberman E, Elliott M, Creasy M, et al: Previous reproductive history in mothers presenting with spontaneous abortions. *Br J Obstet Gynaecol* 1975;82:366-373.

13. Alberman E: The abortus as a predictor of future trisomy 21 pregnancies, in de la Cruz F, Gerald PS (eds): *Trisomy 21: Research Perspectives.* Baltimore, University Park Press, 1981, pp 69-76.

14. Warburton D, Kline J, Stein Z, et al: Does the karyotype of a spontaneous abortion predict the karyotype of a subsequent abortion? *Am J Hum Genet* 1987;41:465-483.

15. Portnoi M-F, Joye N, Van Den Akker J, et al: Karotypes of 1142 couples with recurrent abortion. *Obstet Gynecol* 1988; 72:31-34.

16. Elias S, Simpson JL: Evaluation and clinical management of patients at apparent increased risk for spontaneous abortion, in Porter IH, Hook PB (eds): *Human Embryonic and Fetal Death.* New York, Academic Press, 1980, p 331.

17. Husslein P, Huber J, Wagenbichler P, et al: Chromosome abnormalities in 150 couples with multiple spontaneous abortions. *Fertil Steril* 1982;37:379-383.

18. Coulam CB, Moore BS, O'Fallon WM: Association between major histocompatibility antigen and reproductive performance. *Am J Reprod Immunol Microbiol* 1987;14:54-58.

19. Cauchi MN, Tait B, Wilshire MI, et al: Histocompatibility antigens and habitual abortion. *Am J Repro Immunol Microbiol* 1988;18:28-31.

20. Sargent IL, Wilkins T, Redman CWG: Maternal immune responses to the fetus in early pregnancy and recurrent miscarriage. *Lancet* 1988;2:1099.

21. Mowbray JF, Underwood JL, Michel M, et al: Immunization with paternal lymphocytes in women with recurrent miscarriage. *Lancet* 1987;1:680.

22. Taylor C, Faulk WP: Prevention of recurrent abortion with leukocyte transfusions. *Lancet* 1981;2:68-70.

23. Beer AE, Quebbeman JF, Ayers JW, et al: Major histocompatibility complex antigens, maternal and paternal immune responses and chronic habitual abortions in humans. *Am J Obstet Gynecol* 1981; 141:987-999.

24. Scott JR, Rote NS, Branch DW: Immunologic aspects of recurrent abortion and fetal death. *Obstet Gynecol* 1987;70: 645-656.

25. Cauchi MN, Lim D, Young DE, et al: The treatment of recurrent aborters by immunization with paternal cells—controlled trial. *Am J Repro Immunol* 1991; 25:16-17.

26. Scott JR, Rote NS, Branch DW: Immunologic aspects of recurrent abortion and fetal death. *Obstet Gynecol* 1987;70:645.

27. Cunningham FG: Connective-tissue disorders complicating pregnancy. Suppl 22 to Cunningham FG, MacDonald PC, Gant NF (eds) *Williams Obstetrics,* ed 18. Norwalk, Conn.: Appleton & Lange, 1993.

28. Out HJ, Derksen HWM, Christiaens GCML: Systemic lupus erythematosus and pregnancy. *Obstet Gynecol Surv* 1989;44:585-591.

29. Branch DW, Scott JR, Kochenour NK, Hershgold E: Obstetric complications associated with lupus anticoagulant. *N Engl J Med* 1983;313:1322.

30. Lubbe WF, Butler WS, Palmer SJ, et al: Fetal survival after prednisone suppres-

sion of maternal lupus-anticoagulant. *Lancet* 1983;1:1361-1363.

31. Landy HJ, Kessler C, Kelly WK, Weingold AB: Obstetric performance in patients with the lupus anticoagulant and/or anticardiolipin antibodies. *Am J Perinatol* 1992;9:146.

32. Cowchock FS, Reece EA, Balaban D, et al: Repeated fetal losses associated with antiphospholipid antibodies: A collaborative randomized trial comparing prednisone with low-dose heparin treatment. *Am J Obstet Gynecol* 1992;166:1318.

33. Glass RH, Golbus MS: Habitual abortion. *Fertil Steril* 1978;29:257-265.

34. Crane JP, Wahl N: The role of maternal diabetes in repetitive spontaneous abortion. *Fertil Steril* 1981;36:477-479.

35. Tho PT, Byrd JR, McDonough PG: Etiologies and subsequent reproductive performance of 100 couples with recurrent abortion. *Fertil Steril* 1979;32:389-395.

36. Carson SA: Nongenetic causes of recurrent fetal loss. *Cont OB/GYN* 1991; Feb: 14-26.

37. Jewelewicz R, Khalaf S, Neuwirth RS, et al: Obstetric complications after treatment of intrauterine synechiae (Asherman's syndrome). *Obstet Gynecol* 1976; 47:701-705.

38. Valle RF, Sciarra JJ: Intrauterine adhesions: Hysteroscopic diagnosis, classification, treatment and reproductive outcome. *Am J Obstet Gynecol* 1988;158: 1459-1470.

39. Toth A, Lesser ML, Brooks-Toth CW, et al: Outcome of subsequent pregnancies following antibiotic therapy after primary or multiple spontaneous abortions. *Surg Gynecol Obstet* 1986;163:243.

40. Quinn PA, Shewchuk AB, Shuber J, et al: Efficacy of antibiotic therapy in preventing spontaneous pregnancy loss among couples colonized with genital mycoplasmas. *Am J Obstet Gynecol* 1983;145:239-244.

41. Stray-Pedersen B, Eng J, Reikvan TM: Uterine T-mycoplasma colonization in reproductive failure. *Am J Obstet Gynecol* 1978;130:307.

42. Nederlof KP, Lawson HW, Saftlas AF, et al: Ectopic pregnancy surveillance, United States, 1970-1987. *MMWR* 1989; 39(SS-4):9-17.

43. Strathy JH, Coulam CB, Marchbanks P, et al: Incidence of ectopic pregnancy in Rochester, Minnesota, 1950-1981. *Obstet Gynecol* 1984;64:37-43.

44. DeCherney A, Kase N: The conservative surgical management of unruptured ectopic pregnancy. *Obstet Gynecol* 1979;54:451-455.

45. Mehta L, Young ID: Recurrence risk for common complications of pregnancy: A review. *Obstet Gynecol Surv* 1987;42: 218-223.

46. Hallat JG: Repeat ectopic pregnancy: A study of 123 consecutive cases. *Am J Obstet Gynecol* 1975;122:520-524.

47. Goldenberg RL, Mayberry SK, Cooper RL, et al: Pregnancy outcome following a second-trimester loss. *Obstet Gynecol* 1993;81:444-446.

48. Semmens JP: Congenital anomalies of female genital tract. *Obstet Gynecol* 1962; 19:328-350.

49. Buttram VC Jr, Gibbons WE: Mullerian anomalies: A proposed classification. *Fertil Steril* 1979;32:40-46.

50. Rock JA, Jones HW Jr: The clinical management of a double uterus. *Fertil Steril* 1977;28:798-806.

51. Goldstein DP: Incompetent cervix in offspring exposed to diethylstilbestrol in utero. *Obstet Gynecol* 1978;52:73S-75S.

52. Barnes AB, Colton T, Gunderson J, et al: Fertility and outcome of pregnancy in women exposed in utero to diethylstilbestrol. *N Engl J Med* 1980;302:609-618.

53. Kaufman RH, Adam E, Binder GL, et al: Upper genital tract changes and pregnancy outcome in offspring exposed in

utero to diethylstilbestrol. *Am J Obstet Gynecol* 1980;137:299-308.

54. Schmidt G, Fowler WC Jr, Talbert LM, et al: Reproductive history of women exposed to diethylstilbestrol in utero. *Fertil Steril* 1980;33:21-24.

55. Herbst AL, Hubby MM, Blough RR, et al: A comparison of pregnancy experience in DES-exposed and DES-unexposed daughters. *J Reprod Med* 1980;24: 62-69.

56. Mann EC, McLarn WD, Hayt DB: The physiology and clinical significance of the uterine isthmus. *Am J Obstet Gynecol* 1961;81:209-222.

57. Shirodkar VN: A method of operative treatment for habitual abortions in the second trimester of pregnancy. *Antiseptic* 1955;52:299-303.

58. McDonald IA: Suture of the cervix for inevitable miscarriage. *J Obstet Gynaecol Br Emp* 1957;64:346-350.

59. MRC/RCOG Working Party on Cervical Cerclage. Interim report of the Medical Research Council/Royal College of Obstetricians and Gynaecologists multicentre randomized trial of cervical cerclage. *Br J Obstet Gynaecol* 1988;95: 437-445.

60. Lubbe WF, Liggins GC: Lupus anticoagulant and pregnancy. *Am J Obstet Gynecol* 1985;153:322-327.

61. Feinstein DI: Lupus anticoagulant, thrombosis and fetal loss. *N Engl J Med* 1985;313:1348-1350.

62. Butler NR, Bonham DG: *Perinatal Mortality: The First Report of the British Perinatal Mortality Survey.* Edinburgh, E&S Livingstone, 1963.

63. Newcombe HB: Risks to siblings of stillborn children. *Can Med Assoc J* 1968; 98:189-193.

64. Freeman RK, Dorchester W, Anderson G, et al: The significance of a previous stillbirth. *Am J Obstet Gynecol* 1985; 151:7-13.

65. Carr-Hill RA, Hall MH: The repetition of spontaneous preterm labor. *Br J Obstet Gynaecol* 1985;92:921-928.

66. Rush RW: Incidence of preterm delivery in patients with previous preterm delivery and/or abortion. *S Afr Med J* 1979; 56:1085-1087.

67. Keirse MJ, Rush RW, Anderson AB, et al: Risk of pre-term delivery in patients with previous pre-term delivery and/or abortion. *Br J Obstet Gynaecol* 1978;85: 81-85.

68. Berkowitz GS: An epidemiologic study of preterm delivery. *Am J Epidemiol* 1981;113:81-92.

69. Minkoff H, Grunebaum AN, Schwarz RH, et al: Risk factors for prematurity and premature rupture of membranes: A prospective study of the vaginal flora in pregnancy. *Am J Obstet Gynecol* 1984; 150:965-972.

70. Gravett MG, Hummel D, Eschenbach DA, et al: Preterm labor associated with subclinical amniotic fluid infection and with bacterial vaginosis. *Obstet Gynecol* 1986;67:229-237.

71. Gravett MG: Causes of preterm labor. *Semin Perinatol* 1984;8:246-255.

72. McGregor JA, French JI, Reller LB, et al: Adjunctive erythromycin treatment for idiopathic preterm labor: Results of a randomized, double-blinded, placebo-controlled trial. *Am J Obstet Gynecol* 1986;154:98-103.

73. McGregor JA: Prevention of preterm birth: New initiatives based on microbial-host interactions. *Obstet Gynecol Surv* 1988;43:1-14.

74. Burkedal T: *Occupation and outcome of pregnancy.* Oslo, Norway, Central Bureau of Statistics, 1980.

75. Newton RW, Webster PA, Binu PS, et al: Psychosocial stress in pregnancy and its relation to the onset of premature labor. *Br Med J* 1979;2:411-413.

76. Berkowitz GS, Holford TR, Berkowitz RL: Effects of cigarette smoking, alcohol, coffee and tea consumption on pre-

term delivery. *Early Hum Dec* 1982;7: 239-250.

77. Niswander KR, Gordon M: *The Women and Their Pregnancies: The Collaborative Perinatal Study of the National Institute of Neurologic Diseases and Studies.* Philadelphia, WB Saunders Co, 1972.

78. Socol ML, Dooely SL, Tamura RK, et al: Perinatal outcome following prior delivery in the late second or early third trimester. *Am J Obstet Gynecol* 1984; 150:228-231.

79. Kossmann JC, Bard H: Subsequent pregnancy following the loss of an early preterm newborn infant weighing less than 1000 grams. *Obstet Gynecol* 1982;60: 74-76.

80. MacGillivray I: Some observations on the incidence of pre-eclampsia. *J Obstet Gynaecol Br Emp* 1958;65:536-539.

81. Sibai BM, El-Nazer A, Gonzalez-Ruiz AR: Severe preeclampsia-eclampsia in young primigravidas: subsequent pregnancy outcome and remote prognosis. *Am J Obstet Gynecol* 1986;155:1011.

82. Sibai BM, Mercer B, Sarinoglu C: Severe preeclampsia in the second trimester: recurrence risk and long-term prognosis. *Am J Obstet Gynecol* 1991; 165:1408.

83. Ikedife D: Eclampsia in multipara. *Br Med J* 1980;280:985-986.

84. Sutherland A, Cooper DW, Howie PW, et al: The incidence of severe pre-eclampsia amongst mothers and mothers-in-law of pre-eclamptics and controls. *Br J Obstet Gynaecol* 1981;88: 785-791.

85. Paterson ME: The aetiology and outcome of abruptio placentae. *Acta Obstet Gynecol Scand* 1979;58:34-35.

86. Golditch IM, Boyce NE Jr: Management of abruptio placentae. *JAMA* 1970; 212: 288-293.

87. Egley CE, Cefalo RC: Abruptio placenta, in Studd J (ed): *Progress in Obstetrics and Gynecology.* New York, Churchill Livingston, vol 5, 1985, pp 108-120.

88. Kelly JV, Iffy L: Placenta previa, in Iffy L, Kaminetzky HA (eds): *Principles and Practice of Obstetrics and Perinatology.* New York, John Wiley & Sons, vol 2, 1981, chap 63.

89. Johnson KA: Birth defects and infant mortality. *March of Dimes Birth Defects Foundation Infant Mortality Report*

8

Family History

Although prenatal diagnosis and genetic counseling are ancient skills that date back 3,500 and 1,000 years, respectively,[1] it was not until 1956 that the normal number of chromosomes in the human was firmly established. This discovery and the dramatic developments in biochemical, cellular, and molecular biology that followed it have resulted in our current "golden age of medical genetics."[2]

Important advances in genetic counseling include carrier screening for single gene heterozygosity and chromosomal analysis of the prospective parents, the fetus, and the offspring. Carrier screening is of special preconceptional significance because it allows for relevant counseling before the conception of the first affected child. As a result, couples may now base reproductive decisions on risk data never before imagined. They must realize, however, that only a few genetic abnormalities are recognizable before delivery; fewer still can be identified before pregnancy.[3]

A few well-placed questions and a working knowledge of the basic principles of medical genetics can indicate patterns of inheritance that may prove important to patients who seek preconceptional counseling. Routine family histories should include answers to the following questions:
- Does the patient, her partner, any of their offspring, or any members of their families have
  —hemophilia
  —thalassemia
  —Tay-Sachs disease
  —sickle cell disease or trait
  —phenylketonuria
  —cystic fibrosis
  —a birth defect
  —mental retardation?
- Are the patient and her partner related outside of marriage?
- Do the patient and her partner share the same ethnic background, such as Ashkenazic Jewish, Mediterranean, or black?

BACKGROUND

As the incidence of other causes of infant mortality decreases, the relative contribution of genetic problems to infant mortality increases. In 1940, for example, six children died of infectious diarrhea for every one who died of genetic disease; societal and medical advances have altered the incidence and severity of infectious disease to the extent that, in 1980, seven children died of genetic disease for every one who died of infectious diarrhea.[1(p2)]

The overall incidence of genetic disease is difficult to estimate because many conditions believed to have a genetic component, such as diabetes mellitus and coronary artery disease, do not occur until late in life. In addition, many genetically determined conditions are misdiagnosed or inaccurately reported.[2] The most accurate estimates are believed to be those for the incidence of chromosomal abnormalities in liveborn infants.[2] Examining findings from many nations, Lubs[4] places the overall frequency of chromosomal abnormalities at 5.6 per 1,000 live births. Milunsky[5] reports that chromosomal abnormalities occur in 7.5% of all pregnancies but that 97% of the affected pregnancies do not progress to a liveborn infant. Stenchever[6] states that, of the roughly 40% of fertilized ova that survive the first missed menstrual period, as many as 20% are aborted spontaneously, and 30% to 60% of these losses are attributable to chromosomal abnormalities.

The frequency of single gene disorders is also difficult to estimate. Most of these conditions are extremely rare, making it difficult to compile incidence data. Furthermore, the number of identifications of conditions related to single gene disorders is mushrooming; 2,000 such conditions were known in 1970,[7] but nearly 3,500 had been recognized by 1987.[5(p161)]

The third major cause of inherited disorders, the one believed to be the most common, is called *multifactorial inheritance,* meaning that altered genes and environmental factors combine to produce the outcome. The incidence of multifactorial anomalies is, again, very difficult to estimate in the aggregate.

Patterns of Mendelian Inheritance

Single gene defects or mendelian disorders express themselves through specific patterns of inheritance. By 1983, investigators had identified 1,637 diseases that result from mendelian inheritance and another 1,731 that are probably inherited in this way.[8] The patterns of mendelian inheritance are autosomal dominant, autosomal recessive, X-linked dominant, and X-linked recessive. If a condition is expressed in the heterozygous state (the gene is inherited from one parent), it is dominant; if it is expressed only in the homozygous state (the gene is inherited from both parents), it is recessive.

Autosomal Dominant Inheritance

Among the autosomal dominant conditions are achondroplasia, Huntington's chorea, Ehlers-Danlos syndrome, Marfan syndrome, and pectus excavatum, to name just a few. McKusick[8] listed 934 conditions that are definitely inherited in an autosomal dominant pattern and 893 others in which this pattern of inheritance is possible. In counseling patients about autosomal dominant patterns of inheritance and the risks to future generations, the preconceptional counselor should explain the following:[1,6]

1. The condition follows a vertical pattern, generally appearing in every generation of an affected family. Exceptions occur when there is reduced penetrance.
2. For the offspring to inherit the condition, at least one parent must be affected—unless a new mutation has occurred.
3. Each child in the family has a 50% risk of inheriting the disorder caused by the autosomal dominant gene and a 50% chance of being unaffected.
4. Unaffected persons do not transmit the condition to their offspring unless there is reduced penetrance.
5. The sex of the child does not influence the occurrence or transmission of the condition.

Autosomal Recessive Inheritance

Cystic fibrosis, galactosemia, sickle cell anemia, phenylketonuria, and Tay-Sachs, Wilson's, and Gaucher's diseases are autosomal recessive conditions. McKusick[8] listed 588 conditions that are inherited in an autosomal recessive pattern and 710 that are possibly inherited in this way. The following principles of autosomal recessive inheritance are relevant to preconceptional counseling:[1,6]

1. The disease or condition generally follows a horizontal pattern of inheritance, appearing in siblings but not in parents or other relatives.
2. For the condition to be present in the offspring, both parents must carry the gene.
3. If both parents are heterozygous for the condition (carriers), each child has a 25% chance of being homozygous (affected), a 50% chance of being heterozygous (a carrier), and a 25% chance of not inheriting the gene at all.
4. If both parents are homozygous for the condition (affected), all of their children will be affected.
5. If one parent is homozygous (affected) and one is heterozygous (a carrier), each pregnancy carries a 50% risk that the offspring will be affected and a 50% risk that the offspring will be a carrier.
6. The characteristics or conditions occur equally in both sexes.

Carriers of autosomal recessive genes are usually healthy and may be identified only after the delivery of a homozygous infant. The Council on Scientific Affairs of the American Medical Association notes, however, that identification of the heterozygous state before pregnancy allows the best chance to prevent the birth of a child with an inherited disorder. Couples with the same ethnic background have higher than average risks for autosomal recessive diseases in their offspring, because every group has at least one specific genetic "burden."[5(p201)] Couples who are related to each other also have higher risks.

Carrier tests have been developed for three autosomal recessive diseases that commonly occur in subpopulations in the United States: sickle cell disease, thalassemia, and Tay-Sachs disease. Sickle cell anemia is the most common serious genetic disease in black Americans; approximately 1 in 10 carries the gene. The thalassemia gene is present in approximately 1 in 12 individuals of Mediterranean descent in the United States, and approximately 1 in 30 Ashkenazic Jews (i.e., those with a Central or Eastern European Jewish background) has the gene for Tay-Sachs disease. Thus approximately 1 in 400 black Americans inherits sickle cell disease, 1 in 600 American Mediterraneans inherits thalassemia, and 1 in 3,600 of the Ashkenazic Jewish population inherits Tay-Sachs disease.

Cystic fibrosis is the most common autosomal recessive disease in whites, particularly those of Northern European ancestry.[1] Approximately 1 in 20 white Americans carries the gene, and the incidence in white newborns is 1 in 1,600. The disease is also seen in individuals of other backgrounds. For example, the gene occurs in approximately 1 in 50 blacks; it is less prevalent but does occur in Asians. Genetic screening for cystic fibrosis became possible in 1989 after the cystic fibrosis (CF) gene was cloned. However, the molecular heterogeneity of the disease (over 150 CF alleles have been described) complicates the screening process.[9] In 1991, the American College of Obstetricians and Gynecologists recommended that individuals with a family history of cystic fibrosis be offered screening but that testing not be applied to the general population. The recommendation was based on the likelihood that current methods will not detect a significant proportion of carrier states.[10]

Potentially affected groups have accepted these population-based special risks to varying degrees. For instance, efforts to detect carriers of the sickle cell gene in black communities and the thalassemia gene in Greek communities have been met with suspicion, resentment, and concerns of racism in some cases, but a similar effort to identify carriers of the Tay-Sachs gene has been reported to be well received.[3,11] The variation in response underscores the need for careful, culturally sensitive education and screening programs.

X-Linked Inheritance

Sex-linked traits, referred to as X-linked, are those coded on the sex chromosomes. McKusick[8] listed 115 conditions that are inherited in an X-linked pattern and 128 that may be inherited in this way. Like other genetic traits, X-linked traits are either recessive or dominant. If the condition is recessive, the normal gene overshadows the abnormal gene. Therefore, females who carry the abnormal gene will not be affected. A male conceptus who inherits the abnormal gene on its X chromosome is always affected, however, because there is no other X chromosome with a normal gene to mask the effect of the abnormal gene. If the condition is X-linked dominant, female offspring can also be affected because their other X chromosome is no longer protective.[12]

X-linked recessive conditions include glucose-6-phosphate dehydrogenase (G6PD) deficiency, hemophilia, Duchenne-type muscular dystrophy, and several types of color blindness. General principles of X-linked recessive patterns of inheritance are as follows:[1,6]

1. Affected individuals are almost always male; the female must have the abnormal gene on both of her X chromosomes to manifest the disease.[13]
2. The genes pass from affected males to all of their daughters, who are unaffected carriers. It is never passed directly from father to son.
3. Female carriers have a 25% chance of bearing an affected son, a 25% chance of bearing a normal son, a 25% chance of bearing a carrier daughter, and a 25% chance of bearing a daughter who does not have the gene.

Conditions that result from X-linked dominant patterns of inheritance are extremely rare. They include hyperammonemia, cervico-oculo-acoustic syndrome, and vitamin D–resistant rickets. Features of the X-linked dominant pattern are as follows:[1,6]

1. The condition occurs in both males and females.
2. Affected males transmit the condition to all of their daughters and to none of their sons.
3. Heterozygous females have a 50% chance in each pregnancy of transmitting the condition to their offspring, regardless of sex.
4. Homozygous females transmit the condition to all of their children.
5. X-linked dominant inheritance cannot be distinguished from autosomal dominant inheritance through the progeny of affected females; however, it can be distinguished through the progeny of affected males.

A prenatal karyotype to determine the sex of the fetus makes it possible to state the risks of X-linked disorders with greater precision. For example, if the fetus of a female carrier for an X-linked recessive disease is known to be male, there is a 50% chance that he will inherit the disease. Such information may prove crucial to the parents' desire to continue the pregnancy.

An unusual pattern of inheritance is present in the fragile X syndrome. First explained in 1980, it is now recognized as the most common inherited form of mental retardation. Fragile X syndrome causes mental retardation in 1 of every 1,000 to 1,500 males and milder retardation in 1 of every 2,000 to 2,500 females.[14] An affected male has a characteristic appearance that includes a long, thin face, a prominent jaw, protruberant ears, and macroorchidism. Autistic behavior is also common. The disorder's X-linked mode of inheritance is unique because it is neither recessive nor dominant in its characteristics: approximately 20% of males who inherit the gene are unaffected carriers, whereas 50% of heterozygous females have some characteristics of the disorder, with as many as 30% having mental retardation.[15]

Chromosomal Abnormalities

While it is possible to offer specific odds regarding the risk of single gene defects, chromosomal abnormalities present a somewhat greater challenge. Abnormal chromosomal configurations can lead to malformation syndromes, reproductive loss, or infertility. Generally, infants with multisystem problems are likely to be suffering from some deviation in their chromosomal makeup.

Of the approximately 0.5% of infants born with chromosomal abnormalities, approximately one-third have an abnormal karyotype involving the number of sex chromosomes, one-third have chromosomal aneuploidy (extra or missing chromosomes, as in trisomy 21), and one-third have a chromosomal rearrangement.[1] This distribution is quite different from that observed in spontaneously aborted fetuses; according to Cohen,[16] Turner syndrome, a sex chromosome disorder, accounts for 18% to 23% of the chromosomal abnormalities in these fetuses, trisomies account for as many as 52%, and structural rearrangements for 3% to 7%. Furthermore, Cohen reports that approximately 95% to 97% of all Turner syndrome embryos are spontaneously aborted, as are 95% of those with trisomy 18 and 65% to 75% of those with trisomy 21. Other chromosomal abnormalities, such as triploidy (three sets of 23 chromosomes) and tetraploidy (four sets of 23 chromosomes), have been observed in spontaneous abortuses with an incidence of 55 per 1,000 and 15 per 1,000, respectively. Neither condition results in a viable infant.[12]

Although most chromosomal abnormalities occur sporadically and have a low risk of recurrence, inherited translocations are sometimes transmitted through families.[2] For example, 3% of the cases of Down syndrome are the result of a parental translocation. A previous sporadic event carries little increased risk of recurrence over that of the general population, but an inherited occurrence may carry significantly increased risk. For this reason, chromosome studies should generally be performed on parents who have had repeated pregnancy loss or who have had a child with either a suspected chromosomal abnormality or a diagnosed structural chromosomal rearrangement. In 4.8% to 5.5% of phenotypically normal couples with two or more consecutive spontaneous abortions, one of the parents can be expected to have a chromosomal abnormality, such as reciprocal translocation, Robertsonian translocation, or inversion.[17]

Through cytogenetic studies, the chromosomal makeup of a cell can be determined. Each of the chromosomes differs in size, shape, and staining (known as banding) characteristics.[12] Arrangement of the chromosomes by size and morphology according to a standard classification results in a karyotype. Interpretation of abnormal karyotypes and assignment of risk are best done by genetics specialists.

Multifactorial Inheritance

Many congenital anomalies appear to have a familial basis, but they are associated with neither a mendelian inheritance pattern nor chromosomal abnormalities. It is believed that the occurrence of these anomalies is controlled by a multifactorial model of inheritance. In other words, they are believed to result from a gene-environment interaction. Because multifactorial inheritance involves several genes, the genetic component is regarded as polygenic. Numerous malformations, including cleft lip, pyloric stenosis, congenital dislocations of the hip, neural tube defects, and congenital heart disease, have been identified as multifactorial.[13]

In contrast to the risk of single gene inheritance, which remains constant with each conception,[16] the risk of multifactorial inheritance in subsequent pregnancies increases with the number of affected individuals within the family. For example, the risk of congenital heart disease of multifactorial origin in a child conceived after the birth of one affected child is 2% to 4%; if two previous children have been affected, however, the risk increases to 8%.[16]

Many factors must be considered in multifactorial inheritance before risk data are offered to prospective parents. Such factors include population prevalence of the anomaly and the sex of affected individuals. For example, if a couple has a child with a neural tube defect in Northern Ireland, where the incidence of this anomaly is comparatively high, their risk for recurrence is greater than that of a comparable couple in North America. Similarly, if a female child is born with pyloric stenosis, a condition more common in males, the risk to subsequent children is markedly increased; the recurrence risk for first-degree male relatives in this scenario is 18.2%, compared with 4.6% if the index child was a male.[16] These examples underscore the thoroughness and the attention to detail that must accompany genetic counseling.

PRECONCEPTIONAL COUNSELING

The goal of preconceptional counseling relative to family history is to provide the prospective parents with sufficient information to make informed decisions about their reproductive options. The counseling may be prospective if an affected child has not yet been born or retrospective if a child with a birth defect has been born and the parents seek information about the likelihood of a recurrence.[18]

Genetics involves the health of all family members across generations, not just the health of individuals.[19] The American Society of Human Genetics defines genetic counseling as "a communication process which deals with the occurrence or the risk of occurrence of a genetic disorder in a family."[20(p240)] Garver[18(p89)] states that anyone involved in patient care should counsel on some level: "This would include not only genetic counselors, but also primary care physicians, nurses, social workers, psychologists, and educators." Garver also notes that, of all primary care physicians, obstetricians have the greatest opportunity through premarital and preconceptional visits to provide this type of care to their patients. Recent medical-legal developments underscore the need for all practitioners to counsel their antenatal patients adequately in the area of genetic problems.[12] As antenatal care expands to include the preconceptional period, such medical-legal pressures can be expected to apply to the preconceptional period as well.

The American Public Health Association states that "the primary care team ... must have knowledge and skills in genetics."[19(p14)] Without special training in genetics and in counseling, however, the primary care provider's most appropriate services are likely to be the identification of at-risk patients; an introduction to the services and processes involved in genetic counseling; suggestions regarding the types of information that the genetic counselor is likely to need, such as a detailed family medical history, autopsy reports, and pictures; facilitation of referral; and a sense of optimism. Couples who have genetic disease in their families or who have had a previous child with a birth defect generally have a much better chance of having a normal child in a subsequent pregnancy than they fear.

At the preconceptional counseling session, the family and reproductive histories of both the patient and her partner should be reviewed carefully to identify any indications for prospective or retrospective genetic counseling. At no point during the preconceptional counseling process is the presence of the woman's partner more important than in the gathering of information about family histories. Every effort should be made to include him in the visit. To relieve the patient and her partner of any guilt or anxiety that they are somehow inferior because of their genetic composition, the counselor should explain that all individuals carry many abnormal genes and that one purpose of the family history is to determine whether any of those genes are of identifiable consequence to their offspring.

One common source of error in genetic counseling is called *genetic heterogeneity.*[2] Abnormalities with markedly similar clinical pictures may have different pathogeneses, ranging from a new mutation to single gene, chromosomal, or multifactorial inheritance to a nongenetic origin. Approximately 1% to 2% of congenital heart disease, for example, is of nongenetic origin, 5% is of chromosomal origin, 3% is of single gene origin, and 90% is probably of multifactorial origin.[16] Without adequate investigation of the cause of the problem, risk data are likely to be misleading. A previous child with hypogonadism related to a single gene defect could represent a recurrence risk of 50% for subsequent male conceptuses; if the hypogonadism was not due to a genetic or chromosomal influence, however, the risk of recurrence would be negligible.[2] The marked clinical variability that can occur in presentation may also confuse the tracing of an abnormality in the family tree and again result in inappropriate counseling.

No matter how sophisticated the patient appears, the counselor should never assume that she understands the nature of the disease in question or of the principles of inheritance. The March of Dimes Birth Defects Foundation offers a series of information sheets that cover numerous topics, including cystic fibrosis, Tay-Sachs disease, thalassemia, sickle cell disease, congenital heart disease, and cleft lip and palate. These information sheets explain the significance of each specific disease, modes of inheritance, and the availability of carrier state and prenatal testing. Available through local March of Dimes chapters, these information sheets are a valuable resource for the preconceptional counselor.

Patients often misinterpret the risks associated with patterns of mendelian inheritance. After listening to risk data stated as percentages or fractions, patients often believe that a previous poor outcome protects their future pregnancies. When the preconceptional counselor states that a specific outcome is likely to occur 25% of the time, for example, patients may believe that the three pregnancies that follow a pregnancy with such an outcome are guaranteed to be normal. A crucial counseling principle is that chance has no memory, and a goal for all counselors is to ensure that patients understand this key fact.

The *Guidelines for Perinatal Care,* produced jointly by the American Academy of Pediatrics and the American College of Obstetricians and Gynecologists,[21] identifies many indications for prenatal diagnostic testing. A majority of risk factors are discernible before conception and thus lend themselves to preconceptional counseling. These include advanced maternal age, defined as women expected to be 35 years old or older at the date of delivery; previous offspring with a chromosomal aberration; a chromosomal abnormality in either parent, particularly a translocation; single gene disorders in a previous child or carrier status of the parents; and multifactorial disorders in a first-degree relative. The preconceptional counselor should take care to provide couples who are black or of Ashkenazic Jewish, or Mediterranean ancestry with information on the specific autosomal recessive diseases associated with their ethnic background and then offer appropriate carrier testing.

Every preconceptional counselor should have a strong working relationship with a genetics program. If a risk for genetic abnormalities is identified, the availability of genetic counseling should be discussed with the patient or couple and appropriate referral made. To ensure that the information relayed to the couple is consistent, a follow-up report to the referring provider should be requested. The couple should understand that the purpose of counseling is to define risks, when possible, and to examine reproductive options. Unfortunately, too many people equate genetic counseling with abortion and reject the service on this ground. If the couple rejects genetic counseling, reasons for suggesting referral and the couple's decision should be noted in the record.

The counselor should discuss the various reproductive options with the prospective parents. If a couple has chosen to participate in a genetic counseling program, options will most likely have been introduced at that time.

Decisions regarding the various options will take time and reflection, and patients should have an opportunity to return to their preconceptional counselor for further information. Such options include unchanged plans; foregoing childbearing; artificial insemination; chromosomal analysis and carrier screening of the prospective parents; and prenatal diagnosis through chorionic villus sampling, amniocentesis, α-fetoprotein screening, or ultrasonography. Not all alternatives are appropriate in every situation. For example, chorionic villus sampling does not identify the fetus with a neural tube defect, and ultrasonography does not identify the fetus homozygous for cystic fibrosis. Therefore, the options presented should be appropriate to the risk. In addition, patients must understand that none of the tests or technologies available is 100% predictive.

The moral and ethical beliefs of patients and the degree of risk that they are willing to accept vary markedly. A study of 76 families who underwent genetic counseling after the birth of a child with one of four genetically influenced conditions showed a strong relationship between the parents' perception of the burden of the disease and their plans regarding further reproduction.[22] The authors concluded that burden, as distinct from risk, has a large role in the parents' decisions about future childbearing. Another important factor in making decisions about childbearing may be the comfort associated with decisions made in previous pregnancies. One study indicated that couples who abort a fetus secondary to genetic disease or congenital defects experience more guilt and depression than do couples who abort primarily for social reasons.[23]

The counselor must discuss reproductive options in a nonjudgmental fashion, without interjecting any personal bias.[1] The counselor's mission is to ensure that the couple's decisions, whatever they may be, are informed. Therefore, information on the natural history of the disorder in question, including its associated symptoms, treatment options, and likely effect on functioning and longevity, should be discussed, as well as the potential social and economic ramifications for the family, including risks for lifelong dependency of the offspring or expensive treatments and health insurance exclusions. If the counselor does not feel qualified to provide this information, referral to a pediatric service that specializes in the condition is appropriate. Parents should also be aware of community resources, such as parent-to-parent groups, early stimulation programs, and specialized education facilities, if any of these are relevant to the condition under discussion.

Many women and couples do not view the threat of a genetic disease as sufficient cause for preconceptional screening or prenatal diagnosis. If they have been provided with factual information upon which to base their decision, the preconceptional counselor should support the decision.[24]

In general, couples who have a family history indicative of genetic risk or who have had an anomalous child have an excellent chance of bearing a normal child in the future. Genetic counseling is frequently perceived as a gloomy activity. In actuality, however, it more often offers hope through the careful delineation of risks and, when risks are considered high by the couple, the exploration of a variety of options that can help the couple to realize their reproductive goals, whatever those goals may be.

Patients should be reminded that the occurrence of most birth defects is unpredictable and most often relates to multifactorial causes. The best preventive approach is likely to be the provision of an optimal periconceptional environment for the developing embryo. This can be achieved by practicing good nutrition and avoiding unnecessary exposure to chemicals and drugs, including alcohol and tobacco. Patients should be aware that, although these actions are likely to maximize their chances of a rewarding reproductive experience, they offer no guarantee.

References

1. Garver KL, Marchese SG: *Genetic Counseling for Clinicians.* Chicago, Mosby, 1986.
2. Kaback MM: Medical genetics: An overview. *Pediatr Clin North Am* 1978;25: 395-409.
3. Genetic counseling and prevention of birth defects. Council Report. *JAMA* 1982;248:221-224.
4. Lubs HA: Frequency of genetic disease, in Lubs HA, de la Cruz F (eds): *Genetic Counseling.* New York, Raven Press, 1977.
5. Milunsky A: *How to Have the Healthiest Baby You Can.* New York, Simon & Schuster, 1987.
6. Stenchever MA: Genetics, in Droegemueller W, Herbst AL, Mishell DR, et al (eds): *Comprehensive Gynecology.* St. Louis, Mosby, 1987, chap 2.
7. Lubs HA, Ruddle FH: Chromosomal abnormalities in the human population: Estimation of rates based on New Haven Newborn Study. *Science* 1970;169:495-497.
8. McKusick VA: *Mendelian Inheritance in Man,* ed 6. Baltimore, The Johns Hopkins University Press, 1983.
9. Mennie ME, Geilfillan A, Compton M, et al: Prenatal screening for cystic fibrosis. *Lancet* 1992;340:214.
10. American college of Obstetricians and Gynecologists. Current status of cystic fibrosis carrier screening. *ACOG Committee Opinion 101.* Washington, DC: ACOG, 1991.
11. Rowley PT: Genetic screening: Marvel or menace? *Science* 1984;225:138-144.
12. Beischer NA, MacKay EV: *Obstetrics and the Newborn,* ed 2. Philadelphia, WB Saunders, 1986, pp 132-135.
13. Pritchard JA, MacDonald PC, Gant NF: Injuries and malformations of the fetus and newborn infant, in *Williams Obstetrics,* ed 17. Norwalk, Conn, Appleton-Century-Crofts, 1985, chap 39.
14. Rousseau F, Heitz D, Biancalana V, et al: Direct diagnosis by DNA analysis of the fragile X syndrome of mental retardation. *N Engl J Med* 1991;325:1673-1681.
15. Shapiro LR: The fragile X syndrome—a peculiar pattern of inheritance. *N Engl J Med* 1991;325:1736-1737.
16. Cohen FL: *Clinical Genetics in Nursing Practice.* New York, JB Lippincott, 1984.
17. Portnoi M-F, Joye H, Van Dan Akker J, et al: Karotypes of 1142 couples with recurrent abortion. *Obstet Gynecol* 1988; 72:31-34.
18. Garver KL: Genetic counseling in primary obstetrical care. *Obstet Gynecol Ann* 1979;8:87-123.
19. American Public Health Association: Genetics and public health. *The Nation's Health.* September 1987, pp 14-15.
20. American Society of Human Genetics: Genetic counseling. *Am J Hum Genet* 1975;27:240-242.
21. American Academy of Pediatrics, American College of Obstetricians and Gynecologists: *Guidelines for Perinatal Care,* ed 3. Elk Grove Village, IL: American Academy of Pediatrics, 1992.
22. Leonard CO, Chase GA, Childs B: Genetic counseling: A consumer's view. *N Engl J Med* 1973;287:433-439.
23. Blumberg BD, Golbus MS, Hanson KH: The psychological sequelae of abortions performed for a genetic indication. *Am J Obstet Gynecol* 1975;122:799-808.
24. Cheschier NC, Cefalo RC: Prenatal diagnosis and caring. *Women's Health Issues* 1992;2:123-132.

9

Male Issues in Preconceptional Health

Although it was once common for a woman who had an abnormal baby to blame herself and for the community to echo that blame, it is now acknowledged that men must share some responsibility for abnormalities in the couple's offspring. This realization has prompted a new focus of attention upon male-mediated causes of birth defects.[1]

Even though no strong, consistent human evidence exists that male-mediated factors affect the occurrence of congenital anomalies, this observation should not be misconstrued as evidence that such effects do not occur.[2] The authors of a recent review of male-mediated reproductive outcomes note that experimental evidence is accumulating that paternal exposures during the prefertilization and perifertilization periods can cause a variety of problems.[2] For instance, if the ovum is fertilized by a genetically altered spermatozoon, the resulting conceptus might develop abnormally, resulting in miscarriage or in live birth with malformation, or appear normal at birth but be at increased risk for developing a disease later, such as cancer.[3] Of the 1,491 compounds associated with adverse reproductive outcomes in laboratory animals, 194 relate to paternal exposures.[2] Researchers have associated male exposures in laboratory animals with spontaneous abortion, low birthweight, congenital anomalies, cancer, and developmental delays. Davis and colleagues[2(p290)] hypothesize that the "paucity of [human] evidence on paternally mediated adverse reproductive outcomes represents an imbalance in research efforts rather than a true imbalance in causality."

Blame is not a constructive concept in preconceptional counseling; however, the premise of shared responsibility is. There are biologic limits to a male's influence on reproductive outcomes, but there are no limits to the ways in which he can support his partner. For example, he can control his own alcohol, tobacco, and drug exposures or change his nutritional habits as a means of aiding his partner in doing the same. Such actions not only help the woman to carry through with preconceptional recommendations but also may have a positive effect on spermatogenesis, male fertility, and lifelong health habits.

BACKGROUND
Tobacco

A 1974 study of 3,696 births to nonsmoking women whose partners smoked found that the incidence of severe malformation in the offspring increased significantly with increasing levels of paternal smoking.[4] Malformations in all systems were more frequent if the father smoked more than 10 cigarettes per day; the incidence of facial malformation was particularly influenced by smoking level. Interestingly, the researchers did not identify an association between paternal smoking and reduced birthweight or increased incidence of preterm birth.

Other studies have not associated paternal smoking with an increased incidence of congenital abnormalities but have shown a relationship between paternal smoking and reduced birthweight. A prospective study of 3,891 antenatal patients revealed that 23.6% had not smoked cigarettes during gestation, but they had been exposed to sidestream smoke for at least 2 hours daily.[5] Passive smoke exposure was significantly related to the delivery of full-term low-birthweight infants. The infants of nonsmoking women exposed to passive smoke weighed an average of 24 g less than did those of women not exposed to passive smoke. The reduced birthweights of infants born to women who smoked were not exaggerated by maternal exposure to sidestream smoke.[5] A recent study conducted in Shanghai, China, supports the hypothesis that paternal smoking has a modest effect on birthweight. After adjusting for gestational age, parity, maternal age, and occupation, the average birthweight of infants exposed in utero to paternal smoke was found to be 30 g less than that of nonexposed infants.[6] An advantage to this study is that it is unlikely that maternal smoking confounded the findings: less than 0.5% of women in Shanghai of peak reproductive age smoke, compared with 57% of men in the same age group.

The mechanisms by which passive smoking affects birthweight are not understood. Thiocyanate levels have been investigated, because birthweight has been inversely correlated with elevated levels of thiocyanate in women who smoked during pregnancy. However, two studies of fetal thiocyanate levels in pregnancies of women exposed to passive smoke produced conflicting data: Bottoms and colleagues[7] found that fetal levels of thiocyanate were significantly influenced by sidestream smoke, but Hauth and colleagues[8] found no evidence that passive cigarette smoke exposure resulted in maternal or umbilical cord concentrations higher than those found in nonsmokers.

Preliminary evidence indicates that smoking may affect male fertility by altering spermatogenesis, sperm density, sperm mobility, and sperm morphology.[9] Further study is warranted.

Alcohol

It has been demonstrated in humans that alcohol adversely affects plasma testosterone levels during both acute and chronic use and during the withdrawal period.[10] A common manifestation of chronic alcoholism is a hyperestrogenic state, as evidenced by a female escutcheon, palmar erythema, gynecomastia, or spider angiomas.[11] Both human and animal studies document the significant spermatozoal morphologic changes that alcohol consumption produces.[12] Impotence is another commonly observed complication of alcoholism.

The effects of chronic paternal alcohol ingestion were first observed 70 years ago in the offspring of laboratory animals. Continuing animal research has demonstrated a fairly consistent pattern, including decreased litter size, altered birthweight, increased incidence of stillbirth and neonatal death, increased male to female ratios, and increased incidence of behavioral abnormalities.[13] Little information links paternal alcoholism in humans with poor pregnancy outcomes, however, other than occasional case reports. One exception is a study of 377 infants whose birthweights were analyzed relative to paternal preconceptional drinking. The results indicated a strong correlation between the father's alcohol use in the month before conception and the infant's birthweight.[14] If the father averaged two or more drinks daily or had at least five drinks on one occasion, infant birthweight was reduced by 181 g. A stepwise regression analysis to investigate the effects of other drug use by each parent predicted that paternal alcohol use reduced infant birthweight by an average of 137 g. A study undertaken by Sokol and colleagues[15] of 3,000 women found that the father's height, his frequency of alcohol use, and the infant's sex are significant determinants of infant birthweight percentile. The effect of paternal alcohol use was minimal, however, predicting a 45 g reduction in birthweight at 40 weeks' gestation for infants whose fathers drank nearly every day, compared with infants fathered by nondrinkers. According to Little and Sing,[14] associations between paternal alcohol use and fetal growth can be explained in at least two ways: a direct relationship could exist or drinking could be a surrogate measure for undetermined influences.

Illicit Drug Use

Reductions in birthweight, decreases in litter size, and increases in neonatal mortality have been observed in laboratory animals after paternal exposure to morphine or methadone. However, "structural malformations have not been induced by narcotic treatment of male animals and human effects of paternal narcotic use have not yet been demonstrated."[13(p15)]

Nutrition

In animals, certain nutritional deficiencies have been reported to affect the male gonads directly; others affect spermatogenesis primarily through the endocrine system. Four nutrients reported to be essential for normal spermatogenesis in rats are linoleic acid, vitamin A, vitamin E, and zinc.[16] Much remains unknown about the interaction of nutrition, endocrine activity, and spermatogenesis, but there are good reasons to infer that proper nutrition may be important in ensuring optimal male reproductive health.

Age

The mean age of fathers has been observed to be greater than expected for autosomal dominant disease caused by new mutations.[17] Achondroplasia[18], Marfan syndrome, and fibrodysplasia ossificans progressiva[19] are commonly cited as diseases associated with increased paternal age. According to one mathematical model, the risk that a man older than 40 years of age will father an offspring with an autosomal dominant disease caused by a new mutation is no less than 0.3% to 0.5%.[17] The author concludes that, because one third of babies with such conditions have fathers age 40 or older, the incidence of autosomal dominant disease could be significantly decreased if men completed their families by age 40. The indicated risk, however, is only 3 to 5 per 1,000, which may not be perceived by couples as sufficient to alter their reproductive plans.

Advanced paternal age has also been implicated in the increased incidence of Down syndrome; 20% to 30% of cases are believed to be of paternal origin.[20] Studies to correlate paternal age with the incidence of Down syndrome independent of maternal age have produced conflicting results, however. Some have indicated a twofold effect for men 55 and over,[21,22] whereas others have shown no statistically significant relationship.[23-25]

Analyzing data available from the Metropolitan Atlanta Congenital Defects Program, Lian and colleagues[26] determined that children born to fathers over age 40 are at 20% greater risk of having a birth defect. A tenfold greater risk was observed for chondrodystrophy and situs inversus; less dramatic risks were noted for atrial and ventricular septal defects. A recent analysis of data collected in the early 1960s through the Child Health and Development Studies reveals that paternal age of 35 years and older is associated with increased risk of periauricular cyst, nasal aplasia, cleft palate, hydrocephalus, pulmonic stenosis, urethral stenosis, and hemangioma.[3] The authors caution against over-interpretation of their findings because of the study's imprecision. As have other investigators of male-mediated reproductive effects, they stress the need for additional research.

Medical History

Few male medical conditions have been implicated in adverse reproductive outcomes. Obvious exceptions are those conditions inherited through mendelian principles and those that cause sterility. Some evidence indicates that paternal epilepsy may have a negative effect on fetal development, because the offspring of these men may have a higher incidence of birth defects than do control populations.[13] The increased risk is reported to be less than that in pregnancy complicated by maternal epilepsy, however.[27] It is generally believed that the disease itself, rather than exposure to anticonvulsant drugs, is the significant factor.

The treatment of cancer with chemotherapy that affects DNA has also been suggested as a threat to normal fetal development. Although some authorities have advised termination of pregnancy if conception occurred when the father was recovering from chemotherapy, no evidence shows that these men may not expect to father normal children.[13]

Exposure to Drugs and Chemicals

Reports on the reproductive effects of male chemical exposure are inconclusive. These effects could occur in two ways: paternal exposure could contaminate the maternal environment, resulting in secondary maternal exposure, or exposure could directly affect male germinal tissue.[28] Researchers have suggested that paternal exposure to vinyl chloride, chloroprine, benzene, anesthetic gases, lead, and many other chemicals is detrimental to pregnancy outcome. The adverse outcomes most frequently cited are male infertility and spontaneous abortion in his sexual partner.[29] Some observers have claimed that paternal exposure to certain chemicals causes congenital defects, but conclusive scientific evidence is not always available to support these claims. For example, reports that paternal exposure to Agent Orange caused birth defects in offspring created considerable public anxiety, but epidemiologic evidence for the association is limited.[3,30,31]

Experimental research has been undertaken to investigate the reproductive effects in mammals of at least seven drugs (morphine and related narcotics, alcohol, propoxyphene, thalidomide, anticonvulsant drugs, halothane, and enflurane) and five groups of toxic chemicals (lead, vinyl chloride, dioxin, 2,4-D and 2,4,5-T pesticides, and polychlorinated biphenyls).[32] Unequivocal evidence indicates that poisoning sufficient to cause either a clinically apparent toxic reaction or teratospermia can reduce fertility and the average birthweight of offspring in the laboratory.[32] The evidence does not support a relationship between paternal exposure to these substances and the occurrence of malformation in laboratory animals, however.

Human epidemiologic studies indicate that exposure to many of the substances listed above not only affects fertility but can also, as in the case of vinyl chloride[33] and benzene,[34] increase the frequency of chromosomal abnormalities. Human paternal exposure to lead,[32] vinyl chloride,[35] and anesthetic gases[36] has been demonstrated to increase the spontaneous abortion rate in their partners, but increased incidences of congenital abnormalities have not been definitely established for these paternal exposures.[13,28,32] Because defective conceptuses are selectively aborted, the increased spontaneous abortion rate may reflect a teratogenic effect.

Chemicals may cause mutations that can result in cancer in the offspring (see Chapter 2). Limited information indicates that the incidence of cancer in mice can be increased by paternal exposure to mutagens.[37] A number of case-control studies on the role of parental occupation in the etiology of childhood cancers have been reported[38] but are not conclusive; prospective studies are needed. Given the rarity of childhood cancers, the cohorts would need to be very large. For example, 10,000 workers with an annual birth rate of 20 per 1,000 would need to be followed for 15 years to produce just three cases of childhood carcinoma.[38]

PRECONCEPTIONAL COUNSELING

The goals of preconceptional counseling on male issues are to encourage cooperation and support between the prospective father and mother and to identify male exposures that could adversely affect reproduction.

Including the male partner in the preconceptional counseling session has several advantages. For example, obtaining an adequate family history without both partners present would be cumbersome and most likely unsatisfactory; helping a woman address her feelings about a previous pregnancy loss in isolation would be less than optimal; and decisions regarding pregnancy that could place a woman's life in jeopardy or could affect the couple's lifestyle are best made after both members of the partnership have been fully educated. Including the male partner in the counseling session also has the advantage of allowing the preconceptional counselor to identify any habits or exposures he has had that could jeopardize a healthy pregnancy outcome.

Paternal exposures should be carefully reviewed in instances of repeated pregnancy loss, because animal and human studies indicate that a relationship can exist. The most likely reproductive effects of male exposures are decreased fertility and increased spontaneous abortion rates resulting from damage to the sperm. Because spermatogenesis is continuous, the adverse effects of various chemicals and drugs on the sperm are limited to approximately 12 weeks from the date of exposure. Therefore, the preconceptional counselor should pay particular attention to recent or anticipated drug and chemical contacts. The resources listed in Appendix B should be called upon for the most up-to-date counseling information.

Good principles of health, including optimal nutrition and the avoidance of alcohol, tobacco, and illicit drugs, should be encouraged. Not only will these actions have possible benefits on spermatogenesis, but they will also increase the likelihood that the woman will be successful in managing her own health habits.

References

1. Rogers JG, Danks DM: Birth defects and the father. *Med J Aust* 1983;2:3.
2. Davis DL, Friedler G, Mattison D, Morris R: Male-mediated teratogenesis and other reproductive effects: Biologic and epidemiologic findings and a plea for clinical research. *Repro Toxicol* 1992;6:289-292.
3. Savitz DA, Schwingl PJ, Keels MA: Influence of paternal age, smoking and alcohol consumption on congenital anomalies. *Teratology* 1991;44:429-440.
4. Longo LD: Some health consequences of maternal smoking: Issues without answers. *Birth Defects: Original Article Series* 1982;18(3A):13-31.
5. Martin TR, Bracken MB: Association of low birth weight with passive smoke exposure in pregnancy. *Am J Epidemiol* 1986;124:633-642.
6. Zhang J, Ratcliffe JM: Paternal smoking and birthweight in Shanghai. *AJPH* 1993;83:207-210.
7. Bottoms SF, Kuhnert BR, Kuhnert PM, et al: Maternal passive smoking and fetal serum thiocyanate levels. *Am J Obstet Gynecol* 1982;144:787-791.
8. Hauth JC, Hauth J, Drawbaugh RB, et

al: Passive smoking and thiocyanate concentrations in pregnant women and newborns. *Obstet Gynecol* 1984;63:519-521.

9. Lincoln R: Smoking and reproduction. *Fam Plann Perspect* 1986;18:79-84.

10. Gorden GG, Altman K, Southren LA, et al: Effect of alcohol (ethanol) administration on sex hormones in normal men. *N Engl J Med* 1976;295:793-797.

11. VanThiel DH, Gavaler JS, Eagon P, et al: Effect of alcohol on gonadal function. *Drug Alcohol Depend* 1980;6:41-46.

12. Hadi HA, Hill JA, Castillo RA: Alcohol and reproductive function: A review. *Obstet Gynecol Surv* 1987;42:69-74.

13. Paternally-induced adverse pregnancy effects. *Repro Toxicol* 1984;3:13-16.

14. Little RE, Sing CF: Father's drinking and infant birth weight: Report of an association. *Teratology* 1987;36:59-65.

15. Sokol RJ, Martier SS, Ager JW, et al: Paternal drinking may affect intrauterine growth. *Am J Obstet Gynecol* 1993; 168(3):307.

16. Leathem JH: Nutritional influences on testicular composition and function in animals, in Hamilton DW, Greep RO (eds): *Handbook of Physiology.* Washington, DC, American Physiological Society, 1975, pp 225-232.

17. Friedman JM: Genetic disease in the offspring of older fathers. *Obstet Gynecol* 1981;57.745-749.

18. Thompson JN, Schaefer GB, Conley MC: Achondroplasia and parental age. *N Engl J Med* 1986;314:521-522.

19. Rogers JG, Chase GA: Paternal age effect in fibrodysplasia ossificans progressiva. *J Med Genet* 1979;16:147-148.

20. Hansson A, Mikkelsen M: The origin of the extra chromosome 21 in Down's syndrome. *Cytogenet Cell Genet* 1978;20: 194-203.

21. Stene J, Fischer G, Stene E, et al: Paternal age effect in Down's syndrome. *Ann Hum Genet* 1977;40:299-306.

22. Matsunaga E, Tonomura A, Oishi H, et al: Reexamination of paternal age effect in Down's syndrome. *Hum Genet* 1978; 40:259-268.

23. Erickson JD: Paternal age and Down syndrome. *Am J Hum Genet* 1979;31: 489-497.

24. Regal RR, Cross PK, Lamson SH, et al: A search for evidence for a paternal age effect independent of a maternal age effect in birth certificate reports of Down's syndrome in New York State. *Am J Epidemiol* 1980;112:650-655.

25. Martin RH, Rademaker AW: The effect of age on frequency of sperm chromosomal abnormalities in normal men. *Am J Hum Genet* 1987;41:484-492.

26. Lian Z-H, Zack MM, Erickson JD: Paternal age and the occurrence of birth defects. *Am J Hum Genet* 1986;39:648-660.

27. Shapiro S, Slone D, Hartz SC, et al: Anticonvulsants and parental epilepsy in the development of birth defects. *Lancet* 1976;1:272-275.

28. Haas JF, Schottenfeld D: Risks to the offspring from parental occupational exposures. *J Occup Med* 1979;21:607-613.

29. Stellman JM: The effects of toxic agents on reproduction. *Occup Health Saf* 1979; 36:36-43.

30. Hatch M, Stein ZA: Agent Orange and risks to reproduction. The limits of epidemiology. *Teratog Carcinog Mutagen* 1986;6:185-202.

31. Pearn JH: Teratogens and the male. An analysis with reference to herbicide exposure. *Med J Aust* 1983;2:16-20.

32. Pearn JH: Teratogens and the male: An analysis with special reference to herbicide exposure. *Med J Aust* 1983;2:16-20.

33. Funes-Cravioto F, Lambert B, Lindsten J, et al: Chromosome aberrations in workers exposed to vinyl chloride. *Lancet* 1975;1:459.

34. Trough IM, Court-Brown WM: Chromosome aberrations and exposure to ambient benzene. *Lancet* 1975;1:684.

35. Infante PF, Wagoner JK, McMichael AJ, et al: Genetic risks of vinyl chloride. *Lancet* 1976;1:734-735.

36. Cohen EN, Brown BW, Bruce DL: A survey of anesthetic health hazards among dentists. *J Am Dent Assoc* 1975; 90:1291-1296.

37. Brown NA: Are offspring at risk from their father's exposure to toxins? *Nature* 1985;316:110.

38. Terracini B, Pastore G, Segnan N: Association of father's occupation and cancer in children. *Biol Res Preg Perinatol* 1983;4:40–45.

A
Preconceptional Health Assessment

The following preconceptional health assessment form is derived from the screening questions recommended in the text of this book. This assessment tool can be used in various ways: (1) it can be mailed to the patient before her appointment with instructions to complete it and bring it to her counseling session; (2) it can be completed by the patient in the waiting room just before the session; or (3) it can be completed by the health care professional during the initial interview. The first approach has advantages in that it encourages the patient to organize potentially important information before the counseling session, such as the amounts of vitamin supplementation or the types of chemical exposures, and to review pertinent questions with her partner if he is unable to attend the session with her. If the population being served has limited reading skills, the form or its use should be modified to accommodate patients' abilities.

PRECONCEPTIONAL HEALTH ASSESSMENT*

What is your main interest in seeking preconceptional counseling?

_____

_____

_____

_____

So that we can address your specific interests and concerns, we ask that you complete the following questionnaire. You may use the back of the form to provide additional information when necessary.

_____

*Merry-K. Moos and Robert C. Cefalo, University of North Carolina at Chapel Hill, 1985 (revised 1987).

Place an X next to any item that applies to you.

SOCIAL HISTORY

Do you

_____ drink beer, wine, or hard liquor

_____ smoke cigarettes or use any other tobacco products

_____ use marijuana, cocaine, or any recreational drugs

_____ use lead or chemicals at home or at work
If yes, list the specific chemicals if you know what they are:

_____

_____

_____ work with radiation

_____ participate in an exercise program

Are you

_____ 34 years of age or older

NUTRITION HISTORY

On the back of this sheet, list by meal everything you ate and drank yesterday, including the approximate amount; indicate snacks separately.
Do you

_____ practice vegetarianism

_____ eat unusual substances, such as laundry starch or clay

_____ have a history of bulimia or anorexia

_____ follow a special diet
If yes, describe:

_____

_____

_____ supplement your diet with vitamins
If yes, list vitamins and dosages:

_____

_____

_____ take medications, including oral contraceptives

_____ have an intolerance for milk

MEDICAL HISTORY

Do you now have or have you ever had

_____ diabetes

_____ thyroid disease

_____ phenylketonuria (PKU)

_____ asthma

_____ heart disease

_____ high blood pressure

_____ deep venous thrombosis (blood clots)

_____ kidney disease

_____ systemic lupus erythematosus (SLE)

_____ epilepsy

_____ sickle cell disease

_____ cancer

_____ other health problems that require medical or surgical care
If yes, describe:

_____

_____

INFECTIOUS DISEASE HISTORY

Do you or your partner have a history of

_____ recurrent genital infections

_____ herpes simplex

_____ *Chlamydia* infection

_____ human papillomavirus (genital warts)

_____ gonorrhea

_____ syphilis

_____ viral hepatitis or high-risk behavior, including use of intravenous street drugs, intimate bisexual/homosexual contact, or multiple sexual partners

_____ acquired immunodeficiency syndrome (AIDS) or high-risk behavior, including use of intravenous street drugs, intimate bisexual/homosexual contact, or multiple sexual partners

_____ occupational exposure to the blood or bodily secretions of others

_____ blood transfusions

Do you

_____ own or work with cats

_____ have documented immunity to rubella

MEDICATION HISTORY

Do you

_____ routinely or occasionally take prescribed medications

If yes, list names and dosages:

_____

_____

_____ routinely or occasionally take over-the-counter medications
If yes, list names and dosages:

_____

_____

REPRODUCTIVE HISTORY

Do you have a history of

_____ uterine or cervical abnormalities

_____ two or more pregnancies that ended in first-trimester miscarriages

_____ one or more pregnancies that ended between 14 and 28 weeks of gestation

_____ one or more fetal deaths

_____ one or more infants who weighed less than 5½ lbs. at birth

_____ one or more infants who were admitted to a neonatal intensive care unit

_____ one or more infants with a birth defect

FAMILY HISTORY

Do you, your partner, or members of either of your families, including children, have

_____ hemophilia

_____ thalassemia

_____ Tay-Sachs disease

_____ sickle cell disease or trait

_____ phenylketonuria (PKU)

_____ cystic fibrosis

_____ a birth defect

_____ mental retardation

_____ Are you and your partner related outside of marriage (such as cousins)?

_____ Do you and your partner have the same ethnic or racial background, such as Ashkenazic Jewish, Mediterranean, or black?

Resources for Information on Reproductive Effects of Drugs and Chemicals

Reproductive Toxicology Center. This center markets, at a reasonable fee, an online information database called *Reprotox.* The database includes information on the reproductive effects of industrial and environmental chemicals; prescription, over-the-counter, and recreational drugs; and nutritional agents. 202-293-5137.

Schardein JL: *Chemically Induced Birth Defects.* New York, Marcel Dekker, 1985.

Shepard TH: *Catalog of Teratogenic Agents,* ed 7. Baltimore, The Johns Hopkins University Press, 1992.

Briggs GG, Freeman RK, Yaffe SJ: *Drugs in Pregnancy and Lactation,* ed 3. Baltimore, Williams & Wilkins, 1990.

TERATOLOGY INFORMATION SERVICES FOR THE UNITED STATES AND CANADA
Federal

Environmental Protection Agency Pesticide Hotline
800-858-7378

Arizona

Arizona Teratogen Information Program
800-362-0101 (Ariz. only)

California

California Teratogen Information Service and Clinical Research Program
619-294-6084, 800-532-3749 (Calif. only)

Colorado

Teratogen Information and Education Service
Denver, Colorado
303-861-6395, 800-332-2082 (Colo. only), 800-525-4871 (Wyo. only)

Connecticut

Connecticut Pregnancy Exposure Information Service
203-679-1502, 800-325-5391 (Conn. only)

Florida

Teratogen Information Service
Gainesville, Florida
904-392-3050

Teratogen Information Service
Tampa, Florida
813-975-6905

Georgia

Centers for Disease Control
Atlanta, Georgia
404-488-4967

Illinois

Illinois Teratogen Information Service
312-908-7441, 800-252-4847 (Ill. only)

Indiana

Indiana Teratogen Information Service
317-274-1071

Iowa

University of Iowa Teratogen Information Service
319-356-2674

Kansas

Prenatal Diagnostic and Genetic Clinic
Wichita, Kansas
316-688-2362

Massachusetts

Massachusetts, Teratogen Information Service
617-787-4957, 800-322-5014 (Mass. only)

Embryology Teratology Unit
Massachusetts General Hospital
Boston, Massachusetts
617-726-1742

Teratogen Information System (TERIS), Brigham and Women's Hospital
Boston, Massachusetts
617-732-6507

Occupational and Environmental Reproductive Hazards Center
University of Massachusetts Medical Center
Worcester, Massachusetts
508-856-2818

Nebraska

Nebraska Teratogen Project
402-559-5071

New Jersey

New Jersey Pregnancy Risk Information Service
908-745-6659, 800-287-3015 (N.J. only)

New York

Perinatal Environmental and Drug Consultation Service
Rochester, New York
716-275-3638

Teratogen Information Service
West Seneca, New York
716-634-8132, ext. 265, 800-724-2454 (N.Y. only)

North Dakota

Division of Medical Genetics
Department of Pediatrics
Grand Forks, North Dakota
701-777-4277

Pennsylvania

Pregnancy Healthline
Philadelphia, Pennsylvania
215-829-3601

Pregnancy Safety Hotline
Pittsburgh, Pennsylvania
412-687-SAFE

Department of Reproductive Genetics
Pittsburgh, Pennsylvania
412-647-4168

Utah

Pregnancy Riskline
Salt Lake City, Utah
801-583-2229

Vermont

Vermont Pregnancy Risk Information Service
802-658-4310

Washington

Central Laboratory for Human Embryology
University of Washington
Seattle, Washington
206-543-3373

Teratogen Information System (TERIS)
University of Washington
Seattle, Washington
206-543-2465

Washington, D.C.

Reproductive Toxicology Center
202-293-5137

Wisconsin

Wisconsin Teratogen Project
608-262-4716, 800-442-6692

Great Lakes Genetics
Milwaukee, Wisconsin
414-475-7400, 414-475-7223

Eastern Wisconsin Teratogen Service
Milwaukee, Wisconsin
414-357-6555

Canada

Poison and Drug Information Service
Calgary, Alberta, Canada
403-670-1059

Department of Genetics
Children's Hospital of Eastern Ontario Canada
613-737-2275

Safe Start Program
Hamilton, Ontario, Canada
416-521-2100, ext. 6700

Fetal Risk Assessment from Maternal Exposure Program
London, Ontario, Canada
519-685-8293

Motherisk Program
Toronto, Ontario, Canada
416-813-6780

Department of Medical Genetics
University of British Columbia
Vancouver, British Columbia, Canada
604-875-2157

British Columbia Drug and Poison Information Centre
Vancouver, British Columbia, Canada
604-682-2344, ext. 2126

Estimates of Rates per Thousand of Chromosomal Abnormalities in Live Births by Single-Year Intervals

Maternal Age	Down Syndrome	Edwards' Syndrome (Trisomy 18)	Patau's Syndrome (Trisomy 13)	XXY	XYY	Turner Syndrome Genotype	Other Clinically Significant Abnormality*	Total†
<15	1.0‡	<0.1‡	<0.1-0.1	0.4	0.5	<0.1	0.2	2.2*
15	1.0‡	<0.1‡	<0.1-0.1	0.4	0.5	<0.1	0.2	2.2
16	0.9‡	<0.1‡	-0.1-0.1	0.4	0.5	<0.1	0.2	2.1
17	0.8‡	<0.1‡	-0.1-0.1	0.4	0.5	<0.1	0.2	2.1
18	0.7‡	<0.1‡	-0.1-0.1	0.4	0.5	<0.1	0.2	1.9
19	0.6‡	<0.1‡	-0.1-0.1	0.4	0.5	<0.1	0.2	1.8
20	0.5-0.7	<0.1-0.1	<0.1-0.1	0.4	0.5	<0.1	0.2	1.9
21	0.5-0.7	<0.1-0.1	<0.1-0.1	0.4	0.5	<0.1	0.2	1.9
22	0.6-0.8	<0.1-0.1	<0.1-0.1	0.4	0.5	<0.1	0.2	2.0
23	0.6-0.8	<0.1-0.1	<0.1-0.1	0.4	0.5	<0.1	0.2	2.0
24	0.7-0.9	0.1-0.1	<0.1-0.1	0.4	0.5	<0.1	0.2	2.1
25	0.7-0.9	0.1-0.1	<0.1-0.1	0.4	0.5	<0.1	0.2	2.1
26	0.7-1.0	0.1-0.1	<0.1-0.1	0.4	0.5	<0.1	0.2	2.1
27	0.8-1.0	0.1-0.2	<0.1-0.1	0.4	0.5	<0.1	0.2	2.2
28	0.8-1.1	0.1-0.2	<0.1-0.2	0.4	0.5	<0.1	0.2	2.3
29	0.8-1.2	0.1-0.2	<0.1-0.2	0.5	0.5	<0.1	0.2	2.4
30	0.9-1.2	0.1-0.2	<0.1-0.2	0.5	0.5	<0.1	0.2	2.6
31	0.9-1.3	0.1-0.2	<0.1-0.2	0.5	0.5	<0.1	0.2	2.6

Continued

*XXX is excluded for reasons given in the text.
†Calculation of the total at each age assumes rate for autosomal aneuploidies is at the midpoints of the ranges given.
‡No range may be constructed for those under 20 years by the same methods as for those 20 and over.
Courtesy of Birth Defects Institute, New York State Department of Health, Albany, New York.

Maternal Age	Down Syndrome	Edwards' Syndrome (Trisomy 18)	Patau's Syndrome (Trisomy 13)	XXY	XYY	Turner Syndrome Genotype	Other Clinically Significant Abnormality*	Total†
32	1.1-1.5	0.1-0.2	0.1-0.2	0.6	0.5	<0.1	0.2	3.1
33	1.4-1.9	0.1-0.3	0.1-0.2	0.7	0.5	<0.1	0.2	3.5
34	1.9-2.4	0.2-0.4	0.1-0.3	0.7	0.5	<0.1	0.2	4.1
35	2.5-3.9	0.3-0.5	0.2-0.3	0.9	0.5	<0.1	0.3	5.6
36	3.2-5.0	0.3-0.6	0.2-0.4	1.0	0.5	<0.1	0.3	6.7
37	4.1-6.4	0.4-0.7	0.2-0.5	1.1	0.5	<0.1	0.3	8.1
38	5.2-8.1	0.5-0.9	0.3-0.7	1.3	0.5	<0.1	0.3	9.5
39	6.6-10.5	0.7-1.2	0.4-0.8	1.5	0.5	<0.1	0.3	12.4
40	8.5-13.7	0.9-1.6	0.5-1.1	1.8	0.5	<0.1	0.3	15.8
41	10.8-17.9	1.1-2.1	0.6-1.4	2.2	0.5	<0.1	0.3	20.5
42	13.8-23.4	1.4-2.7	0.7-1.8	2.7	0.5	<0.1	0.3	25.5
43	17.6-30.6	1.8-3.5	0.9-2.4	3.3	0.5	<0.1	0.3	32.6
44	22.5-40.0	2.3-4.6	1.2-3.1	4.1	0.5	<0.1	0.3	41.8
45	28.7-52.3	2.9-6.0	1.5-4.1	5.1	0.5	<0.1	0.3	53.7
46	36.6-68.3	3.7-7.9	1.9-5.3	6.4	0.5	<0.1	0.3	68.9
47	46.6-89.3	4.7-10.3	2.4-6.9	8.2	0.5	<0.1	0.3	89.1
48	59.5-116.8	6.0-13.5	3.0-9.0	10.6	0.5	<0.1	0.3	115.0
49	75.8-152.7	<7.6-17.6	<3.8-11.8	13.8	0.5	<0.1	0.3	149.3

*XXX is excluded for reasons given in the text.

†Calculation of the total at each age assumes rate for autosomal aneuploidies is at the midpoints of the ranges given.

‡No range may be constructed for those under 20 years by the same methods as for those 20 and over.

Courtesy of Birth Defects Institute, New York State Department of Health, Albany, New York.

APPENDIX

Nonmeat Protein Sources

Food	Amount to Equal 20 g Protein
Peanut butter	4½ tablespoons
Dried beans	1⅓ cups
Eggs	3
Milk	2⅓ cups
Cheese	3 oz
Nuts or seeds	7 tablespoons
Tofu	8 oz

Prenatal Nutrient Requirements

Nutrient	Nonpregnant RDA	Pregnant RDA	Dietary Sources
Protein	46-50 g	60 g	Meats, fish, poultry, complementary grains, dairy products
Carbohydrates	100 g	250 g	Grain products, fruits, vegetables, milk
Vitamin A (retinol)	4000 IU	4000 IU	Fortified milk, deep yellow or orange fruits and vegetables, green vegetables
Vitamin D	200 IU	400 IU	Fortified milk, liver, eggs, cod fish, exposure of skin to sunlight
Vitamin E (α-tocopherol)	15 IU	15 IU	Vegetables, oils, milk, eggs, nuts, grain
Vitamin B_1 (thiamine)	1.1 mg	1.5 mg	Enriched grains, pork, wheat germ, lima beans
Vitamin B_6 (pyridoxine)	1.6 mg	2.2 mg	Liver, chicken, potatoes, bananas, wheat germ, spinach, beef, egg yolk, fish
Vitamin C (ascorbic acid)	60 mg	70 mg	Citrus fruits, tomatoes, green peppers, cantaloupe
Folic acid	180 µg	400 µg	Liver, spinach, asparagus, wheat germ, broccoli, grains, leafy vegetables, dried beans and peas
Vitamin B_{12} (cyanocobalamin)	2 µg	2.2 µg	Animal proteins
Vitamin B_2 (riboflavin)	1.3 mg	1.6 mg	Liver, milk and dairy products, enriched cereals, eggs
Niacin (nicotinic acid)	15 mg	17 mg	Fish, liver, meat, poultry, eggs, enriched grains, milk
Iron	15 mg	30 mg	Meats, eggs, enriched grains (See Appendix F)
Calcium	1200 mg	1,200 mg	Dairy products, green vegetables (See Appendix H)
Phosphorus	1200 mg	1,200 mg	Dairy products, grains, eggs, dried beans
Iodine	150 mg	175 mg	Iodized salt, seafood
Zinc	12 mg	15 mg	Oysters, meat, potatoes

Food Sources of Iron

	SERVING SIZE	MG OF IRON
Calf liver, cooked	3½ oz	14.2
Liverwurst	3 oz	8.7
Chicken livers, cooked	3½ oz	8.5
Prune juice	½ cup	5.2
Ground beef, lean, cooked	3½ oz	3.8
Chickpeas	½ cup	3.0
Steak, cooked	3 oz	2.7
Raisins	½ cup	2.5
Molasses	1 tablespoon	2.3
Prunes, large	4	2.2
Kidney beans	½ cup	2.2
Spinach, cooked	½ cup	2.0
Chicken	¼	1.8
Turkey	3 oz	1.5
Apricots, dried	4 halves	1.3
Avocado	½	1.3
Egg	1	1.1
Blueberries	⅝ cup	1.0
Bread, whole wheat	1 slice	0.8
Bread, enriched white	1 slice	0.6
Dry cereal	Read label; varies widely	

G

Iron Supplements

	Amount of Elemental Iron (%)	Dose Containing 60 mg of Elemental Iron (mg)
Ferrous sulfate	20	300
Ferrous fumarate	32.5	185
Ferrous gluconate	11	545

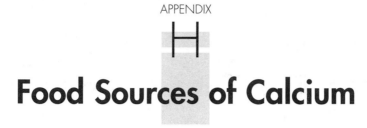

Food Sources of Calcium

	SERVING SIZE	MG OF CALCIUM
Sardines	3 oz	372
Milk, skim	1 cup	300
Milk, whole	1 cup	290
Milk, buttermilk	1 cup	296
Cheese, cheddar	1 oz	210
Cheese, American	1 slice	195
Cheese, mozzarella	1 oz	163
Turnip greens, cooked	⅔ cup	184
Salmon	3 oz	167
Custard	½ cup	161
Tofu	3 oz	128
Ice cream	½ cup	99
Shrimp	3 oz	98
Spinach, cooked	½ cup	88
Broccoli, cooked	½ cup	68
Peanuts, roasted, with husks	⅔ cup	68
Green beans, cooked	½ cup	62
Egg, poached	1 large	51
Beans, cooked	½ cup	50
Cottage cheese	¼ cup	38
Almonds	12 nuts	38
Perrier water	1 cup	32
Cream cheese	1 oz	23
Fish, broiled	4½ oz	20
Bread, enriched white	1 slice	20
Wheat cereal, flakes	1 cup	12

Elemental Calcium Available in Some Over-the-Counter Supplements

Brand	Amount of Calcium Carbonate (mg)	Amount of Elemental Calcium (mg)
Os-Cal 500 (Marion)	1,250	500
Tums (low sodium) (Norcliff-Thayer)	500	200
Tums (extra strength) (Norcliff-Thayer)	750	300

Selected Drug, Vitamin, and Mineral Interactions

DRUG	REDUCTION IN LEVELS OF
Antibiotic	
Tetracycline	Vitamin C
Anticonvulsant	
Diphenylhydantoin (Dilantin)	Folic acid
	Vitamin D
	Vitamin K
Antilipemic	
Cholestyramine	Folic acid
	Vitamin A
	Vitamin D
	Vitamin K
	Vitamin B_{12}
Antituberculous	
Isoniazid	Vitamin B_6
	Niacin
	Vitamin D
Antiinflammatory	
(Aspirin, indomethacin, sulfasalazine)	Folic acid
	Vitamin C
	Iron
	Vitamin K
Diuretic	
Triamterene and hydrochlorothiazide (Dyazide)	Folic acid
Gastrointestinal	
Mineral oil	Vitamin A
	Vitamin D
	Vitamin K
Antacids	Folic acid
Antihypertensive	
Hydralazine (Apresoline)	Vitamin B_6

Continued

263

DRUG	REDUCTION IN LEVELS OF
Tranquilizer	
Chlorpromazine hydrochloride (Thorazine), thioridazine hydrochloride, thioridazine (Mellaril), and other phenothiazines	Riboflavin
Other	
Levodopa	Vitamin B_6
Penicillamine	Vitamin B_6
	Copper
Trimethoprim	Folic acid
Methotrexate	Folic acid

Caffeine Content per 5-oz Cup

Drip percolated coffee	64-150 mg
Instant decaffeinated coffee	2-5 mg
Brewed tea	9-50 mg
Instant tea	12-28 mg
Hot chocolate	8-10 mg

Caffeine Content of Some Prescribed and Over-the-Counter Medications

	Per Tablet (mg)
Over-the-counter cold preparations	15-30
Anacin 3	32
Excedrin	64.8
Fiorinal	40
Caffergot	100
Appetite suppressants	37-325

M

Standard Weight for Women and Deviations of Weight for Height*

Height (No Shoes) (ft/in)	Standard Range (Medium Frame) (lbs)	Standard Weight (Medium Frame) (lbs)	≤85% (Underweight) (lbs)	≥120% (Overweight) (lbs)
4'10"	111-123	117	99	140
4'11"	113-126	120	102	144
5' 0"	115-129	122	104	146
5' 1"	118-132	125	106	150
5' 2"	121-135	128	109	154
5' 3"	124-138	131	111	157
5' 4"	127-141	134	114	161
5' 5"	130-144	137	116	164
5' 6"	133-147	140	119	168
5' 7"	136-150	143	122	172
5' 8"	139-153	146	124	175
5' 9"	142-156	149	127	179
5'10"	145-159	152	129	182
5'11"	148-162	155	132	186
6' 0"	151-165	158	134	190

*Based on data from Metropolitan Life Insurance Company, 1983.

Maternal Phenylketonuria (PKU) Collaborative Study Contributing Centers

NORTHEAST REGION

Connecticut, Delaware, Maine, Maryland, Massachusetts, New Hampshire, New Jersey, New York, Pennsylvania, Rhode Island, Vermont, Virginia, West Virginia, District of Columbia

Principal Investigator:
Harvey Levy, MD
Project Coordinator:
Deborah Lobbregt
Nutritionist: Fran Rohr, MS, RD
Children's Hospital
Gardner 818
300 Longwood Avenue
Boston, MA 02115
617-735-6346

CANADA

Principal Investigator:
William B. Hanley, MD
Project Coordinator:
Wanda Schoonheyt, RN
Nutritionist: Val Austin, RD
The Hospital for Sick Children
555 University Avenue
Toronto, Ontario
Canada M5G 1X8
416-813-6356

SOUTHEAST REGION

Alabama, Arkansas, Florida, Georgia, Louisiana, Mississippi, North Carolina, Puerto Rico, South Carolina, Tennessee, Texas

Principal Investigator:
Bobbye Rouse, MD
Project Coordinator and
Nutritionist:
Lois Castiglioni, MS, RD
Department of Pediatrics
University of Texas Medical Branch
Galveston, TX 77555-0319
409-772-2356

MIDWEST REGION

Illinois, Indiana, Iowa, Kansas, Kentucky, Michigan, Minnesota, Missouri, Nebraska, North Dakota, Ohio, Oklahoma, South Dakota, Wisconsin

Principal Investigator:
Harvey Levy, MD
Co–Principal Investigators:
Reuben Matalon, MD, PhD
Savitri Kamath, PhD
Project Coordinator:
Barbara Goss, MS, RD
Nutritionist:
Kim Matalon, PhD, RD

University of Illinois at Chicago
Department of Nutrition and Medical Dietetics
Mail Code 517
1919 West Taylor
Chicago, IL 60612
312-996-0995

WESTERN REGION

Alaska, Arizona, California, Colorado, Hawaii, Idaho, Montana, Nevada, New Mexico, Oregon, Utah, Washington, Wyoming

Principal Investigators:
Richard Koch, MD
Julian Williams, MD, PhD
Associate Director:
Eva G. Freidman
Project Coordinator:
Cindy Bauman-Frischling, MPH

Nutritionist: Liz Wenz, MS, RD
Maternal PKU Study
Childrens Hospital Los Angeles
4650 Sunset Boulevard
Los Angeles, CA 90027
213-669-2152

GERMANY, AUSTRIA, SWITZERLAND

Principal Investigator:
Friedrich Trefz, MD
Project Coordinator:
Sanja Cipcic-Schmidt, PhD
MPKU Studie
Universitats Kinderklinik
Im Neuenheimer Feld 150
D-6900 Heidelberg, Germany
#011-49-6221-56-37-84

Index

A

Abortion risk in pregnancy after given number of abortions, 206
Abruptio placentae, 215
Accutane; *see* Isotretinoin
Achondroplasia, 225
Acquired immunodeficiency syndrome (AIDS), 185; *see also* Human immunodeficiency syndrome
Age
  maternal, effects of, on pregnancy, 56-62
  paternal, effects of, 238
AIDS; *see* Acquired immunodeficiency syndrome
Alcohol abuse, 18-22
  maternal, effects on fetus, 13-18
  paternal, effects of, 236-237
Amenorrhea, exercise-induced, 50
American College of Obstetricians and Gynecologists, 227
American Public Health Association, 230
American Society of Human Genetics, 230
Anorexia and bulimia, effects of, on pregnancy, 86-87
Anticoagulants, use of, during preconceptional period, 198
Anticonvulsants, use of, during preconceptional period, 198-200
Ascorbic acid; *see* Vitamin C
Aspartame, fetal effects of, 75
Aspirin, 8
Asthma, pregnancy and, 113-115
Autoimmune disorders, reproductive organ abnormalities and, 212
Autosomal dominant inheritance, 225-226
Autosomal recessive inheritance, 226-227
Azathioprine, 130

B

Bromocriptine, 8
Bulimia, anorexia and, effects of, on pregnancy, 86-87

C

Caffeine, pregnancy and, 88-89
Caffeine content
  of some prescribed and over-the-counter medications, 266
  in selected beverages, 265
Calcium, 82
  elemental, in over-the-counter supplements, 262
  food sources of, 261
California Teratogen Registry, 199
Cancer, pregnancy and, 147-154; *see also* specific cancers
Carbamazepine, 199
Carbohydrates, importance of, during pregnancy, 76
Category X drugs, 5
Cervical neoplasia, early, pregnancy and, 148-149
Chemotherapy, pregnancy and, 153
Chlamydia trachomatis, 177, 188
Chlamydial infection, pregnancy and, 177-178
Chromosomal abnormalities, 229
Cigarette smoke, mechanism of action, 26; *see also* Smoking; Tobacco use
Clonazepam, 199
Cocaine use, maternal, effects of, 32-34
Collaborative Perinatal Project of the National Institute of Neurological and Communicative Disorders and Stroke, 58
Congenital malformation
  blood glucose levels and, 99-101
  epilepsy and, 139-140
  fetal and neonatal mortality and, 215-216
  possible causes of, 2
Congenital rubella syndrome (CRS), 167
Contraceptives, use of, during preconceptional period, 200-201
Copper, 84-85
Coumadin; *see* Warfarin
Coumarin, 120

Council of the International Federation of Obstetricians and Gynecologists, 58
Council on Scientific Affairs of the American Medical Association, 226
CRS; *see* Congenital rubella syndrome
Cyanocobalamin, 78
Cystic fibrosis, 227
Cytomegalovirus infection, 175-176

D

Depakene; *see* Valproic acid
DES; *see* Diethylstilbestrol
Diabetes mellitus, pregnancy and, 99-104
Diethylstilbestrol (DES), 211
Digitoxin, 120
Digoxin, 12
Down syndrome, 59, 229
Drinking, heavy, definition of, 14
Drug use, illicit, maternal, 30-37
  cocaine use, 32-34
  heroin use, 34
  lysergic acid diethylamide (LSD) use, 35
  marijuana use, 30-32
  phencyclidine (PCP) use, 34-35
Drug, vitamin, and mineral interactions, selected, 263-264
Drug-alcohol-nutrition interactions, 87-88
Drugs and chemicals, reproductive effects of, resources for information on, 249-253
Drugs in Pregnancy and Lactation, 201

E

Edwards' syndrome, 59
Ehlers-Danlos syndrome, 225
Electromagnetic fields (EMFs), maternal and fetal effects of, 44-46
EMFs; *see* Electromagnetic fields
Environmental exposures at home and work
  maternal effects of, 38-48
  toxic exposures, 39-47
Epilepsy, pregnancy and, 138-142
Epstein-Barr virus, pregnancy and, 175
Erythromycin, 178
Exercise
  beneficial forms of, during pregnancy, 53
  maternal, effects of, 49-55
Exposure to drugs and chemicals, paternal, effects of, 239

F

FAE; *see* Fetal alcohol effects
Family history, 224-242
  chromosomal abnormalities, 228-229
  multifactorial inheritance, 229-230
  mendelian inheritance, patterns of, 225-228
FAS; *see* Fetal alcohol syndrome
Fetal alcohol effects (FAE), 13
Fetal alcohol syndrome (FAS), 13
Fetal and neonatal mortality, reproductive organ abnormalities and, 212-216
Fetus, effects of alcohol on, 13-18
Fluoride, 84
Folic acid, importance of, during pregnancy, 79-81
Food sources of calcium, 261
Food sources of iron, 259

G

GBS; *see* Group B streptococcus
Genetic factors in pregnancy loss, 206-207
Genetic heterogeneity, 231
Glomerulonephritis, chronic, preconceptional guidelines, 133
Gold injections, 8
Gold, 5
Gonorrhea, pregnancy and, 180
Graves' disease; *see* Hyperthyroidism
Gray, 43
Group B streptococcal disease, pregnancy and, 169-170
Group B streptococcus (GBS), 169; *see also* Group B streptococcal disease
Guidelines for Perinatal Care, 232

H

HBeAg; *see* Hepatitis B e antigen
HBsAg; *see* Hepatitis B surface antigen
HBV; *see* Hepatitis B virus
Heart disease
  acquired, 117-118
  congenital, 118-119
  medical and surgical therapies for, 119-121
  pregnancy and, 116-122
Hemoglobinopathies, pregnancy and, 143-146
Heparin therapy, prolonged, risks of, 127
Heparin, 198
Hepatitis, viral, pregnancy and, 183-184

Hepatitis B surface antigen (HBsAg), 183
Hepatitis B virus (HBV), 183; *see also*
  Hepatitis, viral
Hepatitis B e antigen (HBeAg), 183
Heroin use, maternal, effects of, 34
Herpes simplex infection, genital, 173-174
Herpesvirus infections, pregnancy and,
  173-176
HIV; *see* Human immunodeficiency virus
HLAs; *see* Human leukocyte antigens
Hodgkin's disease, pregnancy and, 149-
  151
HPV; *see* Human papillomavirus
Human immunodeficiency virus (HIV)
  pregnancy and, 185-190
  manifestations of, 187-188
  transmission of, 186-187
Human leukocyte antigens (HLAs), 207
Human papillomavirus infection,
  pregnancy and, 179
Huntington's chorea, 225
Hydroxychloroquine, 8
Hyperactivity, maternal alcohol abuse and,
  15
Hyperphenylalaninemia, pregnancy and,
  108-112
Hypertension, chronic, pregnancy and,
  123-125
Hyperthermia, exercise and, effects on
  fetus, 50-52
Hyperthyroidism, 105-106
Hypothyroidism, 105

I

Illicit drug use, paternal, effects of, 237
Infections, maternal; *see* Infectious disease
Infectious disease, pregnancy and, 165-
  194
  chlamydial infection, 177-178
  gonorrhea, 180
  group B streptococcal disease, 169-170
  hepatitis, viral, 183-184
  herpesvirus infections, 173-176
  human inmmunodeficiency virus
    infection, 185-190
  human papilloma virus, 179
  rubella, 176-168
  syphilis, 181-182
  toxoplasmosis, 171-172
Infertility, age-associated, possible causes
  of, 60
Insulin, 8

Intrauterine device (IUD), smoking and,
  25
Iodine, 83
Ionizing radiation, maternal and fetal
  effects of, 43-44
Iron, 81-82
  food sources of, 259
Iron supplements, 260
Isotretinoin, 5, 197

J

*Journal of the American Medical
  Association*, 17

K

Karnofsky's law, 40
Kidney disease, pregnancy and, 129-134
Klinefelter's syndrome, 59

L

Labor induction, fetal and neonatal
  mortality and, 214-215
Levothyroxine, 8
Lipids, importance of, during pregnancy,
  76
Listeria monocytogenes, 210
Low birthweight, maternal exercise levels
  and, 53
LSD: *see* Lysergic acid diethylamide
Lysergic acid diethylamide (LSD), 35

M

Male issues in preconceptional health,
  235-242
March of Dimes Birth Defects
  Foundation, 231
Marfan syndrome, 225
Marijuana, maternal use of, effects of, on
  pregnancy, 30-32
Maternal age, effects of, on pregnancy,
  56-62
Maxzide, 8
Medical history, 98-164
  asthma, 113-115
  cancer, 147-154
  diabetes mellitus, 99-104
  epilepsy, 138-142
  heart disease, 116-122
  hemoglobinopathies, 143-146
  hyperphenylalaninemia, 108-112
  hypertension, chronic, 123-125
  kidney disease, 129-134

Medical history—cont'd
  paternal, effects of, 238-239
  systemic lupus erythematosus, 135-137
  thyroid disorders, 105-107
  venous thrombosis, deep, 126-128
Medication, use of, during
  preconceptional period, 198-201
Medication history, pregnancy and, 195-
  204
Melanoma, malignant, pregnancy and,
  151-152
Menstrual dysfunction, exercise and, 49-
  50
Mental retardation, maternal alcohol abuse
  and, 15
Methimazole, 105
Minerals, importance of, during
  pregnancy, 81-85
Multifactorial inheritance, 225, 229-230
Mycobacterium tuberculosis, 189
Mycoplasma hominis, 210

N

Neisseria gonorrhoeae, 180, 186
Neonatal death, second- and third-
  trimester pregnancy loss and, 210-
  216
Nephrolithiasis, preconceptional
  guidelines, 132
Nephrotic syndrome, preconceptional
  guidelines, 132
Neural tube defects (NTDs), 79
Noise levels, maternal and fetal effects of,
  46-47
Nonmeat protein sources, 257
NTDs; *see* Neural tube defects
Nutrient requirements, prenatal, 258
Nutrients, vitamins, and minerals,
  significance of during pregnancy, 74-
  85
Nutrition, paternal, effects of, 237
Nutrition history, 72-97
  caffeine, pregnancy and, 88-89
  drug-alcohol-nutrition-mineral
    interactions, 87-88
  nutrients, vitamins, and minerals,
    significance of during pregnancy, 74-
    85
  vegetarianism, 87
  weight, pregnancy and, 85-87
  weight, pregnancy outcome and, 85-87

P

Patau's syndrome, 59
PCP; *see* Phencyclidine use
Pectus excavatum, 225
Pelvic inflammatory disease (PID), 177
Phencyclidine (PCP) use, maternal, effects
  of, 34-35
Phenobarbital, 199
Phenylalanine, fetal effects of, 75
Phenylketonuria (PKU), 75
  maternal, collaborative study
    contributing centers, 268-269
Pica, 86
PID; *see* Pelvic inflammatory disease
PKU; *see* Phenylketonuria
Plutarch, 1
Pneumocystis carinii, 187
Polycystic renal disease, preconceptional
  guidelines, 132
PPD test; *see* Purified protein derivative
  (PPD) test
Preconceptional counseling for informed
  decision making, rationale for, 1-10
Preconceptional health assessment form,
  243-248
Preconceptional health care, male issues,
  235-242
Preconceptional health care counseling, 1-
  10
Preeclampsia, 214
Pregnancy
  in older women, maternal health
    considerations, 57-61
  adolescent, maternal health
    considerations, 57
Pregnancy loss, first trimester, 205-210
  anatomic factors, 209-210
  endocrine factors, 208-209
  genetic factors, 206-207
  immunologic factors, 207-208
Prenatal nutrient requirements, 258
Preventing Low Birthweight, 3
Primidone, 199
Propylthiouracil, 105
Protein and amino acids, importance of,
  during pregnancy, 75-76
Purified protein derivative (PPD) test, 9
Pyelonephritis, chronic, preconceptional
  guidelines, 132
Pyridoxine, 78

Q

Quinidine, 120

R

Radiation, ionizing, maternal and fetal effects of, 43-44
Rads, 43
RDA; *see* Recommended Daily Allowance
Recommended Daily Allowance (RDA), 75
Rems, 43
Renal insufficiency, preconceptional guidelines, 133
Renal transplantation, preconceptional guidelines, 134
Reproductive history, 205-223
    pregnancy loss, first-trimester, 205-210
    second- and third-trimester pregnancy loss and neonatal death, 210-216
Reproductive organs, abnormalities in, 211-212
Resources for information on reproductive effects of drugs and chemicals, 249-253
Riboflavin, 78
Roentgens, 43
Rubella, 167-168

S

Seizures during pregnancy, 138-139; *see also* Epilepsy, pregnancy and
Sickle cell disease, 227
Sickling disorders, 143-145; *see also* Hemoglobinopathies
Sievert, 43
SLE; *see* Systemic lupus erythematosus
Smoking cessation, preparation for, 27-28
Smoking, pregnancy and, effects on, 24-26
Smoking, hazards of, sources for information about, 26-27
Smoking, mechanism of action, 26
Smoking, prevalence of, 23-24
Smoking; *see also* Tobacco use
Social history, 11-70
    alcohol abuse, 12-22; *see also* Alcohol abuse
    environmental exposures at home and work, 38-48
    exercise, 49-55

Social history—cont'd
    illicit drug use, 30-37
    maternal age, 56-62
    tobacco use, 23-29
Standard weight table, 267
Synthroid; *see* Levothyroxine
Syphilis, pregnancy and, 181
Systemic lupus erythematosus (SLE), pregnancy and, 135-137

T

Tay-Sachs disease, 227
Tegretol; *see* Carbamazepine
Teratogens, identification of, 196-198
Tetrahydrocannabinol (THC), 31
Thalassemia, pregnancy and, 145
Thalidomide, 196
THC; *see* Tetrahydrocannabinol
The Health Consequences of Smoking for Women, 23
Thiamine, 78
Thrombocytopenia, 127
Thyroid cancer, pregnancy and, 106
Thyroid disorders, pregnancy and, 105-107
Tobacco use
    maternal, pregnancy and, 23-29
    paternal, effects of, 236
Toxic exposures, 38-47
    effects of, 39
    electromagnetic fields, 44-46
    identification of, 39-42
    ionizing radiation, 43-44
    maternal and fetal effects of, 39-47; *see also* Environmental exposures at home and work
    noise levels, 46-47
    sources of, 42-43
Toxoplasma gondii, 171
Toxoplasmosis, pregnancy and, 171-172
Treponema pallidum, 181
Transgenerational carcinogens, 39
Tridione; *see* Trimethalone
Trimethalone, 199
Turner syndrome, 229

U

Ureaplasma urealyticum, 210
Urinary diversion, permanent, preconceptional guidelines, 132-133

V

Valproic acid, 199
Varicella-zoster virus infection, pregnancy and, 174-175
VDTs; *see* Video display terminals
Vegetarianism, effects of, on pregnancy, 87
Venous thrombosis, deep, pregnancy and, 126-128
Video display terminals (VDTs), 45
Vitamin A, 77
Vitamin B, 78-79
Vitamin C, 79
Vitamin D, 77-78
Vitamin E, 78
Vitamin K, 78

Vitamins
fat-soluble, 77-78
importance of, during pregnancy, 77-81
water-soluble, 78-81

W

Warfarin, 5, 127, 198
Weight, maternal, pregnancy outcome and, 85-87

X

X-linked inheritance, 227-228
X-rays; *see* Ionizing radiation

Z

Zinc, 83-84